Small Animal Ophthalmic
Atlas and Guide

Small Animal Ophthalmic Atlas and Guide

Christine C. Lim, DVM

Diplomate of the American College of Veterinary Ophthalmologists
Ophthalmologist, Eye Care For Animals
Chicago, IL, USA

Second Edition

WILEY Blackwell

Registered Office
John Wiley & Sons, Inc., 111 River Street, Hoboken, NJ 07030, USA

Editorial Office
111 River Street, Hoboken, NJ 07030, USA

For details of our global editorial offices, customer services, and more information about Wiley products visit us at www.wiley.com.

Wiley also publishes its books in a variety of electronic formats and by print-on-demand. Some content that appears in standard print versions of this book may not be available in other formats.

Library of Congress Cataloging-in-Publication Data

Names: Lim, Christine C. author.
Title: Small animal ophthalmic atlas and guide / Christine C. Lim.
Description: Second edition. | Hoboken, NJ : Wiley-Blackwell, 2023. |
    Includes index.
Identifiers: LCCN 2022009609 (print) | LCCN 2022009610 (ebook) | ISBN
    9781119804253 (cloth) | ISBN 9781119804260 (adobe pdf) | ISBN
    9781119804277 (epub)
Subjects: MESH: Eye Diseases–veterinary | Animals, Domestic | Eye
    Diseases–diagnosis | Diagnostic Techniques,
    Ophthalmological–veterinary | Atlas
Classification: LCC SF891 (print) | LCC SF891 (ebook) | NLM SF 891 | DDC
    636.089/77–dc23/eng/20220318
LC record available at https://lccn.loc.gov/2022009609
LC ebook record available at https://lccn.loc.gov/2022009610

Cover Design: Wiley
Cover Image: Courtesy of Christine C. Lim

Set in 9.5/12pt MinionPro by Straive, Chennai, India

Printed in Singapore
M116665_280722

This book is dedicated to my mentors, students, colleagues, patients, and especially my family. I am deeply indebted to all of you for your support and for everything you have taught me.

Contents

Preface

Small animal general practice is a high-paced profession that requires the veterinarian to arrive at a diagnosis and formulate diagnostic and therapeutic plans within a 15- to 20-minute appointment window. As a general practitioner, I often found myself in this position. When this happened with ophthalmology cases, I wished for a reference to help me confirm my diagnosis and quickly implement a plan for treatment. Such scenarios provided the idea for this book. The *Small Animal Ophthalmic Atlas and Guide* is designed as a handy reference for the busy general practitioner. The book's goals are to (i) provide an extensive collection of images that practitioners can use to obtain a diagnosis during an outpatient appointment, and (ii) provide just enough information about each disease, relevant diagnostic tests, and treatment to allow for the development of a medically sound management plan.

The majority of ophthalmic conditions selected for inclusion in this book are those that present frequently in general practice. A smaller number of less common conditions are also included because of their significant impact on vision and/or overall health of the eye, or because they can appear similar to (and should be differentiated from) more common conditions. The purpose of this book is not to describe every known small animal ophthalmic disease, nor is it intended to be an exhaustive review of the diseases included in the book. Because this is intended to be a quick reference, each chapter includes only enough background information to facilitate discussion of each ocular disease, most of the information is designed to support immediate management, and ophthalmic procedures are not discussed in detail. (For example, detailed directions for ocular surgeries should be sought from other texts.) As a guide for those who wish to delve more deeply into specific ophthalmic conditions, each chapter contains a list of suggestions for further reading.

For this second edition, each chapter has been updated to include relevant advances in understanding and management of the included ophthalmic diseases. In addition, the number of images has more than doubled. I hope these changes will make this book more valuable for daily practice.

Of course, no reference book can be a substitute for up-to-date education, sound clinical judgment, and the practitioner's individual knowledge of a particular patient. Readers of this book should always think critically about the cases presenting to them, seek advice from and make referrals to veterinary ophthalmologists when warranted, and verify that new research or information from manufacturers has not eclipsed the information in this book. My hope is that this book will make it easier for practitioners to handle ophthalmic cases in their daily practice.

Christine C. Lim

List of abbreviations

CBC	complete blood count		**IV**	intravenous
CsA	cyclosporine A		**KCS**	keratoconjunctivitis sicca
CT	computed tomography		**LIU**	lens-induced uveitis
DLH	domestic longhair		**MRI**	magnetic resonance imaging
DNA	deoxyribonucleic acid		**NSAID**	nonsteroidal anti-inflammatory drug
DSH	domestic shorthair		**PLR**	pupillary light reflex
EK	eosinophilic keratoconjunctivitis		**PO**	by mouth
ERG	electroretinogram		**PPM**	persistent pupillary membrane
FeLV	feline leukemia virus		**PRA**	progressive retinal atrophy
FIP	feline infectious peritonitis		**RPE**	retinal pigmented epithelium
FHV-1	feline herpesvirus		**SARDS**	sudden acquired retinal degeneration syndrome
FIV	feline immunodeficiency virus		**STT**	Schirmer tear test
IOP	intraocular pressure		**TFBUT**	Tear film breakup time

Glossary

Accommodation—the process by which the eye changes its focus (e.g., from near objects to far objects, or vice versa).

Anisocoria—unequal pupil size between eyes.

Anterior uvea—iris and ciliary body.

Anterior uveitis—inflammation of the iris and ciliary body.

Aphakic crescent—a crescent shape that becomes visible within the pupil when a lens subluxates or luxates. In health, the equator of the lens is not visible. When the lens dislocates, the change of position of the lens causes the equator to become visible within the pupil. The borders of the aphakic crescent are the pupillary margin and the equator of the lens.

Blepharitis—inflammation of the eyelids.

Blepharospasm—squinting. This is a sign of ocular pain. It is due to spasm of the orbicularis oculi muscle. Marked blepharospasm can cause the eyelids to roll inward (referred to as entropion).

Blood-aqueous barrier—tight junctions within the anterior uvea, which limit the entrance of blood-borne substances into the eye. For example, systemically administered medications may not penetrate into the eye when the blood-aqueous barrier is intact. In the presence of uveitis, the blood-aqueous barrier is compromised. In addition to the blood-aqueous barrier anteriorly, the blood-retina barrier functions similarly posteriorly.

Brachycephalic ocular syndrome—a set of conformational abnormalities most commonly seen in brachycephalic dogs. These abnormalities are bilateral and include exophthalmos (due to shallow orbits), macropalpebral fissure, ventromedial entropion, and medial trichiasis.

Buphthalmos—enlargement of the eye as a result of increased intraocular pressure.

Cataract—an opacity of the lens. The size of the opacity can range from small and focal to encompassing the entire lens.

Chalazion—retention of inspissated Meibomian gland secretions within the eyelid, usually accompanied by eyelid inflammation.

Chemosis—edema of the conjunctiva.

"Cherry eye"—prolapse of the gland of the third eyelid.

Chorioretinitis—inflammation of the choroid and retina, also referred to as posterior uveitis.

Choroid—the posterior portion of the vascular tunic of the eye, also known as the posterior uvea.

Ciliary body—a portion of the anterior uvea. The ciliary body is not visible on ophthalmic examination because it is posterior to the iris. Functions of the ciliary body include aqueous humor production and accommodation, and it also forms a part of the blood-aqueous barrier.

Coloboma—congenital absence of tissue. For example, an optic nerve coloboma refers to an area of the optic nerve that is missing tissue because it did not form completely.

Conjunctivitis—inflammation of the conjunctiva.

Cyclitis—inflammation of the ciliary body.

Cyclophotocoagulation—destruction of the ciliary body with laser energy. This procedure is most often performed in patients with glaucoma. The goal of this procedure is to decrease aqueous humor production (thereby lowering IOP).

Cycloplegia—paralysis of the ciliary body.

Dacryocystitis—inflammation of the nasolacrimal canaliculi and lacrimal sac, usually due to nasolacrimal duct obstruction.

Distichia—an aberrant hair that arises from a Meibomian gland and emerges from the Meibomian gland openings.

Dyscoria—abnormal shape of the pupil.

Ectopic cilium—an aberrant hair that arises from a Meibomian gland and emerges through the palpebral conjunctiva. Because the ectopic cilium emerges through the palpebral conjunctiva, it is in constant contact with the ocular surface.

Ectropion—outward rolling of the eyelids.

Electroretinogram (ERG)—a test that measures the response of the retina to light; that is, it is a test of retinal function.

Enophthalmos—the position of the globe when it is set more posteriorly, or deeply, than normal within the orbit.

Entropion—inward rolling of the eyelids that results in eyelid hairs directly rubbing against the cornea.

Enucleation—surgical removal of the eye, third eyelid, conjunctiva, and eyelid margins.

Epiphora—spillage of tears onto the face due to excessive production.

Exenteration—surgical removal of all orbital contents (i.e., removal of all other orbital soft tissues in addition to enucleation). This is usually performed to remove ocular or orbital neoplasia.

Exophthalmos—the position of the globe when it is set more anteriorly, or shallowly, than normal within the orbit.

Fundus—the image obtained when the posterior segment is viewed through the pupil with an ophthalmoscope. The image is created by a superimposition of the retina and optic nerve upon the choroid (which includes the tapetum) and sclera.

Glaucoma—optic nerve damage as a result of increased intraocular pressure (intraocular pressure greater than 25 mm Hg).

Goniodysgenesis—congenital malformation of the iridocorneal angle. Also referred to as pectinate ligament dysplasia.

Gonioscopy—visual examination of the iridocorneal angle. This test is performed by a veterinary ophthalmologist. It is most often used to help determine if glaucoma is primary or secondary.

Hyphema—blood in the anterior chamber. Presence of hyphema indicates anterior uveitis.

Hypopyon—pus in the anterior chamber. Presence of hypopyon indicates anterior uveitis.

Hypotony—decreased IOP. This is often a symptom of anterior uveitis.

Iridocorneal angle—the angle created by the iris and the cornea. This is the main exit pathway for aqueous humor from the eye. This aqueous outflow pathway is referred to as the conventional pathway.

Iridocyclitis—inflammation of the iris and ciliary body.

Iridodonesis—visible movement of the iris seen as a result of zonular breakdown (indicates lens instability).

Keratectomy—surgical removal of a portion of the cornea.

Keratitis—inflammation of the cornea.

Keratoconjunctivitis—inflammation of the cornea and conjunctiva.

Keratoconjunctivitis sicca (KCS)—inflammation of the cornea and conjunctiva due to insufficient production of the aqueous component of the precorneal tear film. This is diagnosed when the tear production is less than 15 mm/min in dogs and less than 9 mm/min in cats, as measured by the STT.

Keratotomy—incision into the cornea without removal of tissue.

Lacrimomimetic—tear film substitute (artificial tears).

Lagophthalmos—incomplete blink. Lagophthalmos causes exposure and drying of the cornea (usually the central cornea). This is a common finding in exophthalmic eyes.

Luxation—complete dislocation of a structure. In ophthalmology, the term luxation is most often used in reference to the lens. Lens luxation occurs when all zonules break down and the lens fully dislocates from its normal position.

Macroblepharon—abnormally large eyelid openings. This is often seen in dogs with brachycephalic ocular syndrome. Also referred to as macropalpebral fissure.

Macropalpebral fissure—abnormally large eyelid openings. This is often seen in dogs with brachycephalic ocular syndrome. Also referred to as macroblepharon.

Miosis—small pupil due to constriction of the pupillary sphincter muscle. Miosis occurs as a normal response to light. It also occurs in the presence of uveitis or in response to certain drugs.

Mucinomimetic—having properties similar to precorneal tear film mucin. This term is used to describe how closely artificial tears approximate tears made by the body. Mucinomimetic properties are desired when there is a deficiency of mucin in the precorneal tear film (a qualitative tear film abnormality).

Mydriasis—pupil dilation, as a result of constriction of the iris dilator muscle. Mydriasis occurs as a normal response to decreased ambient light. It also occurs as a result of retina and optic nerve disease or in response to certain medications (such as tropicamide and atropine).

Nictitans—the third eyelid. Also referred to as the nictitating membrane.

Ophthalmoplegia—paralysis of the ocular muscles. External ophthalmoplegia refers to paralysis of the extraocular muscles (which results in lack of globe movement). Internal ophthalmoplegia refers to paralysis of muscles inside of the eye (which results in fixed, dilated pupils).

Optic neuritis—inflammation of the optic nerve.

Pannus—also referred to as chronic superficial keratitis. This is immune-mediated inflammation that can involve the conjunctiva, cornea, and third eyelid. It is commonly seen in German shepherds and related breeds.

Pectinate ligament dysplasia—congenital malformation of the iridocorneal angle. Also referred to as goniodysgenesis.

Peripapillary—the region of the fundus immediately surrounding the optic nerve.

Phacodonesis—visible movement of the lens seen as a result of zonular breakdown (indicates lens instability).

Phthisis bulbi—an atrophied eye. This eye is smaller than normal and is no longer functional. Phthisis bulbi occurs as a sequela to chronic inflammation and chronic glaucoma.

Pigmentary keratitis—a syndrome of corneal melanosis and vascularization that preferentially affects the medial and central cornea. It most commonly affects dogs with brachycephalic ocular syndrome.

Posterior uveitis—inflammation of the choroid. Since inflammation of the retina usually occurs in the presence of choroidal inflammation, posterior uveitis usually refers to inflammation of both the choroid and the retina. This is also referred to as chorioretinitis.

Ptosis—drooping of the upper eyelid. This is one abnormality consistently found in Horner's syndrome.

Qualitative tear film abnormality—deficiency of the lipid or mucin portion of the tears.

Quantitative tear film abnormality—deficiency of the aqueous portion of the tears (KCS).

Retropulsion—gentle, posteriorly directed pressure placed onto the eyes. It is used to assess orbital disease. Retropulsion is performed by placing the index and/or middle fingers over the eyes, through closed eyelids. Gentle pressure is then used to push the eyes in the posterior direction (into the orbit). The amount of resistance by the eyes should feel equal on both sides. In the presence of orbital disease, the resistance noted by this action could be increased or decreased compared to normal. Unilateral orbital disease will show asymmetric resistance to retropulsion.

Schirmer tear test (STT)—a measurement of tear production. The test is performed by placing an STT strip (commercially available adsorbent paper strip) into the ventrolateral conjunctival sac and leaving it in place for 1 minute. During this minute, tears are taken up by the test strip. After 1 minute, the strip is removed from the conjunctival sac and the length of wet strip is measured. Tear production is expressed in the units of millimeters per minute. Normal STT values are above 15 mm/min in the dog and above 9 mm/min in the cat.

Sequestrum—usually used to describe a corneal sequestrum, which is necrotic corneal tissue resulting from chronic irritation. This condition is most commonly seen in cats. It rarely occurs in dogs.

Strabismus—misalignment of the eyes relative to one another. Strabismus can be congenital or acquired. An example of acquired strabismus is lateral deviation of the globe following proptosis. When the globe is proptosed, tearing of the medial rectus muscle can occur, allowing unopposed action of the lateral rectus muscle. This causes the direction of gaze of the affected eye to become deviated laterally.

Subluxation—partial dislocation of a structure. In ophthalmology, the term subluxation is most often used in reference to the lens. Lens subluxation means that the lens has partially dislocated from its normal position as a result of zonular breakdown.

Synechia—adhesion of the iris to an adjacent ocular structure, resulting from inflammation. Anterior synechia refers to an adhesion between the iris and the cornea. Posterior synechia refers to an adhesion between the iris and the lens.

Tapetum—reflective layer that is part of the choroid. The tapetum is found in the innermost layer of the dorsal half of the choroid.

Tarsorrhaphy—a procedure that partially or completely closes the palpebral fissure by suturing the upper and lower eyelids to each other.

Tear film breakup time (TFBUT)—measures the amount of time the precorneal tear film remains as a stable film over the corneal surface. Therefore, it is a measure of tear film stability, with shorter TFBUTs indicating less stability of the tear film (earlier evaporation of the tears). The TFBUT is considered an indirect measure of the mucin content of the tears. Normal TFBUTs in the cat fall between 12 and 21 seconds, while normal values in the dog fall between 15 and 25 seconds.

Tonometry—measurement of intraocular pressure.

Transillumination—the act of shining light through a structure during the ophthalmic examination.

Uvea—the vascular tunic of the eye. This can be divided into the anterior uvea (which is made up of the iris and ciliary body) and the posterior uvea (which is made up of the choroid).

Uveitis—inflammation of all or part of the uveal tract. See anterior uveitis, cyclitis, iridocyclitis, chorioretinitis, posterior uveitis.

Zonule—a thin ligament that runs radially between the ciliary body and the lens. Zonules hold the lens in correct position. Breakdown of the zonules results in lens subluxation or luxation.

About the companion website

This book is accompanied by a companion website:

www.wiley.com/go/lim/atlas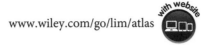

This website includes:
- Images from the book as downloadable PowerPoint slides
- Supplementary videos

Atlas

1 Orbit

Please see Chapter 10 for more information about diseases, diagnostic testing, and treatment plans related to the orbit.

Figure 1.1 Orbital adenocarcinoma in a 14-year-old, castrated male Pomeranian. Left-sided abnormalities, which developed slowly, include exophthalmos, lateral and dorsal displacement of the eye, third eyelid elevation, and conjunctival vascular engorgement. Retropulsion of the left globe was reduced. Discussion of orbital neoplasia can be found in Chapter 10.

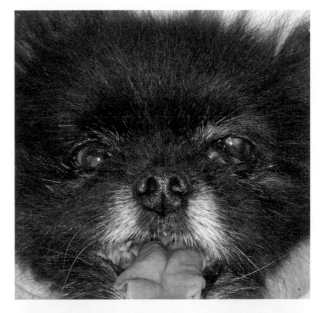

Figure 1.2a Right-sided buphthalmos, exophthalmos, and periocular swelling in a 2-year-old castrated male mixed breed dog. The IOP of the right eye was 56 mm Hg at the time of the photograph. This patient was diagnosed with endophthalmitis and secondary glaucoma resulting from systemic blastomycosis. Signs of orbital disease, including exophthalmos, are discussed in Chapter 10. Anterior uveitis is discussed in Chapter 15. Glaucoma is discussed in Chapter 18.

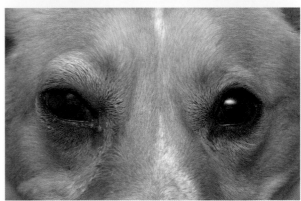

Small Animal Ophthalmic Atlas and Guide, Second Edition. Christine C. Lim.
© 2023 John Wiley & Sons, Inc. Published 2023 by John Wiley & Sons, Inc.
Companion website: www.wiley.com/go/lim/atlas

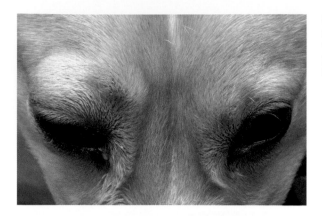

Figure 1.2b The same patient as in the previous figure, viewed from above. In many cases of orbital disease, assessing facial symmetry from above the head as well as from in front of the patient helps to identify changes that are present. In this patient, periocular swelling is more noticeable when viewed from above. Signs of orbital disease, including exophthalmos, are discussed in Chapter 10.

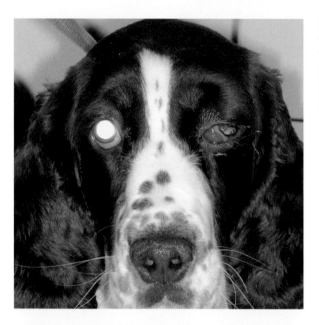

Figure 1.3 Orbital cellulitis in a 1-year-old, castrated male English springer spaniel. Left-sided abnormalities, which developed overnight, include exophthalmos, third eyelid elevation, chemosis and hyperemia of the conjunctiva overlying the third eyelid, and swelling of soft tissues around the left eye. This patient had stopped chewing on toys and had difficulty eating. *Enterococcus faecalis* was cultured from the left orbit. Clinical signs resolved with oral antibiotic therapy. Discussion of orbital cellulitis/abscess can be found in Chapter 10.

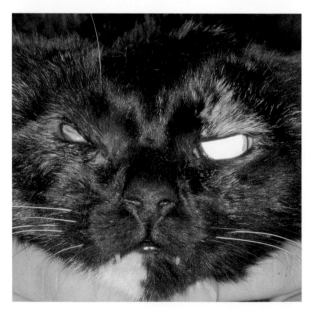

Figure 1.4 Orbital squamous cell carcinoma in a 12-year-old, spayed female DSH. The right eye is enophthalmic. The right palpebral fissure is distorted and the eyelids thickened and immobile. As a result of exposure, the right cornea became ulcerated. Orbital neoplasia is discussed in Chapter 10.

Figure 1.5 Left-sided orbital disease in a 5-year-old DSH. This patient presented for difficulty breathing and had a history of nasal discharge. The left globe was exophthalmic on presentation. Note the dorsal and lateral displacement of the globe, which corresponds to displacement caused by a mass in the nasal cavity. Necropsy revealed lymphoma. Orbital disease is discussed in Chapter 10.

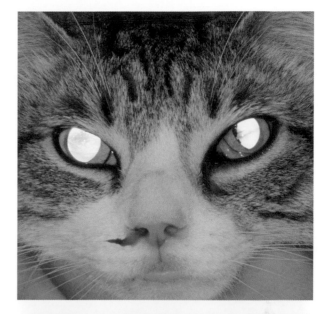

Figure 1.6 Bilateral enophthalmos, more pronounced in the left eye, in an elderly collie. Both third eyelids are raised, secondary to enophthalmos, and the left third eyelid almost completely obscures the globe. This patient had a recent history of weight loss; therefore, the enophthalmos was presumed to be due to atrophy of the orbital fat pads. Discussion of orbital disease is found in Chapter 10.

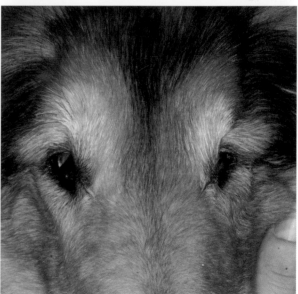

Figure 1.7 Brachycephalic ocular syndrome in a shih tzu. Note the excessive scleral show resulting from breed-related exophthalmos and enlarged palpebral fissures. Brachycephalic ocular syndrome is discussed in Chapter 10.

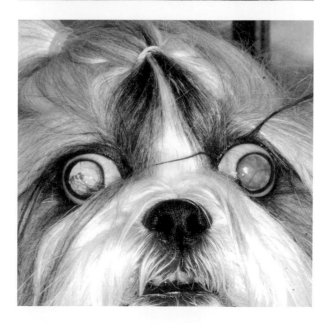

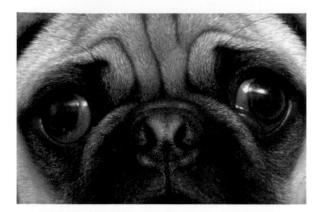

Figure 1.8 Bilateral exophthalmos and enlarged palpebral fissures in a pug puppy. Note the excessive exposure of the sclerae bilaterally. This patient also has central fibrosis on the right cornea and a prolapsed left third eyelid gland. Brachycephalic ocular syndrome is discussed in Chapter 10. Prolapse of the third eyelid gland is discussed in Chapter 12.

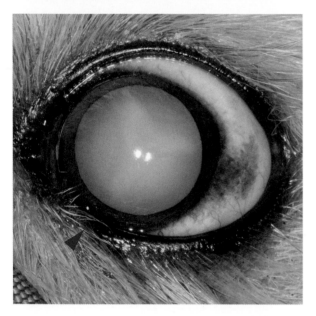

Figure 1.9 Left eye of a lhasa apso with brachycephalic ocular syndrome. Entropion affects the ventral eyelid between the medial canthus and the red arrowhead. Entropion is recognized by the inability to see the black eyelid margin medial to the red arrowhead (the margin is rolled under the haired skin.) Instead of eyelid margin, haired eyelid skin contacts the globe. Note the excessive scleral show resulting from enlarged palpebral fissures. This dog also has a complete cataract. Brachycephalic ocular syndrome is discussed in Chapter 10.

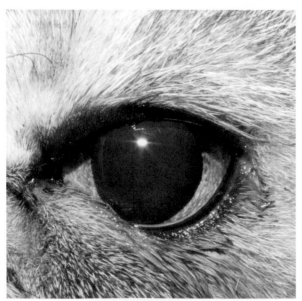

Figure 1.10 Left eye of a Himalayan cat, a breed with brachycephalic conformation. Note the contact between the nasal hairs and the cornea, referred to as nasal fold trichiasis. Brachycephalic ocular syndrome is discussed in Chapter 10. Trichiasis is discussed in Chapter 11.

Figure 1.11 Idiopathic, postganglionic Horner's syndrome. There is right-sided enophthalmos, miosis, third eyelid elevation, and ptosis. Horner's syndrome is discussed in Chapter 10.

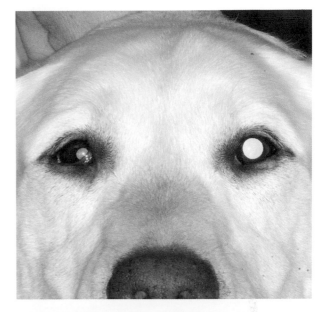

Figure 1.12a Left-sided, idiopathic, postganglionic Horner's syndrome. Ptosis and third eyelid elevation completely obscure the eye. Horner's syndrome is discussed in Chapter 10.

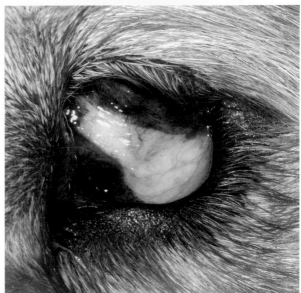

Figure 1.12b The same eye as in the previous figure, less than 20 minutes after instillation of phenylephrine into the conjunctival sac. Ptosis and third eyelid elevation are still present, but are less severe than prior to phenylephrine administration (as shown in the previous figure). The speed of clinical improvement led to a diagnosis of postganglionic Horner's syndrome. Horner's syndrome is discussed in Chapter 10.

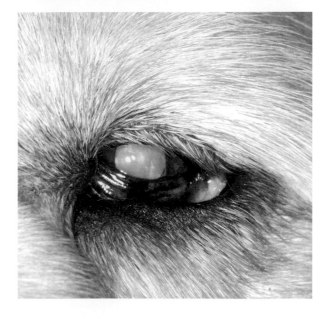

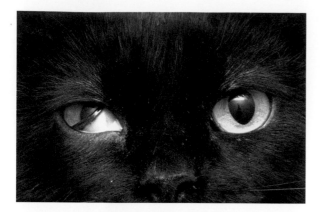

Figure 1.13a Right-sided ptosis, enophthalmos, and raised third eyelid in a 5-year-old American shorthair. The right pupil, which is partially obscured by the third eyelid, was smaller than the left pupil. Based on the ophthalmic abnormalities, Horner's syndrome was suspected and pharmacologic testing was performed. Horner's syndrome is discussed in Chapter 10.

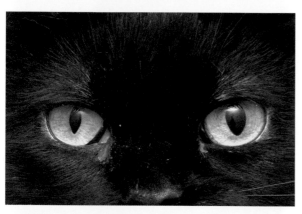

Figure 1.13b The same patient as in the previous figure, 5 minutes after application of phenylephrine. Although the abnormalities (ptosis, enophthalmos, raised third eyelid, and miosis) are still present in the right eye, they are reduced in severity when compared to before phenylephrine application. Because the ocular lesions improved in a short time frame, this patient was diagnosed with postganglionic Horner's syndrome. Horner's syndrome is discussed in Chapter 10.

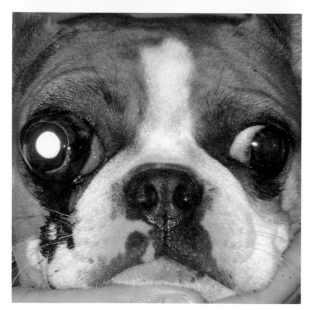

Figure 1.14 Proptosis in a 4-year-old, spayed female Boston terrier cross. The right eyelid margins are partially visible. Along with anterior displacement of the right eye, there is marked subconjunctival hemorrhage. The right pupil is miotic compared with the left pupil. Proptosis is discussed in Chapter 10.

Figure 1.15 Left-sided proptosis. Lubricating ointment had been applied to the ocular surface prior to taking this photograph. Almost the entire globe is anterior to the orbit and eyelid margins (which are not visible because they are trapped posterior to the globe). There is marked subconjunctival hemorrhage. Due to the distance of the globe displacement, there was significant rectus muscle avulsion and optic nerve trauma. The right pupil did not constrict when light was directed into the left eye. Due to the poor prognosis for return to vision, enucleation was elected. Proptosis is discussed in Chapter 10.

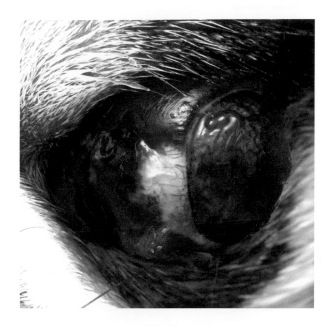

2 Eyelids

Please see Chapter 11 for more information about diseases, diagnostic testing, and treatment plans related to the eyelids.

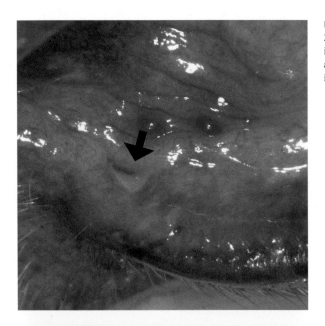

Figure 2.1 Ventral left punctum of a dog (arrow). The punctum is approximately 2 mm lateral to the medial canthus and is visible as a small, triangular irregularity in the eyelid margin. When eyelids are more deeply pigmented, puncta often appear as small, less pigmented foci within the brown to black skin. For more information, please see Chapter 11.

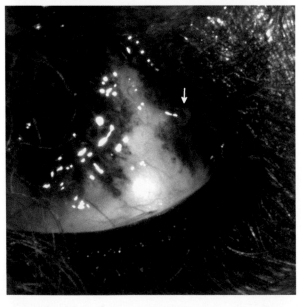

Figure 2.2 Photograph of the lower right eyelid, showing the normal appearance of the punctum (white arrow). The eyelids in this dog are darkly pigmented. In these cases, the punctum can often be found by looking for an irregularity to the pigment around the eyelid margin, approximately 2 mm from the medial aspect of the eyelid. A red arrow indicates one Meibomian gland opening; the remainder form a line of regularly spaced pale dots along the eyelid margin (gray line). Eyelids are discussed in Chapter 11.

Small Animal Ophthalmic Atlas and Guide, Second Edition. Christine C. Lim.
© 2023 John Wiley & Sons, Inc. Published 2023 by John Wiley & Sons, Inc.
Companion website: www.wiley.com/go/lim/atlas

Figure 2.3 Dorsal right eyelid of an 8-month-old miniature poodle. This patient presented for evaluation of right corneal ulceration with severe blepharospasm and epiphora, which did not improve during 4 weeks of medical treatment by the referring veterinarian. Ophthalmic examination found one ectopic cilium (arrow). This was presumed to be the cause of the ulcer and ocular pain, as the blepharospasm resolved immediately following the removal of the cilium and the ulcer resolved shortly thereafter. An arrowhead indicates one Meibomian gland opening; the remainder form a line of regularly spaced pale dots along the eyelid margin (gray line). Ectopic cilia are discussed in Chapter 11.

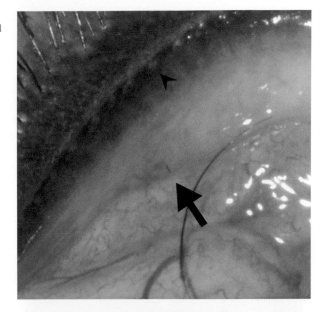

Figure 2.4 Ectopic cilium in the upper eyelid of a French bulldog puppy. The eyelid has been everted for this photograph so that the palpebral conjunctiva is visible. The ectopic cilium (arrow) is a black hair emerging from the surface of the palpebral conjunctiva. It is visible immediately proximal to the brown eyelid margin. Note how short the hair is; magnification was needed to identify it on examination. This patient had a history of chronic blepharospasm and epiphora that was sometimes associated with a corneal ulcer. Ocular discomfort resolved following removal of the ectopic cilium. Ectopic cilia are discussed in Chapter 11.

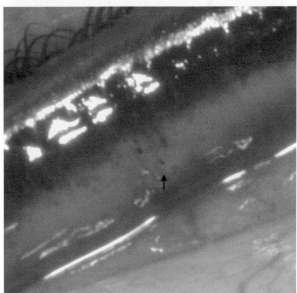

Figure 2.5 Distichiae in the dorsal right eyelid of an English bulldog (arrows). These dark, coarse hairs arise from the Meibomian gland openings. Distichiae are discussed in Chapter 11.

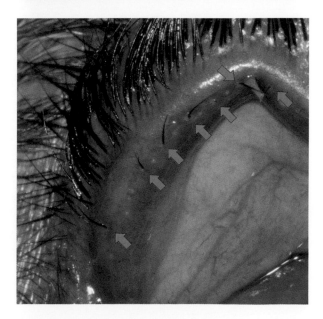

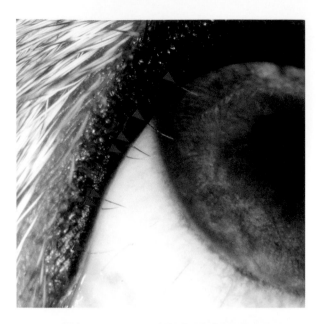

Figure 2.6 Several brown distichiae (arrowheads) along the dorsal right eyelid margin of a 3-year-old, spayed female Alaskan malamute. Distichiae are discussed in Chapter 11.

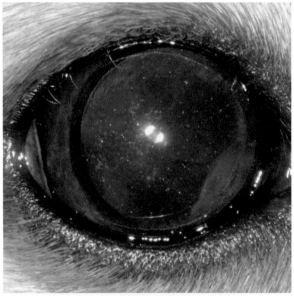

Figure 2.7 Multiple distichiae arising from the margin of the upper eyelid. Distichiae are discussed in Chapter 11.

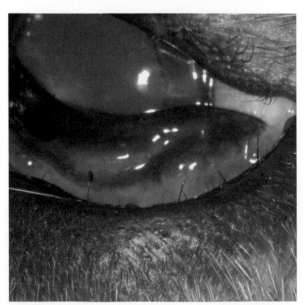

Figure 2.8 Multiple lower eyelid distichiae in a young golden retriever. Distichiae are discussed in Chapter 11.

Figure 2.9 Upper eyelid distichiae. The hairs can be seen arising from Meibomian gland openings. Distichiae are discussed in Chapter 11.

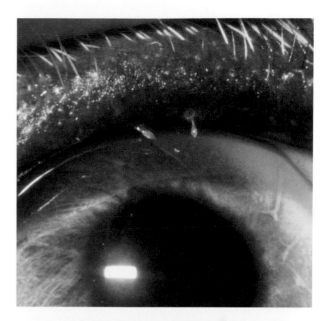

Figure 2.10 Multiple ectopic cilia (arrows) in the upper eyelid of a shih tzu. This patient suffered from chronic superficial keratitis, to which the ectopic cilia were likely contributing. Contrast the length of these ectopic cilia with that seen in Figures 2.3 and 2.4. A chalazion is also visible within the palpebral conjunctiva (arrowhead). The appearance of this chalazion is typical; it is white, round, and adjacent to the eyelid margin. Ectopic cilia and chalazia are discussed in Chapter 11.

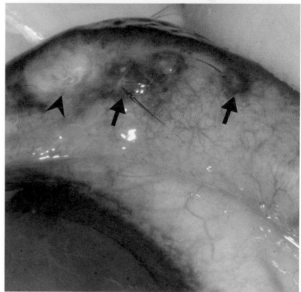

Figure 2.11 Long periocular hairs rub the medial cornea of this shih tzu. This chronic corneal trauma has caused the medial cornea to become melanotic (pigmentary keratitis). Trichiasis is discussed in Chapter 11. Pigmentary keratitis is discussed in Chapter 14.

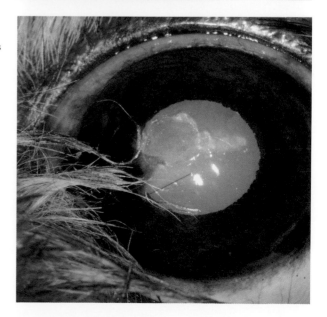

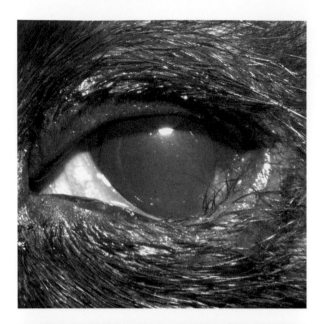

Figure 2.12 Lower eyelid entropion in a DSH. Chronic contact between the eyelid hairs and the cornea has led to development of superficial corneal vascularization. Entropion is discussed in Chapter 11.

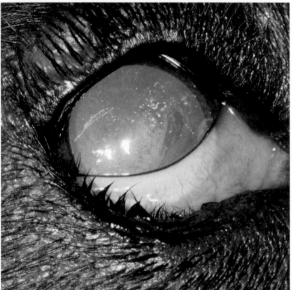

Figure 2.13 Conformational entropion affecting the entire ventral right eyelid. The eyelid margin of the ventral eyelid is not visible due to inward rolling of the eyelid. Instead, wet eyelid hairs can be seen contacting the ocular surface. Entropion is discussed in Chapter 11.

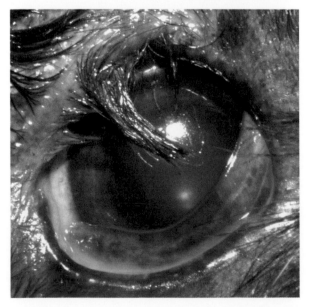

Figure 2.14 Entropion of the right upper eyelid of an elderly Portuguese water dog. The upper left eyelid was similarly affected. The entropion was secondary to enophthalmos, which was caused by age-related atrophy of the orbital fat pads. Note the elevated third eyelid, which was another consequence of enophthalmos. Entropion is discussed in Chapter 11.

Figure 2.15 Lower eyelid entropion in an English bulldog. Due to inward rolling of the lower eyelid, the eyelid margin is not visible. Haired skin is in contact with the ocular surface. As in most cases of entropion, the hairs and skin of the affected eyelid are wet with tears. Entropion is discussed in Chapter 11.

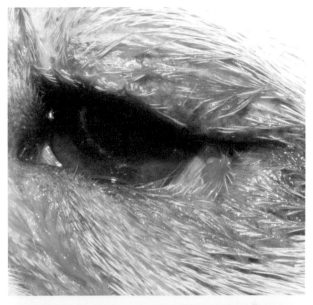

Figure 2.16 Upper and lower eyelid entropion in a 15-month-old great Dane. Entropion affects the lateral half of the upper eyelid and the lateral two-thirds of the lower eyelid. Conjunctival hyperemia is present as a result of chronic surface ocular irritation. As in most cases of entropion, the hairs and skin of the affected eyelids are wet with tears. Entropion is discussed in Chapter 11.

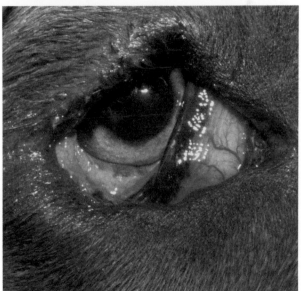

Figure 2.17 Tacking sutures were placed in the lower eyelid, upper eyelid, and lateral canthus to correct spastic entropion. The source of ocular pain was a corneal ulcer. The tacking sutures were left in place until the corneal ulcer resolved. Entropion is discussed in Chapter 11. Corneal ulcers are discussed in Chapter 14.

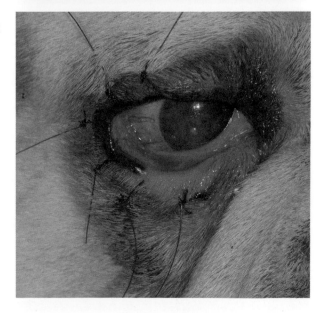

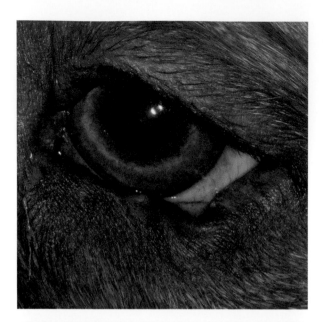

Figure 2.18 Very mild ectropion of the central lower left eyelid. This was not associated with any ocular pathology and was therefore not treated. Ectropion is further discussed in Chapter 11.

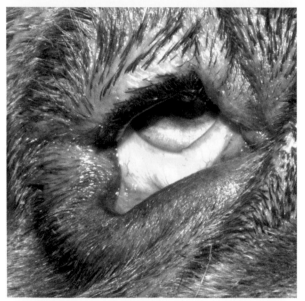

Figure 2.19 Lower right eyelid ectropion in a Neapolitan mastiff. The lower eyelid is everted due to excessive length (part of the normal conformation for this breed). The result is exposure and irritation of the conjunctiva, seen as conjunctival hyperemia and ocular discharge. Ectropion is discussed in Chapter 11.

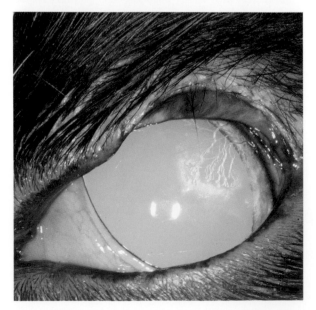

Figure 2.20 Eyelid agenesis in a DSH. Just over half of the upper eyelid margin is absent. As a result of the eyelid defect, lagophthalmos and trichiasis are present. Superficial vascularization of the lateral cornea corresponds to the area of corneal exposure and trichiasis. Eyelid agenesis is discussed in Chapter 11.

Figure 2.21a Left eye of a DSH with upper eyelid agenesis. Note the lack of eyelid margin for all but the most medial aspect of the upper eyelid (between the medial canthus and the arrow). Superficial vasculature and fibrosis affect the dorsolateral cornea. Eyelid agenesis is discussed in Chapter 11.

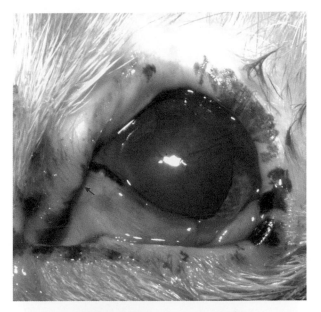

Figure 2.21b The same eye as in the previous figure. This photograph shows how the eyelid defect leaves the cornea exposed even when the eyelids are closed. The corneal lesions (see Figure 2.21a) correlate with the area that is exposed when the eyelids are closed. Eyelid agenesis is discussed in Chapter 11.

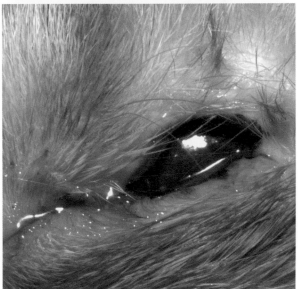

Figure 2.22 Right eye of a DSH. The upper eyelid margin is present medially, but is missing for approximately half of the eyelid length laterally. The defect is milder than for the patient in the previous figures as there is complete corneal coverage when the eyelids are closed. However, the lack of eyelid margin allows hairs from the upper eyelid to contact the corneal surface (trichiasis). Over time, this trichiasis can lead to keratitis. Eyelid agenesis is discussed in Chapter 11.

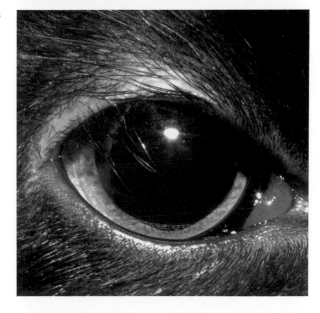

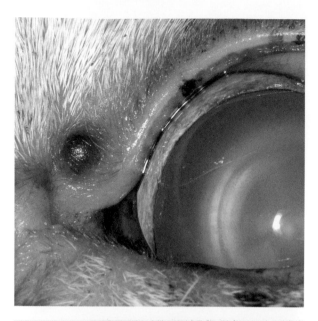

Figure 2.23 Medial canthal mass in a DSH. Because of the dark, circular appearance, and because the patient was a cat, apocrine hidrocystoma was suspected. Eyelid masses are discussed in Chapter 11.

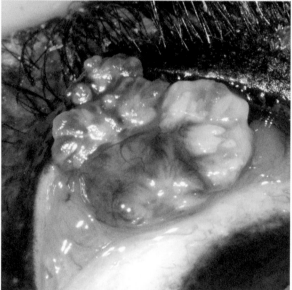

Figure 2.24 Typical appearance of a Meibomian adenoma. The mass is lightly pigmented, hairless, has a rough surface, and arises from the eyelid margin. Eyelid neoplasia is discussed in Chapter 11.

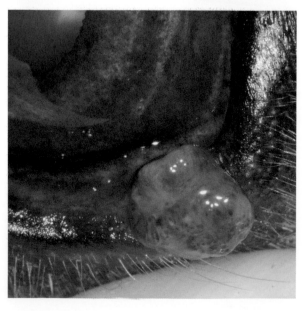

Figure 2.25 Meibomian adenoma in a 10-year-old, spayed female golden retriever. The tumor is nonpigmented, hairless, has a rough surface, and arises from the eyelid margin. The vessels within the tumor and the surrounding conjunctiva are hyperemic, indicating concurrent conjunctivitis. Eyelid neoplasia is discussed in Chapter 11.

Figure 2.26 Upper left eyelid mass in a 10-year old spayed female Labrador retriever. Although histopathology was declined, the characteristic appearance of the mass was highly suggestive of Meibomian adenoma. The most visible portion of the mass is the inflamed and ulcerated tissue ventral to the upper eyelid margin. Dorsal to this, the skin proximal to the eyelid margin is swollen and erythemic. Eversion of the upper eyelid revealed that the mass extended into the palpebral conjunctiva under the swollen area of skin. The dried blood in the periocular hairs is a result of periodic bleeding from the mass. Eyelid masses are discussed in Chapter 11.

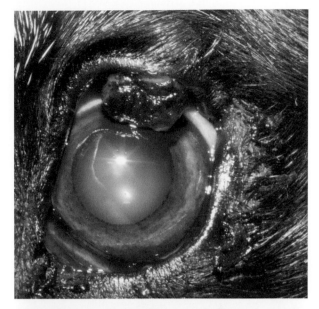

Figure 2.27 Suspected upper eyelid melanoma in 10-year-old basset hound. The mass was attached to the eyelid margin by a thin strand of tissue. A melanoma rather than an adenoma was suspected due to the color and thin attachment to the eyelid. Eyelid masses are discussed in Chapter 11.

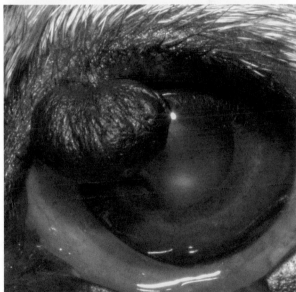

Figure 2.28 Upper right eyelid of an elderly German shepherd cross. The mass was visible in the palpebral conjunctiva (black arrow) as well as protruding from a Meibomian gland opening (white arrow). The conjunctival portion of the mass was not visible without everting the upper eyelid. The bulbar conjunctiva is hyperemic due to irritation caused by contact between the mass and the ocular surface. Following removal of the mass, histopathology confirmed it to be Meibomian adenoma. Eyelid masses are discussed in Chapter 11.

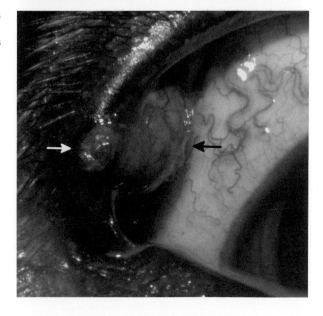

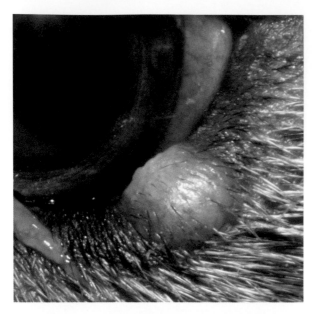

Figure 2.29 Lower left eyelid of a 3-year-old, spayed female English bulldog. There is a pink mass at the eyelid margin that had been present for approximately 2 weeks prior to presentation. It was removed and identified by histopathology to be plasmacytoma. Eyelid masses are discussed in Chapter 11.

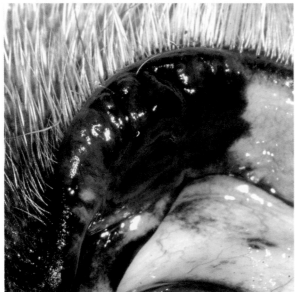

Figure 2.30 Upper eyelid melanocytoma. Rather than forming a discrete mass, this neoplasm was associated with diffuse thickening and melanosis of the eyelid. Eyelid neoplasia is discussed in Chapter 11.

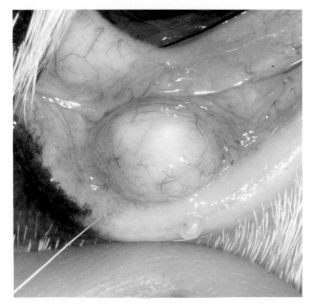

Figure 2.31 Typical appearance of a chalazion. Chalazia tend to be round, white (due to the accumulation of lipid secretions), and variably raised from the surface of the palpebral conjunctiva. Their proximity to the eyelid margins corresponds to the location of the Meibomian glands. Chalazia are discussed in Chapter 11.

Figure 2.32 Another example of the typical appearance of a chalazion: round, white, and located adjacent to the eyelid margin (where Meibomian glands are found). Chalazia are discussed in Chapter 11.

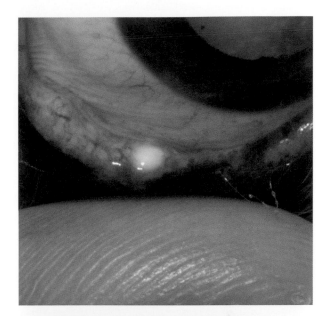

Figure 2.33 Two adjacent chalazia. These chalazia are associated with mild conjunctivitis, as seen by engorgement of the conjunctival blood vessels immediately surrounding the chalazion. Chalazia are discussed in Chapter 11.

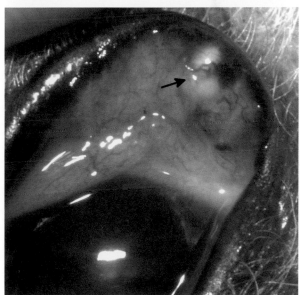

Figure 2.34 Idiopathic pyogranulomatous Meibomian adenitis and conjunctivitis. The eyelids are thickened, erythematous, and ulcerated. The blepharitis resolved following a course of oral prednisone. Blepharitis is discussed in Chapter 11.

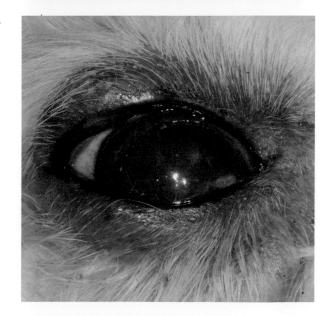

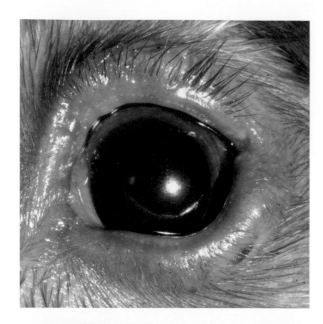

Figure 2.35 The typical appearance of Meibomitis is swelling and erythema concentrated at the eyelid margins. Blepharitis is discussed in Chapter 11.

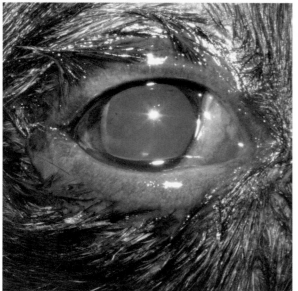

Figure 2.36 Alopecia, edema, erythema, and depigmentation of the eyelid margins. This blepharitis developed acutely after several weeks of topical cidofovir therapy and was suspected to be a drug reaction. Blepharitis is discussed in Chapter 11.

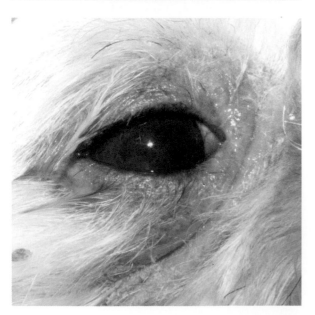

Figure 2.37 Right eye of a 9-year-old, spayed female shih tzu. There is periocular alopecia, erythema, and thickening of the eyelid skin. Mucoid ocular discharge is present. These changes were suspected to be a reaction to a topically-applied carbonic anhydrase inhibitor; clinical signs resolved when the medication was discontinued. Blepharitis is discussed in Chapter 11.

Figure 2.38 Right eye of a 1-year-old, spayed female pug whose owner noticed a bump in the upper right eyelid. There is alopecia, erythema, and thickening of the central upper eyelid. When pressure was applied to this swelling, the palpebral conjunctiva ruptured and a thick, white discharge was released. Cytology indicated suppurative inflammation. Culture and sensitivity isolated *Streptococcus pseudointermedius*. The lesion resolved with oral carprofen and cefpodoxime treatment. Blepharitis is discussed in Chapter 11.

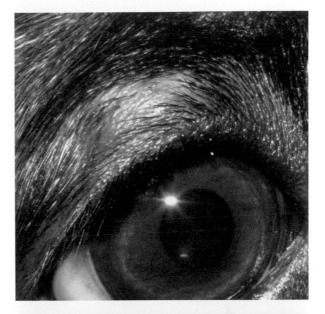

Figure 2.39 Steroid-responsive blepharitis in a 7-year-old, castrated male standard poodle. There is a moist dermatitis with depigmentation, alopecia, ulceration, and crusting of the eyelids. There are erosive changes to the eyelid margins. Neomycin polymyxin B dexamethasone ophthalmic ointment, to be applied to the affected skin, was prescribed after diagnostics were declined. Treatment was associated with complete resolution of clinical signs. Blepharitis is discussed in Chapter 11.

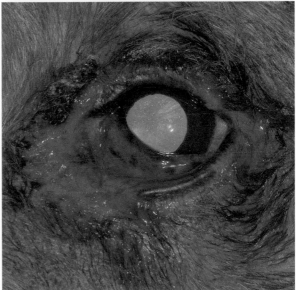

Figure 2.40 Blepharitis in a DSH. The eyelids are thickened and erythematous. There is also alopecia and crusting. Cytology detected 2+ cocci and inflammatory cells. The blepharitis resolved following treatment with tobramycin/dexamethasone ophthalmic ointment and erythromycin ophthalmic ointment applied to the affected skin twice daily. Blepharitis is discussed in Chapter 11.

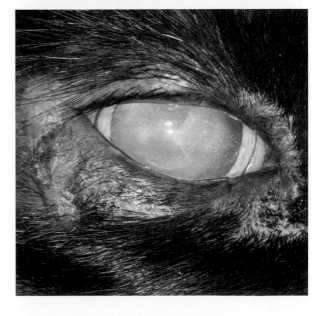

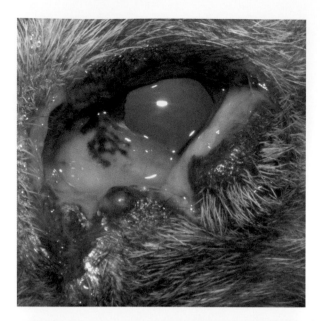

Figure 2.41 Chronic lower left eyelid laceration. The patient was a previously stray DSH of unknown age. Note the discontinuity of the lower eyelid margin, resulting in a wedge-shaped defect in the lower eyelid. Conjunctival hyperemia, chemosis, and mucopurulent ocular discharge are also present and reflect chronic surface ocular inflammation. Eyelid lacerations are discussed in Chapter 11.

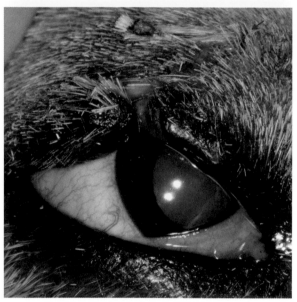

Figure 2.42 Upper right eyelid laceration. The periocular hairs have been clipped to aid in cleaning and evaluation. Note the discontinuity in the central upper eyelid; the laceration extends from the eyelid margin to the red arrow. It is crucial to examine underneath the injured eyelid to rule out concurrent injury to the globe. Eyelid lacerations are discussed in Chapter 11.

3 Third eyelid, nasolacrimal system, and precorneal tear film

Please see Chapter 12 for more information about diseases, diagnostic testing, and treatment plans related to the third eyelid, naso-lacrimal system, and precorneal tear film.

Figure 3.1 Left eye of a 2-year-old spayed female standard poodle. The third eyelid has been elevated for this photograph. This is the typical, normal appearance of a third eyelid. In this individual, the leading edge of the third eyelid is pigmented. The surface of the third eyelid is smooth, and it sits flat against the globe. Ventral to the leading edge, the anterior surface of the third eyelid is smooth and is covered by less pigmented conjunctiva. Diseases of the third eyelid are discussed in Chapter 12.

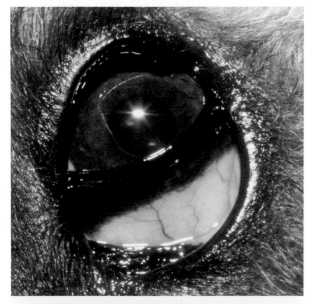

Figure 3.2 Positive Jones test in a cat. Fluorescein appeared within the mouth on the tongue, but not at the nares. The Jones test is discussed in Chapter 12.

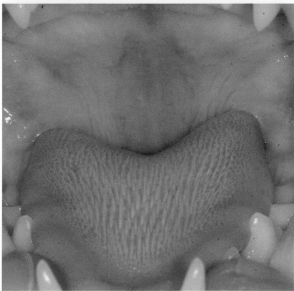

Small Animal Ophthalmic Atlas and Guide, Second Edition. Christine C. Lim.
© 2023 John Wiley & Sons, Inc. Published 2023 by John Wiley & Sons, Inc.
Companion website: www.wiley.com/go/lim/atlas

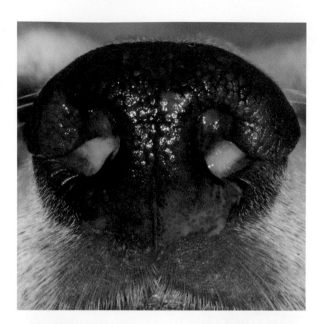

Figure 3.3 Fluorescein is not visualized at the right nare (negative Jones test) but is seen on the left side (positive Jones test). This is consistent with obstruction of the right nasolacrimal drainage apparatus and patency of the left nasolacrimal drainage apparatus. Nasolacrimal duct obstruction is discussed in Chapter 12.

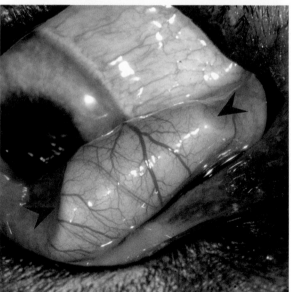

Figure 3.4 Everted right third eyelid cartilage. The vertical cartilage is bent outward, causing the third eyelid to fold upon itself. The medial and lateral edges of the vertical cartilage are visible (arrowheads). Note the more linear appearance of these edges compared with the rounded edges typical of prolapsed third eyelid glands (Figures 3.7–3.11). Mild conjunctivitis is present. This patient later developed prolapse of the third eyelid gland in the same eye. Scrolled cartilage and third eyelid gland prolapse are discussed in Chapter 12.

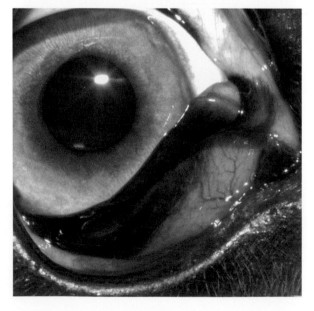

Figure 3.5 Right eye of a great Dane puppy. The medial aspect of the horizontal third eyelid cartilage is bent, causing the leading edge of the third eyelid to evert in this area. Cartilage eversion and prolapse of the third eyelid are discussed in Chapter 12.

Figure 3.6 Right eye of a Newfoundland puppy. The vertical portion of the third eyelid cartilage is bent, as are the medial and lateral tips of the horizontal cartilage. The bend in the vertical cartilage has caused eversion of the third eyelid and exposure of its bulbar surface (between the red and black arrows). The black arrow shows the leading edge of the third eyelid. Cartilage eversion and prolapse of the third eyelid are discussed in Chapter 12.

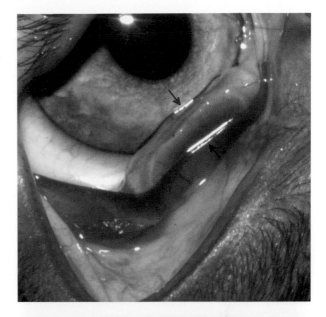

Figure 3.7 Prolapsed right third eyelid gland in a Burmese cat. The leading edge of the nictitans is not visible. The prolapsed gland is the pink, rounded structure protruding from the medial canthus. Prolapse of the third eyelid gland is discussed in Chapter 12.

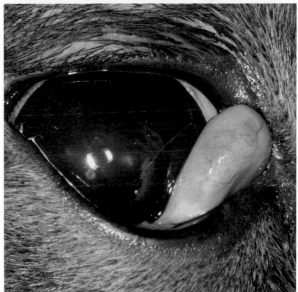

Figure 3.8 Right eye of a 3-month-old female Persian mix. The third eyelid gland had been prolapsed since the time of adoption. The moderate conjunctival hyperemia and mucoid ocular discharge are consistent with irritation induced by exposure of the gland. Prolapse of the third eyelid gland is discussed in Chapter 12.

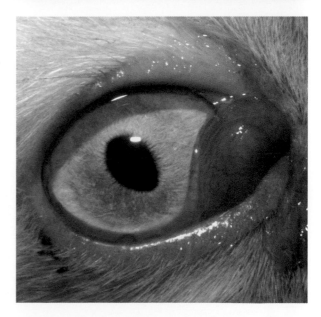

CHAPTER 3

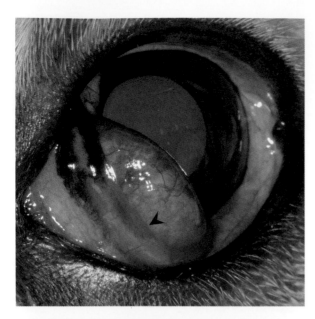

Figure 3.9 Prolapsed left third eyelid gland in a 5-month-old female Labrador retriever. The lightly pigmented leading edge of the third eyelid (arrowhead) is ventral and anterior to the prolapsed gland. The gland itself is rounded and pink and brown, with a smooth surface. Mild conjunctivitis is present. Prolapse of the third eyelid gland is discussed in Chapter 12.

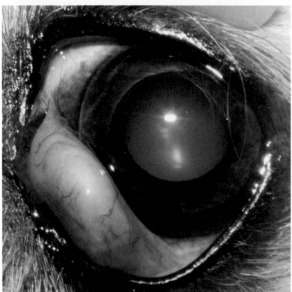

Figure 3.10 In this photograph, the left third eyelid gland is prolapsed, mildly hyperemic, and mildly swollen. The leading edge of the third eyelid is not visible in this photograph because it is below the prolapsed gland and behind the lower eyelid. Prolapse of the third eyelid gland is discussed in Chapter 12.

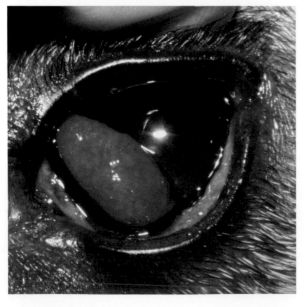

Figure 3.11 Left third eyelid gland prolapse. The gland is swollen and hyperemic, and located dorsal and posterior to the leading edge of the third eyelid (which is darkly pigmented in this individual). Prolapse of the third eyelid gland is discussed in Chapter 12.

Figure 3.12 Left third eyelid gland prolapse. The patient was a 6-month-old male English bulldog with a history of previous gland replacement surgeries. The thickened, hyperemic third eyelid gland is visible dorsal and posterior to the leading edge of the third eyelid (arrow). Conjunctival hyperemia and chemosis are also present. Tear production was decreased at 10 mm/min, likely secondary to chronic inflammation of the gland. Prolapse of the third eyelid gland is discussed in Chapter 12.

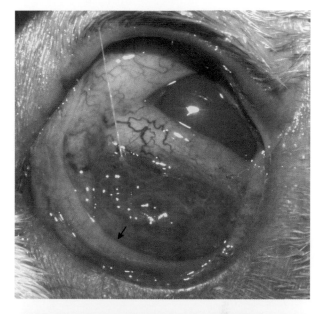

Figure 3.13 Raised, brown mass on the conjunctiva lining the bulbar surface of the third eyelid. This was an incidental finding on ophthalmic examination. Excisional biopsy and histopathology revealed squamous papilloma. Third eyelid neoplasia is discussed in Chapter 12, and conjunctival neoplasia is discussed in Chapter 13.

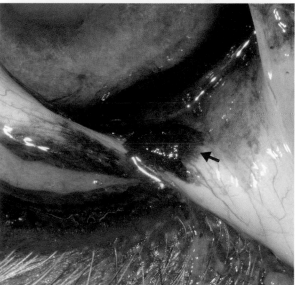

Figure 3.14 Right third eyelid mass (arrow) of an elderly Labrador retriever. The mass is melanotic and raised from the anterior surface of the third eyelid. Third eyelid neoplasia is discussed in Chapter 12 and conjunctival neoplasia is discussed in Chapter 13.

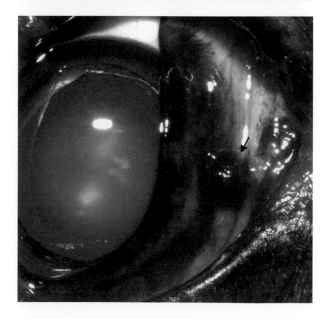

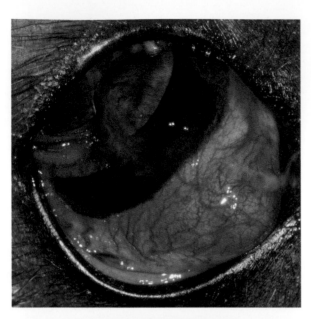

Figure 3.15 Right third eyelid gland adenocarcinoma. The mass is between the eye and the third eyelid. It displaces the eye caudally, causing enophthalmos. Conjunctival hyperemia is also visible. Due to the size of the mass, exenteration was required in order to completely excise the mass. Note the similar appearance to third eyelid gland prolapses in Figures 3.9, 3.11, and 3.12. Because of this, third eyelid gland neoplasia and other orbital neoplasia should always be considered when an older individual presents with a prolapsed gland. Third eyelid neoplasia is discussed in Chapter 12.

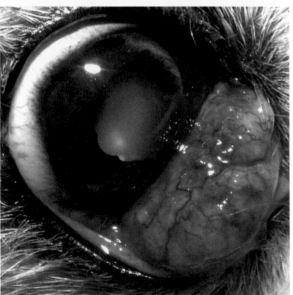

Figure 3.16 Right third eyelid of a 16-year-old poodle mix. The third eyelid gland is enlarged, thickened, and prolapsed. An arrow indicates the leading edge of the third eyelid, which is ventral to the prolapsed gland. The surface of the gland is irregular and the overlying conjunctival vessels are engorged. Areas of darker pigmentation are visible within the gland. Because of the appearance of the gland and because the prolapse occurred in an older individual, neoplasia was suspected and the third eyelid was excised. Histopathology confirmed adenocarcinoma arising from the gland of the third eyelid. As with Figure 3.15, note the similar appearance to third eyelid gland prolapses in Figures 3.9, 3.11, and 3.12. Third eyelid gland neoplasia and other orbital neoplasia should always be considered when an older individual presents with a prolapsed gland. Third eyelid neoplasia is discussed in Chapter 12.

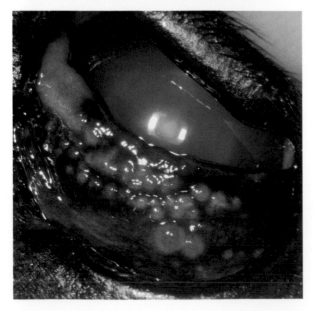

Figure 3.17 Left third eyelid of a 12-year-old, spayed female German shepherd. The third eyelid is depigmented, thickened, and irregular. These changes are typical of pannus, which is discussed in Chapter 14.

Figure 3.18 Right third eyelid of a German shepherd. The conjunctiva overlying the third eyelid is hyperemic. The leading edge of the third eyelid is mildly depigmented and its surface is uneven. These findings were present bilaterally, which is consistent with a diagnosis of third eyelid pannus. Incidentally, an upper eyelid mass is present. Pannus is discussed in Chapter 14.

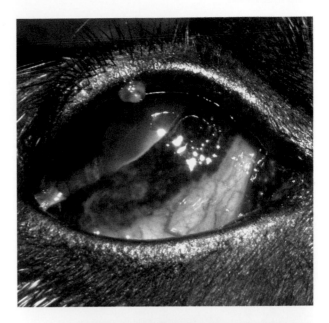

Figure 3.19 Right eye of a Belgian malinois. There is conjunctival hyperemia, depigmentation of the leading edge of the third eyelid, and irregular thickening of the leading edge of the third eyelid. These findings were present bilaterally, which is consistent with a diagnosis of third eyelid pannus. Pannus is discussed in Chapter 14.

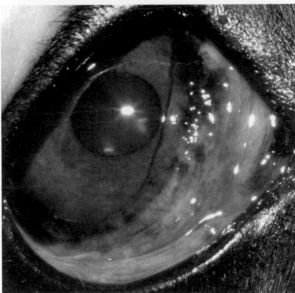

4 Conjunctiva

Please see Chapter 13 for more information about diseases, diagnostic testing, and treatment plans related to the conjunctiva.

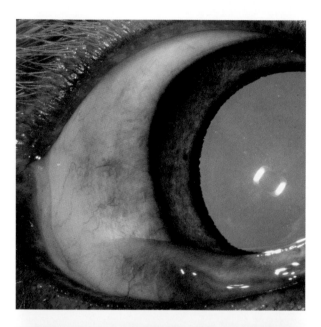

Figure 4.1 Lateral bulbar conjunctiva in a dog. Normal conjunctiva appears smooth and moist, is light pink due to blood vessels, and contains varying levels of melanin. Because conjunctiva is elastic, folds are sometimes seen in the tissue, particularly in the conjunctival fornices. For more information, please see Chapter 13.

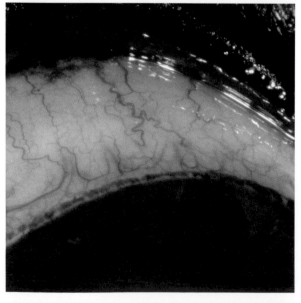

Figure 4.2 Conjunctival hyperemia. Compared with Figure 4.1, each vessel is wider, more visible, and the conjunctiva appears more reddened overall. Canine conjunctivitis is discussed in Chapter 13.

Figure 4.3 Left blepharitis and keratoconjunctivitis in a DSH. There is mild erythema and crusting of the eyelids, conjunctival hyperemia, chemosis, and superficial corneal vascularization. Feline conjunctivitis is discussed in Chapter 13.

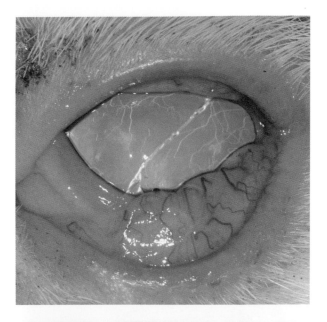

Figure 4.4 Conjunctival hyperemia, chemosis, and mucopurulent ocular discharge in a DLH. Because the ocular signs manifested acutely following subcutaneous steroid injection, recrudescent herpetic disease following immunosuppression was suspected as the cause. Clinical signs improved with antibiotic and antiviral therapy. Feline conjunctivitis is discussed in Chapter 13.

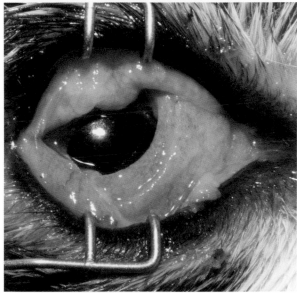

Figure 4.5 Chemosis, conjunctival hyperemia, conjunctival follicle development (arrow), and mucoid ocular discharge in a young DSH. Clinical signs resolved with oral famciclovir treatment. Feline conjunctivitis is discussed in Chapter 13.

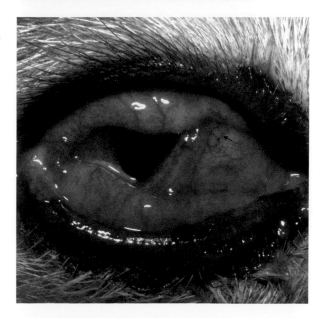

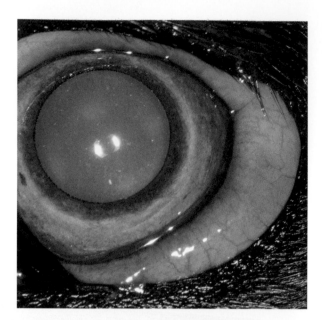

Figure 4.6 Chemosis often causes a "puffy" appearance of the conjunctiva. The swelling often results in protrusion of the conjunctiva from the palpebral fissure. Conjunctivitis is discussed in Chapter 13.

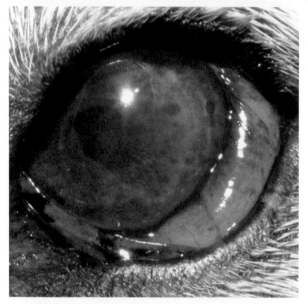

Figure 4.7 Chemosis in a 12-year-old, castrated male Labrador retriever. The chemosis makes the conjunctiva appear "puffy" and has caused the conjunctiva to protrude above the margin of the lower eyelid. Conjunctivitis is discussed in Chapter 13.

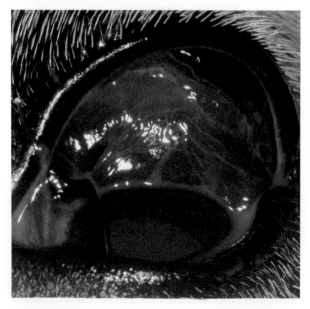

Figure 4.8 Marked subconjunctival hemorrhage in a stray dog. Note the swelling of the conjunctiva and inability to distinguish individual conjunctival vessels. Fluorescein stain has been applied to the eye. For more information, please see Chapter 13.

Figure 4.9 Subconjunctival hemorrhage, periocular swelling, serosanguineous ocular discharge, and hyphema as a result of a car accident. In spite of anti-inflammatory therapy, this eye continued to experience pain and inflammation and did not regain vision. Subconjunctival hemorrhage is discussed in Chapter 13. Uveitis and hyphema are discussed in Chapter 15.

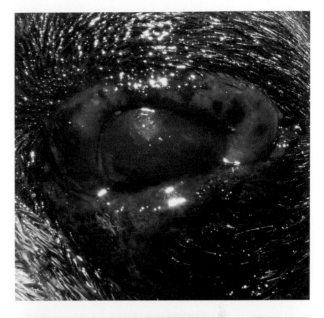

Figure 4.10 Follicles in the ventral conjunctival fornix of a dog. Follicles typically appear round and pink. They occur singly or in clusters, as in this photograph. Diffuse conjunctival hyperemia is also shown in this photograph. Conjunctivitis is discussed in Chapter 13.

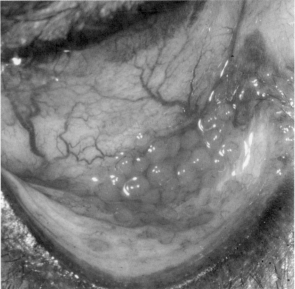

Figure 4.11 Multiple conjunctival follicles in the ventral conjunctival fornix of a Siberian husky. This eye was being treated for an indolent corneal ulcer. The follicles are unpigmented while the surrounding conjunctiva is melanotic. Conjunctivitis is discussed in Chapter 13.

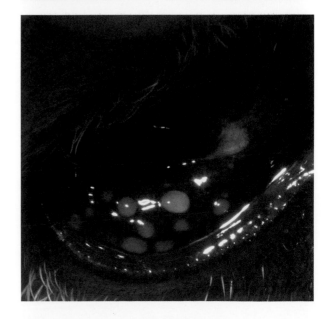

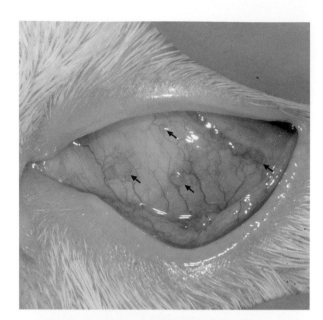

Figure 4.12 Left eye of a 7-month-old, spayed female DSH. There is mild erythema of the eyelids, diffuse conjunctival hyperemia, and conjunctival follicle development (arrows) on the anterior surface of the third eyelid. Feline conjunctivitis is discussed in Chapter 13.

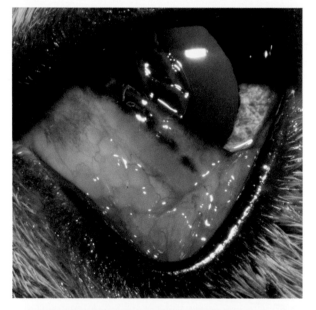

Figure 4.13 Multiple conjunctival follicles are visible in the ventral conjunctival fornix of this 10-year-old DSH. This patient had brachycephalic conformation, a chronic source of ocular surface irritation. Conjunctivitis is discussed in Chapter 13.

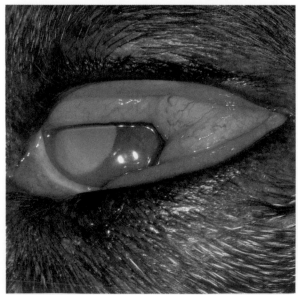

Figure 4.14 Left eye of an 8-year-old, spayed female blue heeler dog. Both eyes and periocular structures were similar in appearance. The conjunctiva is diffusely thickened and hyperemic. While chemosis is present, the conjunctiva is much firmer than if the thickening were due to fluid alone. Mild corneal edema is also present, most prominent in the ventromedial quadrant. A conjunctival biopsy revealed lymphoma. Concurrent cutaneous lesions were also diagnosed as lymphoma. Conjunctival neoplasia is discussed in Chapter 13.

CHAPTER 4

Figure 4.15 Raised, melanotic conjunctival mass posterior to the dorsal limbus. Surgical removal was declined; therefore, a diagnosis was not obtained. Conjunctival neoplasia is discussed in Chapter 13.

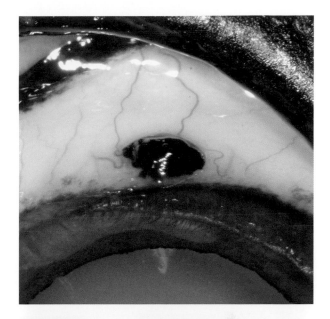

Figure 4.16 Nonpigmented mass arising from the ventral conjunctival fornix. The mass was not visible unless the lower eyelid was everted. The mass was not removed, so a diagnosis was not obtained. Other abnormalities in this photograph include conjunctival hyperemia, superficial corneal vascularization, and corneal fibrosis. Conjunctival masses are discussed in Chapter 13.

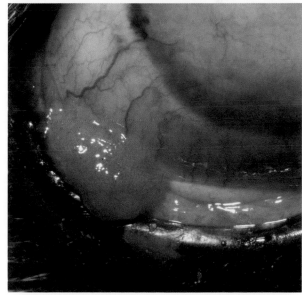

Figure 4.17 Raised, melanotic mass posterior to the lateral limbus. The histopathologic diagnosis was squamous papilloma and excision was curative. Conjunctival masses are discussed in Chapter 13.

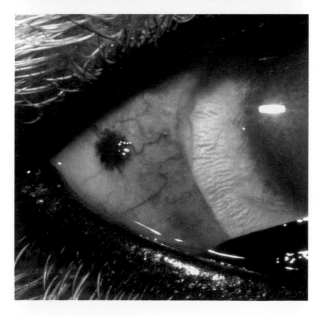

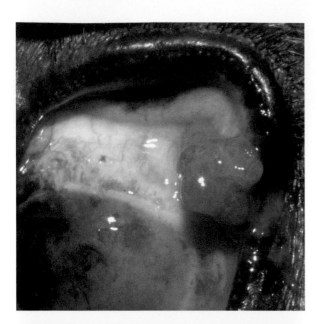

Figure 4.18 Mass arising from the dorsal conjunctival fornix. Because this was rubbing on the ocular surface, it was removed. A histopathologic diagnosis was not obtained. Conjunctival masses are discussed in Chapter 13.

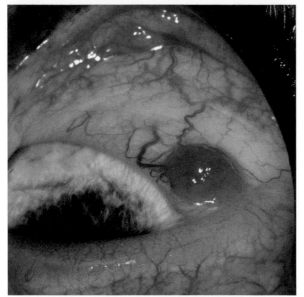

Figure 4.19 Raised, pink mass on the perilimbal bulbar conjunctiva. Surrounding conjunctiva is diffusely hyperemic. Histopathology revealed this to be a squamous papilloma. Conjunctival neoplasia is discussed in Chapter 13.

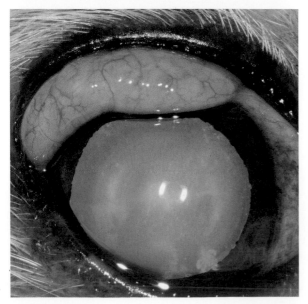

Figure 4.20 Canine conjunctival mast cell tumor. Note the swelling and hyperemia of the conjunctiva dorsal to the right eye. Conjunctival neoplasia is discussed in Chapter 13.

5 Cornea

Please see Chapter 14 for more information about diseases, diagnostic testing, and treatment plans related to the cornea.

Figure 5.1 Chronic, superficial, nonulcerative keratoconjunctivitis due to KCS. The STT was 0 mm/min. The corneal surface is rough, dry, and lackluster. This is evidenced by scattering of the camera flash on this cornea (compare with Figures 3.1, 4.1, and 5.23, where the corneas are smooth and hydrated and the flash is easily discernible). The appearance of the cornea, the mucoid discharge (in this photograph, the mucous is yellow due to the application of fluorescein stain), and the adherence of the discharge to the cornea are characteristic of KCS. Keratitis and KCS are discussed in Chapter 14.

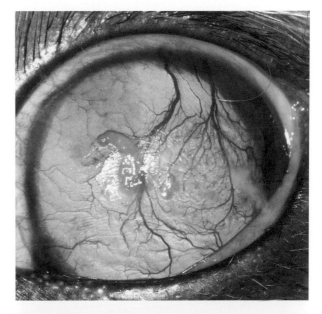

Figure 5.2 Superficial corneal ulceration, KCS, and anterior uveitis in the right eye of a dog. The STT was 0 mm/min. Note the uneven, dry corneal surface; indistinct camera flash; and adherent mucous that are typical of KCS. Anterior uveitis is indicated by hypopyon and red blood cells settled in the ventral anterior chamber. KCS is discussed in Chapter 14. Anterior uveitis is discussed in Chapter 15.

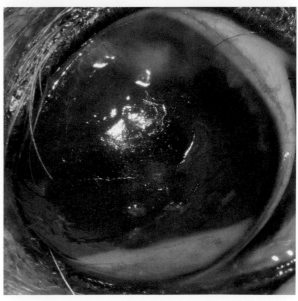

Small Animal Ophthalmic Atlas and Guide, Second Edition. Christine C. Lim.
© 2023 John Wiley & Sons, Inc. Published 2023 by John Wiley & Sons, Inc.
Companion website: www.wiley.com/go/lim/atlas

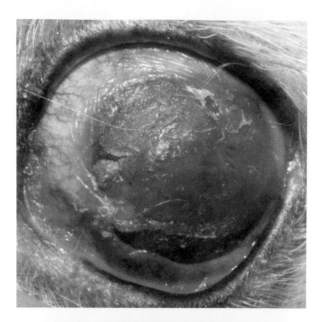

Figure 5.3 Left eye of an elderly shih tzu with chronic KCS. The tear production had been 0 mm/min bilaterally for many years. Note the dry ocular surface and adherence of crusted discharge to the cornea. The cornea itself is diffusely fibrotic with superficial vasculature. Conjunctival hyperemia is present. KCS is discussed in Chapter 14.

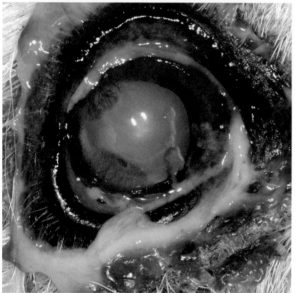

Figure 5.4 Chronic, superficial nonulcerative keratitis due to KCS. The copious and tenacious mucoid discharge is characteristic of KCS. Superficial corneal vascularization is another characteristic of KCS. The STT in this eye was 8 mm/min. KCS is discussed in Chapter 14.

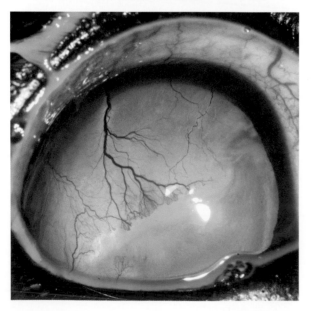

Figure 5.5 Right conjunctival hyperemia, superficial corneal vascularization, and corneal fibrosis (chronic, superficial, nonulcerative keratoconjunctivitis). Fluorescein has been applied but is not retained by the cornea. The extensive branching of the corneal vessels indicates their location in the superficial corneal stroma. The fibrosis affects the dorsal and lateral portions (approximately two-thirds) of the visible cornea. Because the fibrosis is causing mild corneal opacification, the pupillary margin immediately behind the fibrosis is less distinct than medially, where the cornea is unaffected. An eyelid mass is also present on the medial aspect of the lower eyelid. Keratitis is discussed in Chapter 14.

Figure 5.6 Left eye of a young, mixed breed rescue dog. The right cornea appeared similar. Neither cornea retained fluorescein stain. The length of the superficial corneal vessels indicates that the surface ocular irritation is chronic. The reflections on the central cornea are irregular due to the uneven surface of the cornea. These changes are consistent with chronic, nonulcerative superficial keratitis. Keratitis is discussed in Chapter 14.

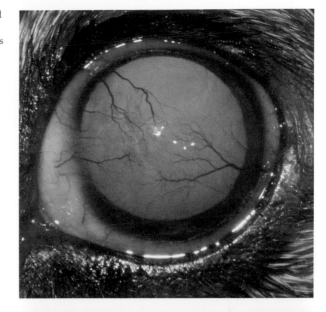

Figure 5.7 Right eye of a shih tzu with a long history of KCS. There is conjunctival hyperemia, superficial corneal vascularization, corneal edema, and mucoid ocular discharge. The STT was 13 mm/min. Keratitis is discussed in Chapter 14.

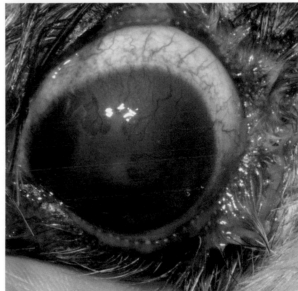

CHAPTER 5

Figure 5.8 Right eye of a DLH with chronic, nonulcerative superficial keratitis. Fibrosis is present within the central and ventral cornea. Superficial vascularization is also visible in this photograph and indicates a chronic process. Keratitis is discussed in Chapter 14.

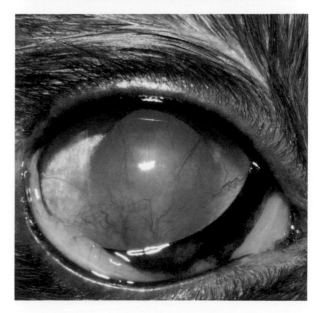

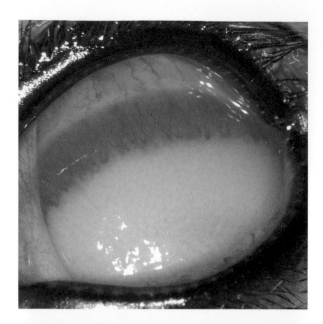

Figure 5.9 Chronic, stromal keratoconjunctivitis. Abnormalities include episcleral congestion, deep corneal vascularization, and diffuse corneal edema. The yellow tinge to the cornea is suggestive of white cell infiltrate in addition to edema. The dense grouping of the vessels and lack of branching are characteristic for vessels in the deep corneal stroma. For more information on corneal changes consistent with keratoconjunctivitis, please see Chapter 14.

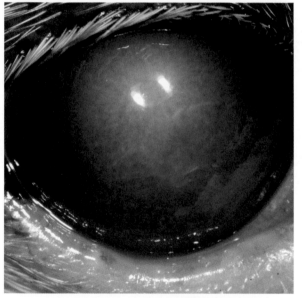

Figure 5.10 Classic appearance of corneal edema. Note the bluish-white discoloration of the cornea. A regular pattern, often referred to as a "chicken wire" or "cobblestone" pattern, can be seen within the cornea and is also considered a characteristic finding of corneal edema. The white, amorphous shape adjacent to the limbus from 3 to 6 o'clock is a reflection and not a true corneal change. Corneal edema is discussed in Chapter 14.

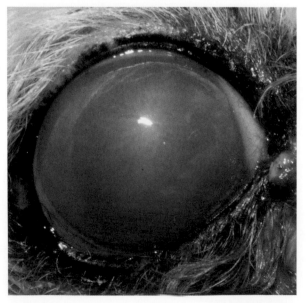

Figure 5.11 Diffuse corneal edema showing the typical bluish-white discoloration and "chicken wire" or "cobblestone" pattern. Corneal edema is discussed in Chapter 14.

Figure 5.12 Diffuse corneal edema. Fluid accumulation has led to development of corneal bullae (arrowheads) within the corneal stroma. Corneal edema is discussed in Chapter 14.

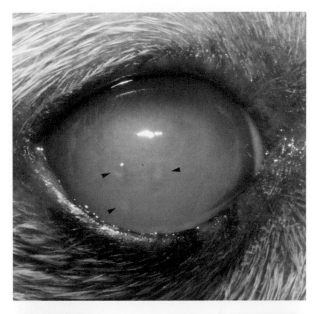

Figure 5.13 Superficial corneal vascularization, corneal melanosis, and absence of fluorescein retention (chronic, superficial, nonulcerative keratitis) in a dog with chronic KCS. The STT was 13 mm/min with medical therapy. Keratitis and KCS are discussed in Chapter 14.

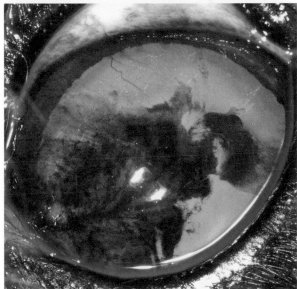

Figure 5.14 Right eye of a 5-year-old, castrated male pug. Note the corneal melanosis in the medial corneal quadrant. Melanosis results from chronic corneal irritation, which is caused in this case by ventromedial entropion, corneal contact with the nasal fold (nasal fold trichiasis), lagophthalmos, macropalpebral fissure, and exophthalmos. The lesions are bilateral and symmetrical. Pigmentary keratitis is discussed in Chapter 14 and brachycephalic ocular syndrome is discussed in Chapter 10.

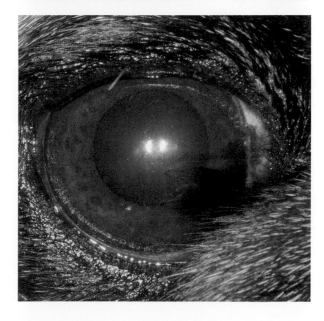

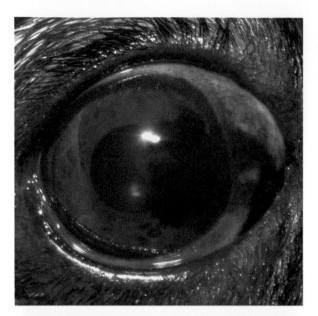

Figure 5.15 Right eye of a 4-year-old castrated male pug. There is melanosis of the medial corneal quadrant, as is typical of pigmentary keratitis. Note the ventromedial entropion and trichiasis, which contributes to the medial distribution of the pigment. Also note the excessive amount of visible sclera; the exposure is due to enlarged eyelid openings (macropalpebral fissure) and contributes to chronic corneal exposure. Pigmentary keratitis is discussed in Chapter 14 and brachycephalic ocular syndrome is discussed in Chapter 10.

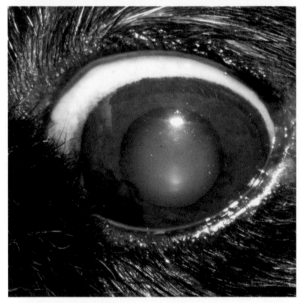

Figure 5.16 Left eye of an elderly Pekingese. There is melanosis of the ventromedial cornea. Note the nasal fold trichiasis, which contributes to the medial location of the pigment. Pigmentary keratitis is discussed in Chapter 14.

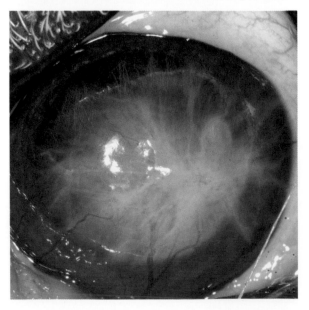

Figure 5.17 Conjunctival hyperemia, superficial corneal vascularization, and corneal fibrosis (chronic, superficial keratoconjunctivitis) resulting from previous corneal ulceration. The corneal fibrosis is dense, white, and linear in this photograph. It is associated with irregularities of the corneal surface (as evidenced by the indistinct borders of the camera flash in the central cornea). Keratitis is discussed in Chapter 14.

Figure 5.18 Chronic, superficial keratitis suspected to be due to previous injury. The central corneal fibrosis is circular and gray. Also shown in this photograph are corneal melanosis and superficial vascularization. Corneal lesions are discussed in Chapter 14.

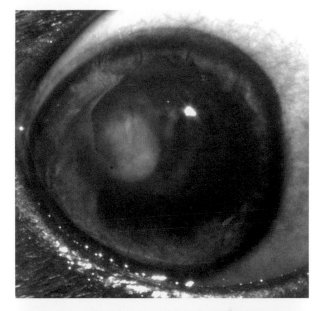

Figure 5.19 Left conjunctival hyperemia, deep corneal vascularization, corneal edema, and corneal white cell infiltrate (chronic, stromal keratitis) following left ocular proptosis and corneal ulceration. Unlike superficial corneal vessels, deep vessels rarely branch. The corneal edema is responsible for the blue change in the lateral cornea, and the white cell infiltrate is responsible for the yellow discoloration of the medial cornea. Keratitis and corneal white cell infiltrates are discussed in Chapter 14. Proptosis is discussed in Chapter 10.

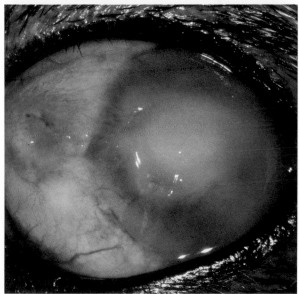

Figure 5.20 Left eye of a shih tzu. This patient presented for evaluation of acute squinting. Examination revealed mucoid ocular discharge, moderate conjunctival hyperemia, diffuse corneal edema, and focal corneal white cell infiltrate (arrow). Samples were taken from the area of white cell infiltrate and submitted for cytology and culture and sensitivity, and aggressive medical management was started. Cytology was consistent with bacterial proliferation. Results of culture and sensitivity indicated the presence of *E. coli*, beta hemolytic streptococcus, and *Staphylococcus pseudointermedius*. The ocular lesions resolved after a few weeks of medical therapy. Corneal white cell infiltrates are discussed in Chapter 14.

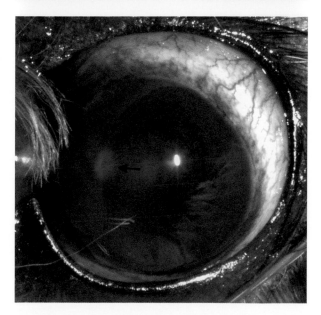

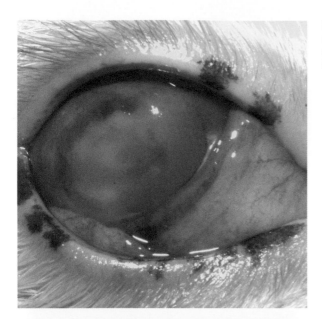

Figure 5.21 Chronic, deep ulcerative keratitis in a DSH. There is a central stromal defect surrounded by corneal edema and deep corneal vascularization. Some of the areas within the affected cornea are yellowish, consistent with white blood cell infiltrate. Corneal ulcers and feline keratitis are discussed in Chapter 14.

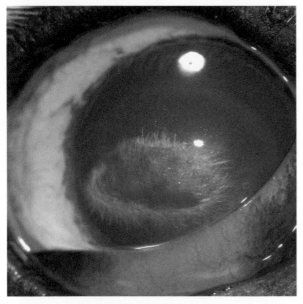

Figure 5.22 Corneal dystrophy in a Siberian husky. White, refractile deposits without any associated keratitis are characteristic. Also characteristic are the overall oval shape and the central location. This condition is bilateral and symmetrical and is not associated with detectable visual compromise or other ocular pathology. Corneal dystrophy is discussed in Chapter 14.

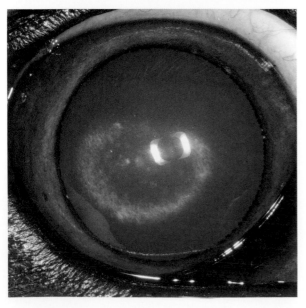

Figure 5.23 White, crystalline opacities in the central cornea. The lesions were bilateral and symmetrical. The oval shape, crystalline white color, central location, symmetry between eyes, and lack of concurrent ocular pathology are supportive of corneal dystrophy. This dog did not show any signs of ocular discomfort or visual compromise. Corneal dystrophy is discussed in Chapter 14.

Figure 5.24 Refractile, white deposits in the central cornea. The patient did not show signs of visual compromise or ocular discomfort. The lesions, which were bilateral and symmetrical, were suspected to be lipid and secondary to corneal dystrophy. Corneal lesions and corneal dystrophy specifically are discussed in Chapter 14.

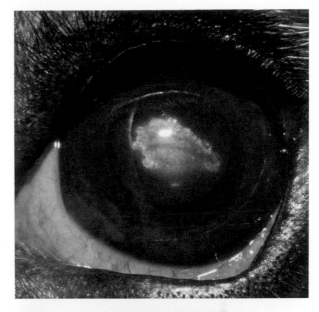

Figure 5.25 Refractile, white deposits in the central cornea, suspected to be lipid. These lesions were bilateral and symmetrical. Corneal lesions and corneal dystrophy specifically are discussed in Chapter 14.

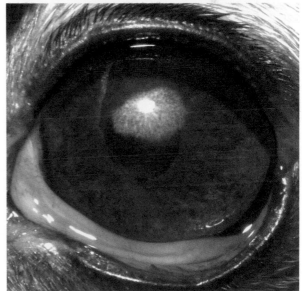

Figure 5.26 Chronic, superficial keratitis in an elderly terrier with recent corneal ulceration. The brighter, white lesions in the paracentral cornea were thought to be mineral. In addition to corneal mineral, there is diffuse corneal edema and superficial corneal vascularization. The combination of corneal mineralization and inflammation is consistent with a diagnosis of corneal degeneration. Keratitis is discussed in Chapter 14.

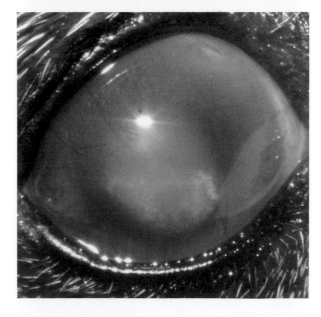

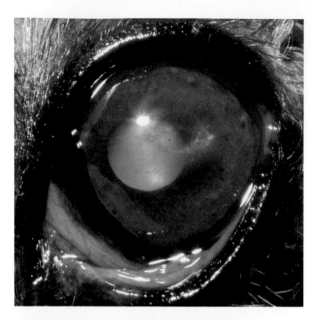

Figure 5.27 Refractile, white deposits within the cornea of a 15-year-old Havanese. The lesions were unilateral and consistent in appearance with mineral. Keratitis is discussed in Chapter 14.

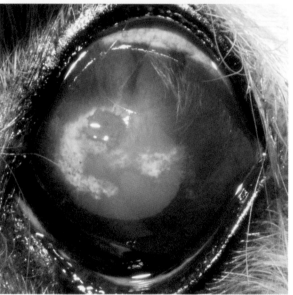

Figure 5.28 Chronic, superficial keratitis in an elderly poodle showing signs of ocular irritation. The mineral deposits are the dense, white lesions in the central cornea. The bluish discoloration dorsal to these lesions is corneal edema. Also shown in this photograph are corneal melanosis and superficial vascularization. The irregular reflections on the corneal surface indicate that the surface of the cornea is not smooth. Because of the association with surface ocular inflammation and the unilateral nature of lesions, the patient was diagnosed with corneal degeneration. Please see Chapter 14 for more information about keratitis.

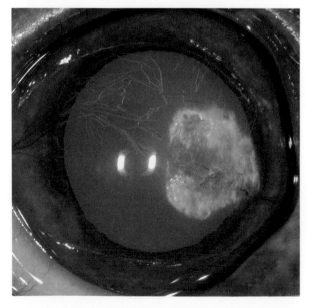

Figure 5.29 Chronic, superficial keratitis. Dense, refractile, white deposits are associated with superficial corneal vascularization. Although the deposits were present bilaterally, they were not symmetrical between eyes. The asymmetry and the associated keratitis were not consistent with corneal dystrophy; a diagnosis of corneal degeneration is more appropriate. Corneal dystrophy and corneal degeneration are both discussed in Chapter 14.

Figure 5.30 Typical appearance of pannus, or chronic superficial keratitis, in the left eye of a German shepherd. Corneal melanosis affects the ventrolateral peripheral cornea. In pannus, this is the typical location for melanosis to arise from (in contrast to pigmentary keratitis). Pannus is discussed in Chapter 14.

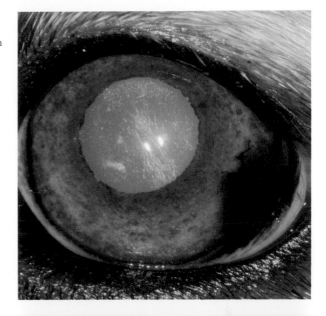

Figure 5.31 Left eye of a 7-year-old castrated male German shepherd cross. Corneal fibrosis, melanosis, and superficial vascularization are present. Although these changes were predominantly in the ventral and medial cornea, their appearance, combined with the breed and response to treatment, supported a diagnosis of pannus (chronic superficial keratitis). Pannus is discussed in Chapter 14.

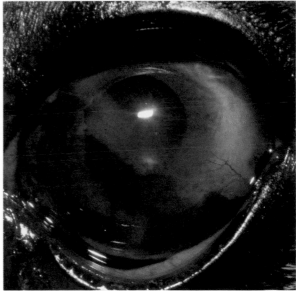

Figure 5.32 Pannus with a more fibrovascular component than in the previous figures. Corneal melanosis is present in the ventrolateral cornea. However, the predominant feature in this case is superficial corneal vascularization, also located ventrolaterally. The leading edge of the third eyelid is mildly depigmented. Pannus is discussed in Chapter 14.

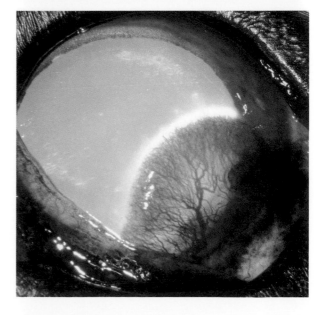

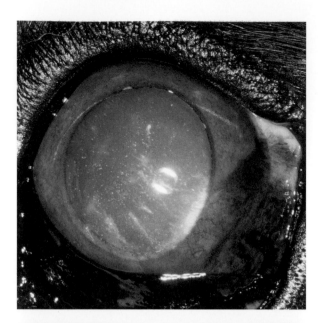

Figure 5.33 Pannus in the left eye of a German shepherd. Corneal melanosis and superficial vascularization affect the ventrolateral corneal quadrant. Linear, white wisps are visible in the central and ventral cornea; these are likely lymphocytes infiltrating the cornea (Williams, 1999; see Chapter 14). Pannus is discussed in Chapter 14.

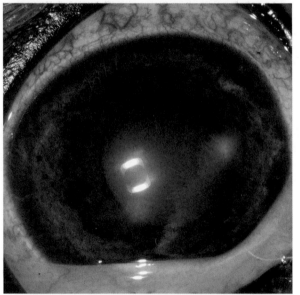

Figure 5.34 Right eye of a shih tzu presenting with a 1-day history of a red eye and excessive tearing. There is moderate conjunctival hyperemia and superficial corneal fluorescein retention. This ulcer is considered simple because it is acute, superficial, and there are no signs of white cell infiltrate or melting. The white opacity extending from the ulcer to the 6 o'clock limbus is a reflection. Simple corneal ulcers are discussed in Chapter 14.

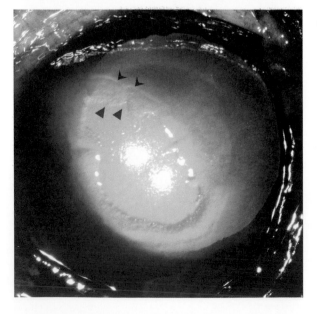

Figure 5.35 Indolent corneal ulcer of the right eye of a 9-year-old, spayed female boxer. Red arrowheads indicate the edges of the epithelial defect. However, because the epithelium is not adhering to the underlying stroma, fluorescein has been taken up by stroma beyond the epithelial edge (underneath epithelium) up to the area indicated by the black arrowheads. Mild corneal edema and superficial corneal vascularization obscure the ventrolateral iris. Also note the indistinct edges of the camera flash, indicating a roughened corneal surface. Indolent corneal ulcers are discussed in Chapter 14.

Figure 5.36a Indolent corneal ulcer with nonadherent epithelium. The red arrowhead indicates the edge of the epithelial defect. The epithelium is present but nonadherent to the underlying stroma between the red and the black arrowheads. Similar changes can be seen arounsd the entire circumference of the ulcer. The disrupted reflection of the camera flash indicates that the central cornea, near the edge of the defect, is uneven. Indolent corneal ulcers are discussed in Chapter 14.

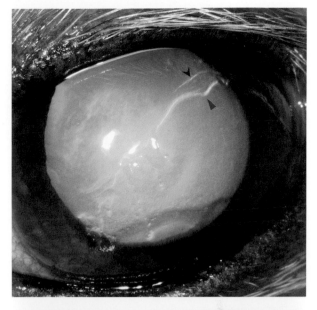

Figure 5.36b The same ulcer as in the previous figure (with similar arrowhead placement) after application of fluorescein stain. This photograph shows fluorescein retention by stroma that has overlying but nonadherent epithelium (between the red and the black arrowheads). Similar patterns of fluorescein retention are visible around the circumference of the ulcer. Indolent corneal ulcers are discussed in Chapter 14.

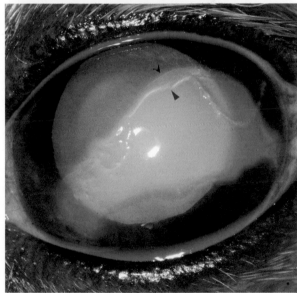

Figure 5.37 Chronic, superficial, ulcerative keratitis in a boxer. There is corneal edema and superficial vascularization. The arrow indicates one edge of the ulcer, which is elevated from the corneal surface because it is not adherent to the underlying stroma. This ulcer was classified as indolent because the ulcer was superficial, chronic, had nonadherent epithelium, and did not have signs of white cell infiltrate or malacia. In addition, the patient was of a predisposed breed. Indolent ulcers are discussed in Chapter 14.

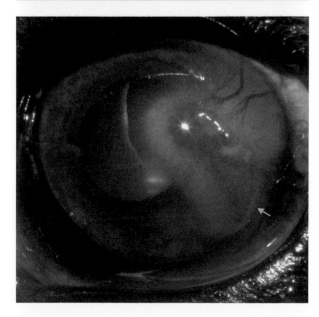

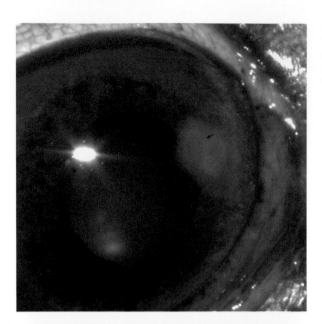

Figure 5.38 Due to lack of adhesion between the corneal epithelium and stroma, fluorescein stain applied to indolent ulcers can often be seen underneath the corneal epithelium. In this photograph, fluorescein can be seen extending beyond the epithelial margin of the ulcer (arrow). Indolent ulcers are discussed in Chapter 14.

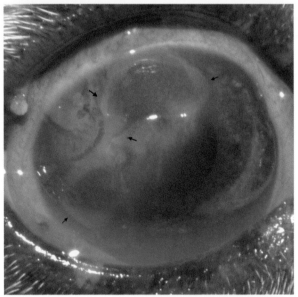

Figure 5.39 Chronic, superficial, ulcerative keratitis associated with an indolent ulcer. There is corneal edema and superficial vascularization. Arrows indicate various points of the ulcer periphery where nonadherent epithelium is most visible. Indolent ulcers are discussed in Chapter 14.

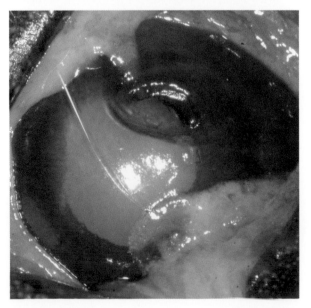

Figure 5.40 Chronic, deep ulcerative keratitis. In addition to the deep ulcer, KCS was diagnosed because the STT was 0 mm/min. The visible crater in the cornea indicates stromal loss; the cornea within the defect is clearer than the surrounding cornea because it is much thinner. This defect retained fluorescein stain when it was applied. The surrounding cornea is edematous, with deep vascular ingrowth. Chemosis and conjunctival hyperemia are also present. The copious amount of mucoid ocular discharge is a common finding with low tear production. Deep corneal ulcers and KCS are both discussed in Chapter 14.

Figure 5.41 Chronic, deep ulcerative keratitis in the right eye of a Boston terrier. A circular stromal defect is present within the central cornea. The length of the superficial corneal vessels suggests corneal disease has been present chronically. Conjunctival and episcleral hyperemia are also present in this photograph. Corneal ulcers are discussed in Chapter 14.

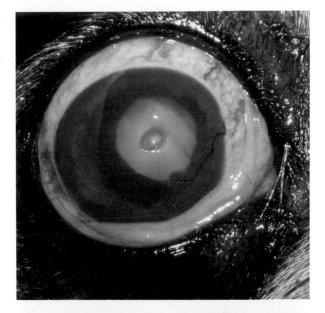

Figure 5.42 Stromal ulcer of the left eye of an 18-year-old poodle. The ulcer is an ovoid depression within the central cornea. The cornea dorsolateral to the ulcer is melanotic. Intrastromal hemorrhage is visible lateral and ventral to the ulcer. The cornea is diffusely edematous, with superficial vascularization present in the dorsal half of the cornea. In addition to the corneal lesions, episcleral hyperemia and mucopurulent ocular discharge are present. Corneal ulcers are discussed in Chapter 14.

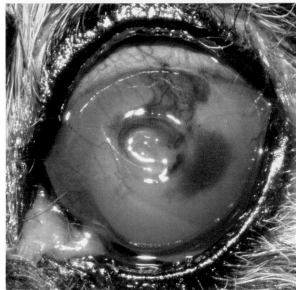

Figure 5.43 Chronic, deep ulcerative keratitis in a 21-year-old spayed female DSH. There is a stromal defect in the central cornea. The surrounding cornea is edematous. Superficial corneal vessels extend from the limbus into the margins of the defect. Corneal ulcers are discussed in Chapter 14.

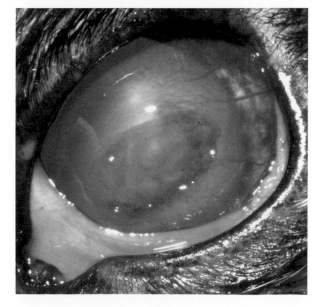

CHAPTER 5

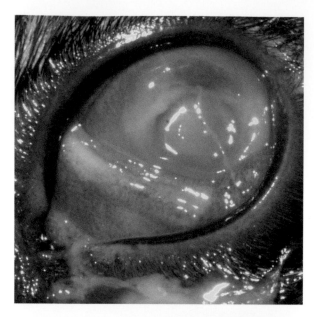

Figure 5.44 Chronic, deep ulcerative keratitis in a DSH. A circular stromal defect is visible in the central cornea. The cornea at the dorsal rim of the ulcer is yellow, consistent with white blood cell infiltrate. The remainder of the cornea shows deep vascularization and edema. Chemosis, conjunctival hyperemia, and mucopurulent ocular discharge are also present. This patient was treated with a conjunctival graft in addition to medical therapy. Corneal ulcers are discussed in Chapter 14.

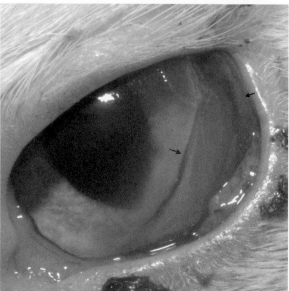

Figure 5.45 Deep corneal ulcer in the left eye of a DLH. This ulcer was not visible until the lower eyelid was lowered during ophthalmic examination. The red arrow marks the abrupt change from the nonulcerated, edematous cornea to the ulcerated cornea. The stroma in the ulcerated area was significantly thinned, and was therefore at risk of rupture. Deep vasculature is present at the limbal edge (black arrow) of the ulcer. Conjunctival hyperemia and chemosis are also present. This patient was treated with a conjunctival graft in addition to medications. Corneal ulcers are discussed in Chapter 14.

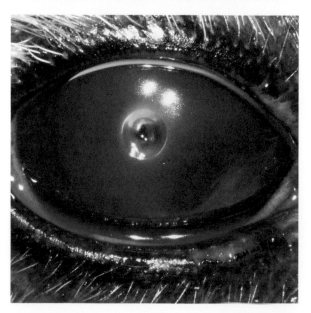

Figure 5.46 Descemetocele. Note the deep, central corneal defect. Fluorescein stain is retained by corneal stroma exposed at the periphery of this defect. However, fluorescein is not retained in the center of the defect, which appears black. This indicates loss of the entire corneal stroma centrally, with only hydrophobic Descemet's membrane and corneal endothelium intact. Deep corneal ulcers are discussed in Chapter 14.

Figure 5.47a Central corneal Descemetocele. The cornea is diffusely edematous, but this is most pronounced at the periphery of the ulcer. Superficial corneal vessels are present dorsal to the ulcer. Conjunctival changes include hyperemia and chemosis. Corneal ulcers are discussed in Chapter 14.

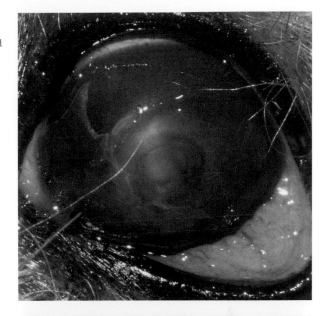

Figure 5.47b The same ulcer as in the previous figure. In this picture, fluorescein stain has been applied. It is retained at the margins of the ulcer but not in the ulcer bed due to the hydrophobic nature of Descemet's membrane. Corneal ulcers are discussed in Chapter 14.

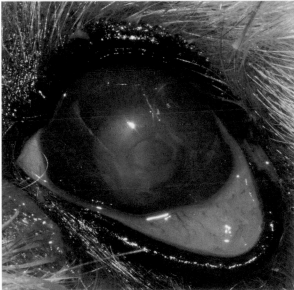

Figure 5.48 Right eye of an 8-year-old castrated male Cavalier King Charles spaniel. A Descemetocele is present in the central cornea. Although the cornea is diffusely edematous, the ventral pupillary margin is clearly visible because the cornea within the Descemetocele is extremely thin. Superficial corneal vessels are visible at the dorsal limbus and deep corneal vessels are visible at the ventrolateral limbus. Also shown in this photo are conjunctival hyperemia, a raised third eyelid, and mucoid ocular discharge. Corneal ulcers are discussed in Chapter 14.

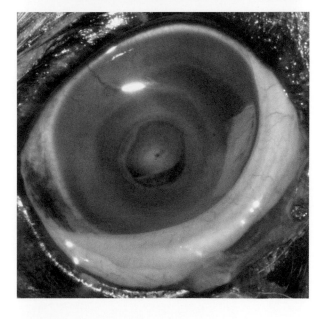

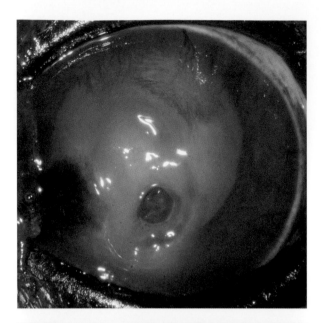

Figure 5.49 Perforated left cornea. The brown, central lesion is iris plugging a full-thickness corneal defect. Immediately surrounding the perforation, there is corneal stromal loss. The remainder of the cornea is edematous (most pronounced around the area of stromal loss). Superficial and deep corneal vessels, indicating chronicity, can be seen arising from all limbus visible in this photograph. Corneal melanosis is visible medial to the perforation. This patient was treated with a conjunctival graft. Deep and perforating corneal ulcers are discussed in Chapter 14.

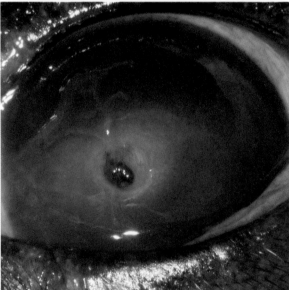

Figure 5.50 Corneal perforation. The iris is the red object in the central cornea. The surrounding cornea is edematous. Deep corneal vessels (indicating chronicity, in addition to depth) are visible at the limbus dorsally and laterally; the remainder of the red discoloration is hyphema viewed through the cornea. Deep and perforating corneal ulcers are discussed in Chapter 14.

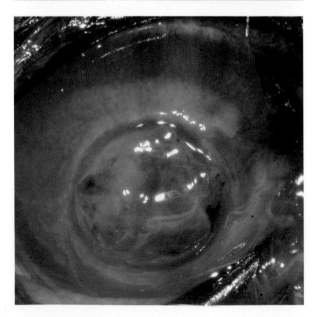

Figure 5.51 The large brown and pink structure protruding from the central cornea is the iris. The surrounding cornea is edematous with ingrowth of deep corneal vessels. Due to the severity of this injury, the globe was enucleated. Deep and perforating corneal ulcers are discussed in Chapter 14.

Figure 5.52 Central corneal malacia and rupture. The ruptured surface of the malacic cornea is uneven. The cornea surrounding this is edematous, with blood vessels that are both superficial and deep. This eye was enucleated. Corneal ulcers are discussed in Chapter 14.

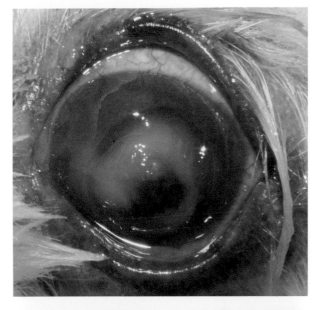

Figure 5.53 Central corneal rupture and uveal prolapse. There is white blood cell infiltrate of the cornea at the ventromedial ulcer periphery. The remaining cornea is edematous with deep vessels. Episcleral hyperemia is also shown in this photo. Corneal ulcers are discussed in Chapter 14.

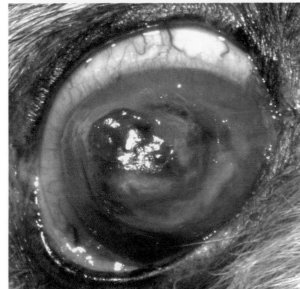

Figure 5.54 Central corneal rupture and uveal prolapse. There is fibrin adhered to the prolapsed uvea. The surrounding cornea is edematous with deep corneal vascularization visible at the limbus. Although the pupil isn't visible, miosis can be inferred from the amount of iris that is visible. Episcleral and conjunctival hyperemia are also shown. This eye was enucleated. Corneal ulcers are discussed in Chapter 14.

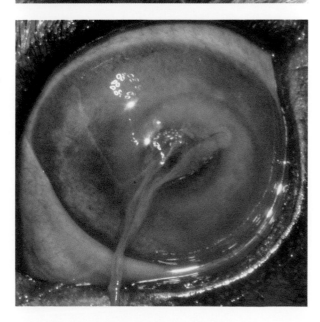

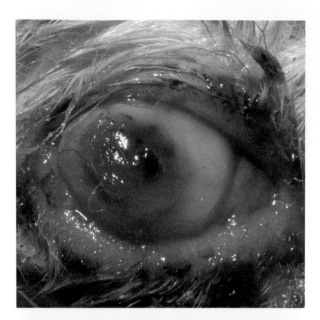

Figure 5.55 Ruptured globe in a kitten. The central cornea is dark due to a combination of uveal prolapse and fibrin. The cornea surrounding the rupture is yellow due to white cell infiltrate. This eye was enucleated. Corneal ulcers are discussed in Chapter 14.

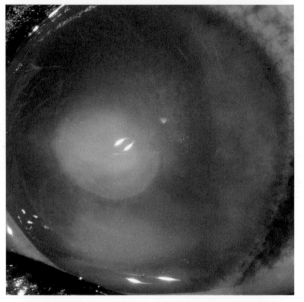

Figure 5.56 Melting corneal ulcer. There is diffuse corneal edema, and deep corneal vessels are present near the limbus. The central, white lesion is protruding from the corneal surface and appears soft. This is the area of corneal melting. It is raised from the corneal surface because as the malacic cornea becomes less firm, it deforms. The creamy appearance of the melting cornea is highly suggestive of white cell infiltrate in addition to the malacia. A second white lesion ventral to this is hypopyon. Melting corneal ulcers are discussed in Chapter 14.

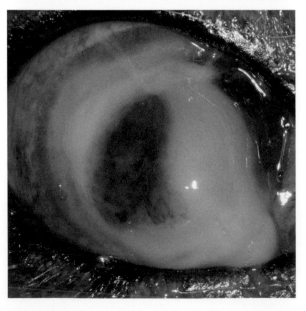

Figure 5.57 Perforated melting corneal ulcer. The central, red lesion is iris that has protruded through a corneal perforation. Malacic cornea is visible around the iris and exuding over the surface of the iris. Some areas of the malacic cornea are yellow, suggestive of white cell infiltrate. Episcleral hyperemia and deep corneal vascularization are also visible in this photograph. Due to the severity of ocular disease and grave prognosis, the eye was enucleated. Melting corneal ulcers are discussed in Chapter 14.

Figure 5.58 Melting corneal ulcer of the left eye in a bichon frise. There is lateral corneal white blood cell infiltrate and stromal loss. Corneal edema is also present, most pronounced in the lateral cornea. The lateral cornea was less solid than in other areas, supportive of corneal malacia. Hypopyon is visible in the ventral anterior chamber. Although it is difficult to visualize the pupil, miosis can be inferred from the amount of visible iris. Conjunctiva hyperemia and chemosis are also visible. This ulcer resolved with aggressive medical therapy. Corneal ulcers are discussed in Chapter 14.

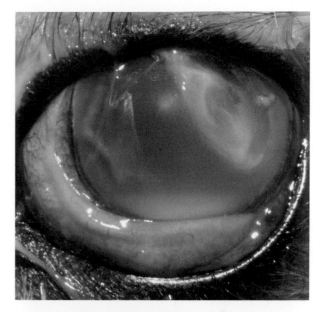

Figure 5.59 Left eye of an elderly mixed breed dog that was diabetic and Cushingoid. There is a corneal perforation immediately ventral to the limbus at 12 o'clock, through which uvea is protruding. The cornea ventral to the perforation is cream-colored due to white cell infiltrate. It is also malacic. This photograph also shows episcleral congestion, deep corneal vascularization, and corneal edema. This eye was enucleated. Corneal ulcers are discussed in Chapter 14.

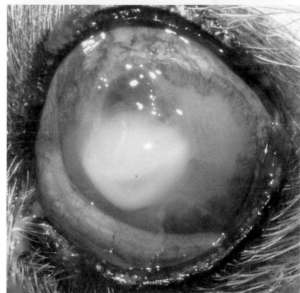

Figure 5.60 Dendritic refers to the linear nature of the superficial corneal ulcers shown here. These are pathognomonic for FHV-1 infection. The cobalt blue filter of the direct ophthalmoscope enhances visualization of fluorescein. See Chapter 14 for discussion of feline corneal ulcers.

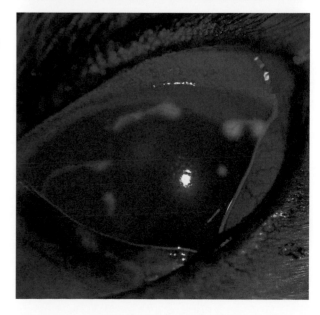

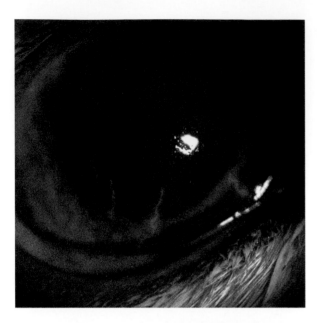

Figure 5.61 Dendritic corneal ulcers in a British shorthair kitten. These ulcers appeared during chronic steroid treatment for endophthalmitis. They resolved with cessation of the steroid and use of a topical antiviral. Corneal ulcers are discussed in Chapter 14.

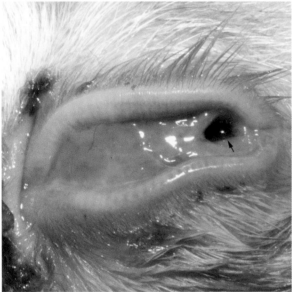

Figure 5.62 Left eye of a rescue kitten with unknown history. The upper and lower eyelids are fused together by adhesions with the conjunctiva. The arrow indicates a small opening within the adhesions, through which a small area of cornea is seen. Periocular discharge is also present. Symblepharon is mentioned in Chapter 14, under the discussion for feline keratitis, nonulcerative and ulcerative.

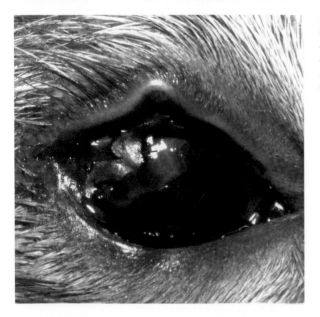

Figure 5.63 Right eye of a DSH. The cornea is diffusely melanotic and fibrotic. Symblepharon between the upper eyelid and the cornea (arrows) is visible dorsolaterally. These adhesions prevented normal movement of the upper eyelid and are also responsible for the notch in the central upper eyelid. Symblepharon is mentioned in Chapter 14, under the discussion for feline keratitis, nonulcerative and ulcerative.

Figure 5.64 Left eye of a DSH. There is corneal fibrosis, melanosis, and vascularization. The third eyelid is persistently elevated as a result of adhesions between it and the cornea. The arrow indicates the lateral extent of the leading edge of the third eyelid, where it is adhered to the melanotic cornea. Symblepharon is mentioned in Chapter 14, under the discussion for feline keratitis, nonulcerative and ulcerative.

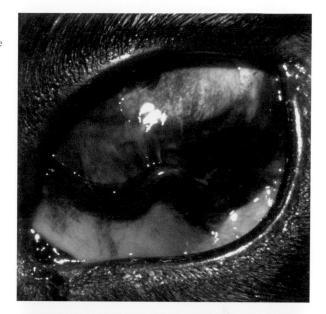

Figure 5.65 Chronic, superficial keratoconjunctivitis (chemosis, conjunctival hyperemia, superficial corneal vascularization, and corneal edema) due to EK. The raised, round, white structures on the cornea and conjunctiva near the dorsolateral limbus are white cell plaques. EK is discussed in Chapter 14.

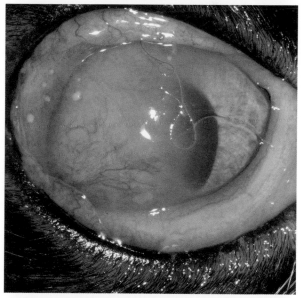

Figure 5.66 Eyelid depigmentation, chemosis, conjunctival hyperemia, superficial corneal vascularization, and corneal plaques due to EK. The plaques in this photo are larger and more diffuse than in the previous figure. However, regardless of plaque appearance, the association of white cell plaques with chronic superficial keratoconjunctivitis in cats should raise clinical suspicion for EK. EK is discussed in Chapter 14.

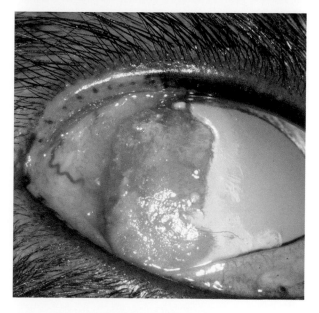

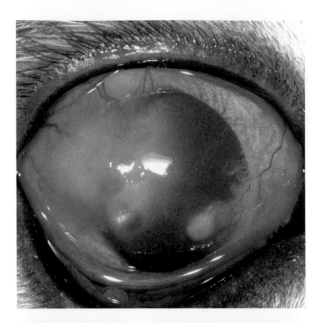

Figure 5.67 Chronic, superficial keratitis, diagnosed via corneal cytology as EK. In contrast to the Figures 5.65 and 5.66, the white cell infiltrate has not formed discrete, raised plaques on the cornea. This underscores the importance of cytology for obtaining a diagnosis. EK is discussed in Chapter 14.

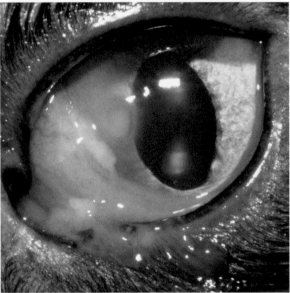

Figure 5.68 Left eye of a 10-year-old castrated male DSH with a history of chronic ocular irritation and color change. The medial and dorsomedial cornea is edematous with circular area of white cell infiltrate. The third eyelid is thickened, hyperemic, and raised. There is mucopurulent ocular discharge. Eosinophils were identified on corneal cytology, consistent with a diagnosis of EK. The lesions resolved with topical antibiotic and steroid therapy. EK is discussed in Chapter 14.

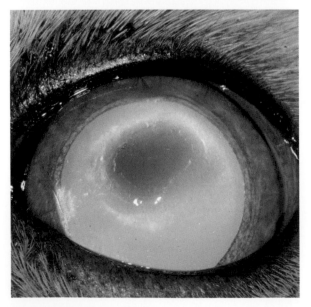

Figure 5.69 Chronic, superficial ulcerative keratoconjunctivitis and corneal sequestrum of the left eye of a Persian cat. Conjunctival hyperemia is present, and superficial corneal vessels extend from the dorsal and medial limbus. The sequestrum is the bronze to light brown discoloration in the central cornea. Corneal sequestra are discussed in Chapter 14.

Figure 5.70 Chronic, superficial ulcerative keratoconjunctivitis and corneal sequestrum. There is chemosis, conjunctival hyperemia, and superficial corneal vascularization. The vessels extend from the dorsal limbus to the sequestrum. In contrast to Figure 5.69, the sequestrum is dark brown. Mild corneal edema is present immediately around the sequestrum. Fluorescein stain has been applied to the eye. However, it is not retained over the sequestrum in spite of an epithelial defect due to the hydrophobic nature of the sequestrum. Corneal sequestra are discussed in Chapter 14.

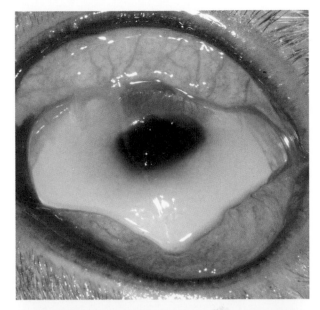

Figure 5.71 Chronic, superficial ulcerative keratitis and corneal sequestrum. There is diffuse, superficial corneal vascularization. The sequestrum is the black, central corneal lesion. The cornea around the sequestrum is ulcerated. However, fluorescein is retained only at the periphery of the sequestrum because the sequestrum is hydrophobic. Corneal sequestra are discussed in Chapter 14.

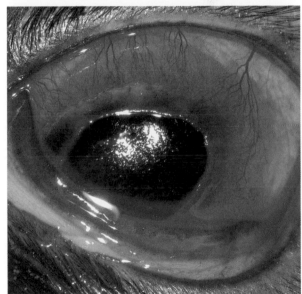

Figure 5.72 Chronic, superficial, ulcerative keratitis associated with a corneal sequestrum. Superficial corneal vessels are visible extending from the lateral and ventrolateral limbus to the central sequestrum. Corneal edema is visible dorsal and lateral to the sequestrum. In this patient, the ulcer and sequestrum are likely in part caused by lower eyelid entropion. Note the hairs of the lower eyelid directly contacting the cornea along its entire length. In contrast, the hairless eyelid margin is visible along the entire length of the dorsal eyelid, where entropion is absent. Corneal sequestra are discussed in Chapter 14.

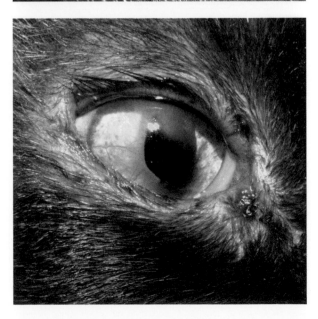

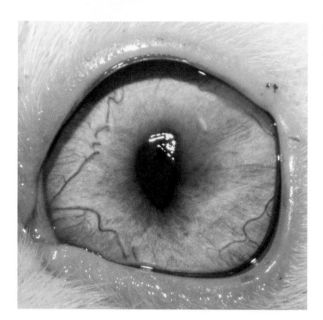

Figure 5.73 The appearance of this sequestrum ranges from light bronze to black (arrow). The scattered reflections indicate that the central cornea has an uneven surface. Corneal sequestra are discussed in Chapter 14.

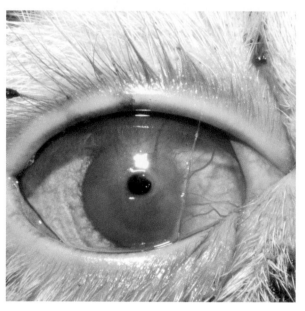

Figure 5.74 Chronic, superficial, ulcerative keratitis associated with a corneal sequestrum. Corneal edema is present dorsal to the sequestrum. Multiple superficial corneal vessels are present in the dorsal and medial cornea. Corneal sequestra are discussed in Chapter 14.

CHAPTER 5

6 Anterior uvea

Please see Chapter 15 for more information about diseases, diagnostic testing, and treatment plans related to the anterior uvea.

Figure 6.1 Right eye of a Himalayan cat showing the normal appearance of the iris. Some variation in color throughout the iris can be normal. The photograph depicts the normal shape of the pupil midway between complete miosis and mydriasis. When fully constricted, the feline pupil is a vertical slit and when fully dilated, it is almost perfectly round. Iridal vasculature is more visible in eyes with light irides and should not be mistaken for pathology. The anterior uvea and its diseases are discussed in Chapter 15.

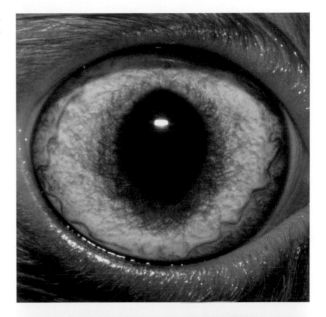

Figure 6.2 Left eye of a young standard poodle showing the normal appearance of the iris. Regional variation in the degree of pigmentation in different areas of the iris is common. The canine pupil is round at all sizes. The anterior uvea and its diseases are discussed in Chapter 15.

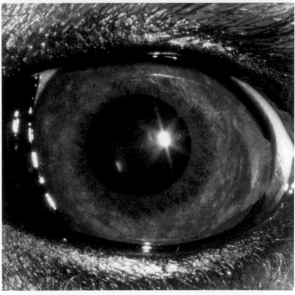

Small Animal Ophthalmic Atlas and Guide, Second Edition. Christine C. Lim.
© 2023 John Wiley & Sons, Inc. Published 2023 by John Wiley & Sons, Inc.
Companion website: www.wiley.com/go/lim/atlas

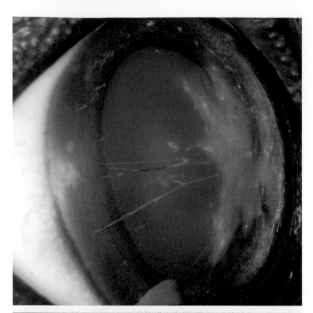

Figure 6.3 This photo was taken from the right side of the dog's head to show iris-to-cornea PPMs spanning the anterior chamber of the right eye. The PPMs are the thin, brown and white strands extending from the lateral iris collarette to the large, white opacity that obscures the view of the nasal pupillary margin. This opacity is corneal fibrosis at the PPM insertion. Discussion of PPMs can be found in Chapter 15.

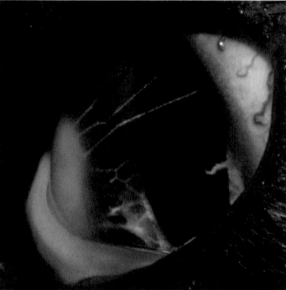

Figure 6.4 Left eye of a young DSH with multiple congenital ocular anomalies, viewed from the left side of his head. The yellow strands in this photograph are iris-to-cornea PPMs. They extend from the iris collarette to the posterior cornea. The cornea is fibrotic at the site of their insertion. In addition, the globe was microphthalmic. PPMs are discussed in Chapter 15.

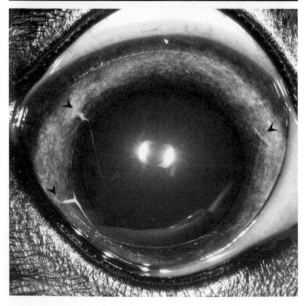

Figure 6.5 These iris-to-iris PPMs were an incidental finding. The black arrowheads indicate PPMs on the iris (thin white strands). The PPMs at 2 and 8 o'clock lie flat on the iris, while the PPM at 10 o'clock crosses the pupillary aperture (red arrowhead) to insert onto the ventral iris collarette. Discussion of PPMs can be found in Chapter 15.

Figure 6.6 Right eye of a young wire fox terrier. The iris-to-iris PPMs (arrow) are thin strands of uveal tissue lying flat against the iris collarette. In this photograph they are visible in the ventral half of the iris. They were incidental findings on ophthalmic examination. Persistent pupillary membranes are discussed in Chapter 15.

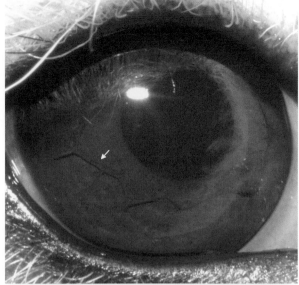

Figure 6.7 Left eye of a young mountain cur. This patient had multiple congenital abnormalities that included iris-to-lens PPMs. The PPM is a thin strand of uveal tissue that extends from the iris collarette (arrow) to the anterior lens capsule. Melanotic and fibrotic changes are present on the lens capsule at the site of PPM insertion. In addition to the intraocular changes, corneal fibrosis and melanosis are present laterally. PPMs are discussed in Chapter 15.

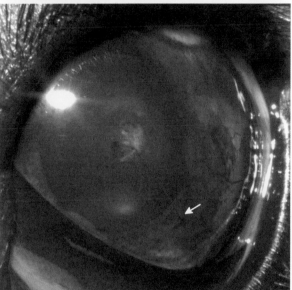

Figure 6.8 Anterior chamber uveal cysts. Two free-floating, circular brown objects were seen in the ventral anterior chamber. The horizontal white line overlying the larger, more dorsal cyst is a reflection of the eyelid margin. Transillumination confirmed both of these structures to be thin-walled uveal cysts, and no diagnostics or therapeutics were needed. Discussion of uveal cysts can be found in Chapter 15.

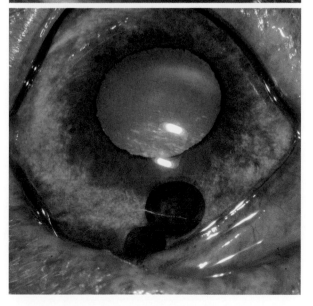

CHAPTER 6

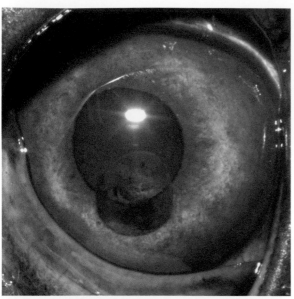

Figure 6.9 Left eye of a golden retriever. A uveal cyst is in the anterior chamber and is also adhered to the ventral pupillary margin. The cyst wall is thin, allowing visualization of the iris behind it. Uveal cysts are discussed in Chapter 15.

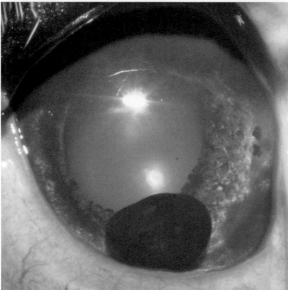

Figure 6.10 Left eye of an American bulldog. A uveal cyst is in the ventral anterior chamber. Its appearance is typical, with smooth, rounded edges. Although the cyst wall is dark, there are areas that are less brown; these are areas where the cyst wall is thinner. Uveal cysts are discussed in Chapter 15.

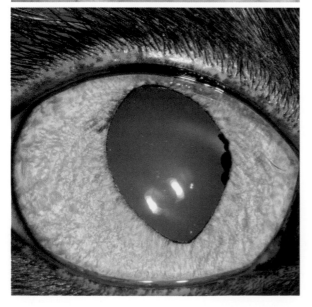

Figure 6.11 Right eye of a DSH. Uveal cysts are attached to the medial pupillary margin. These cysts are dark due to their thick walls. The smooth, rounded edges of the cysts are characteristic. Feline uveal cysts are typically adhered to the pupil margins. Uveal cysts are discussed in Chapter 15.

Figure 6.12 Left eye of a Siberian cat. Two uveal cysts are visible in this photograph. One is attached to the medial pupil margin and the other is attached to the lateral pupil margin. Both have dark brown walls with smooth edges. The medial cyst is more round while the lateral cyst is more elongated. Uveal cysts are discussed in Chapter 15.

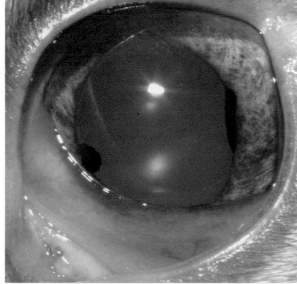

Figure 6.13 Transillumination of multiple posterior chamber cysts. The cysts are rounded objects visible at the pupillary margin from 3 to 11 o'clock. Transillumination causes the cysts to appear yellow; this is the effect of light passing through the thin walls of the cyst (which appear light brown in ambient light). Discussion of uveal cysts can be found in Chapter 15.

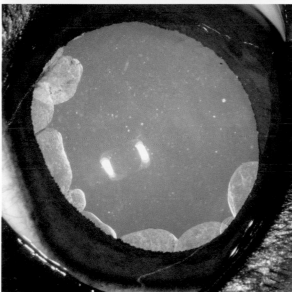

Figure 6.14 Scalloped pupillary margin due to age-related iris atrophy. The atrophy is more severe at the 5–6 o'clock pupillary margin, where there is a full-thickness defect of the iris. Discussion of iris atrophy can be found in Chapter 15.

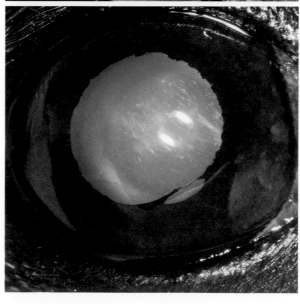

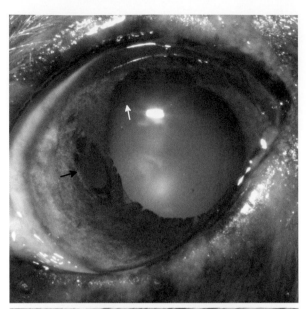

Figure 6.15 Right eye of a 12-year-old, castrated male mixed breed dog. Iris atrophy is most notable adjacent to the lateral pupillary margin, where there is a full-thickness defect within the iris (black arrow). Iris atrophy has also caused irregularity of the pupillary margin and resulting dyscoria. A white arrow indicates a small strand of iridal tissue that remains at the dorsal pupil after significant atrophy of iris tissue in that area. Iris atrophy is discussed in Chapter 15.

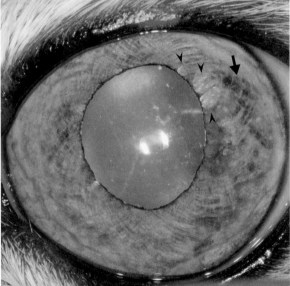

Figure 6.16 Iris atrophy in the left eye of a 14-year-old, spayed female Persian. Thinning of the iris along the pupillary margin from 1 to 2 o'clock allows tapetal reflection to be visible through the iris tissue (arrowheads), giving the iris a moth-eaten appearance. At the adjacent iris collarette (arrow), the black posterior pigmented epithelium is visible through the thinned anterior iris stroma. Discussion of iris atrophy can be found in Chapter 15.

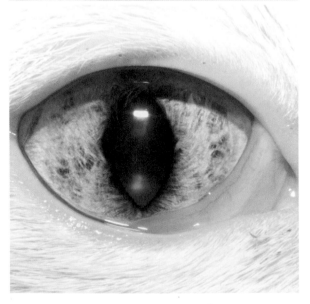

Figure 6.17 Right eye of a 14-year-old, castrated male DSH. The black posterior pigmented epithelium is visible through the thinned anterior iris stroma, which appears blue. Iris atrophy is discussed in Chapter 15.

Figure 6.18 Marked iris atrophy in the right eye of a 15-year-old, spayed female Chihuahua. The tapetal reflection is clearly visible through full-thickness iris defects. Dyscoria is also present as result of atrophy affecting the muscles of the iris. Discussion of iris atrophy can be found in Chapter 15.

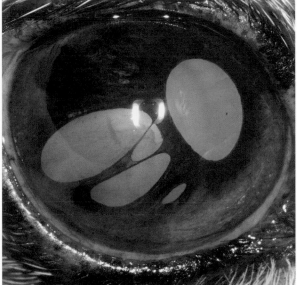

Figure 6.19 Focal, flat iridal hyperpigmentation (arrow) in a DSH. This was found incidentally during ophthalmic examination. The lesion was photographed at each visit, and at last examination, had not appreciably changed. A histopathologic diagnosis was therefore not obtained. Feline iris melanoma is further discussed in Chapter 15.

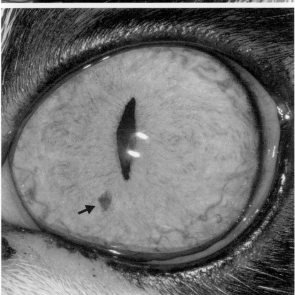

Figure 6.20 Focal iridal hyperpigmentation in the right eye of a DSH. Due to increasing size noted over multiple examinations, the client elected for enucleation. Histopathology confirmed iris melanoma. Feline iris melanoma is discussed in Chapter 15.

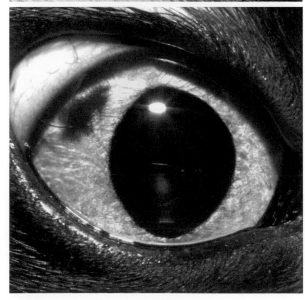

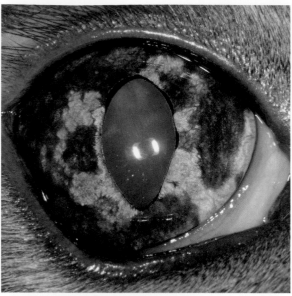

Figure 6.21 Histopathology confirmed iris melanoma in this 6-year-old, castrated male DSH. The iris is mildly thickened in the melanotic areas. Very mild dyscoria is present. Eversion of the pupillary margin, which allows visualization of the posterior pigmented epithelium, is present along the dorsal, medial, and ventral pupillary margins. Feline iris melanoma is discussed in Chapter 15.

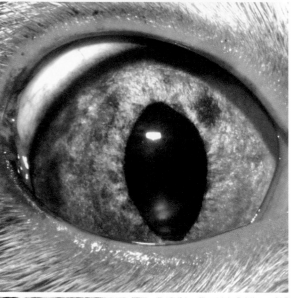

Figure 6.22 Multiple areas of iridal hyperpigmentation in the right eye of a DSH. Note the variation in degree of pigmentation. This patient was lost to follow-up. Feline iris melanoma is discussed in Chapter 15.

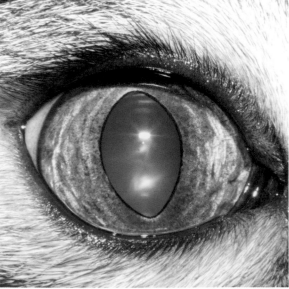

Figure 6.23 Right eye of a DSH. The iris is diffusely hyperpigmented. The clients elected to monitor the lesions so histopathology was not obtained. Feline iris melanoma is discussed in Chapter 15.

Figure 6.24 This cat presented for evaluation of brown discoloration of the iris, which was previously yellow. Due to the considerable iris involvement, raised iridal surface, dyscoria, altered pupillary constriction, and IOP of 30 mm Hg, melanoma was suspected and enucleation recommended. Histopathology confirmed extensive iris melanoma. Feline iris melanoma is discussed in Chapter 15.

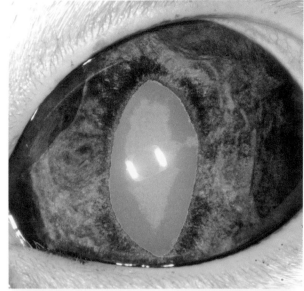

Figure 6.25 Histopathology-confirmed iris melanoma, uveitis, and secondary glaucoma. This photograph shows episcleral hyperemia, corneal edema, iridal hyperpigmentation, dyscoria, mydriasis, and anterior lens capsule pigmentation. On ophthalmic examination, aqueous flare and melanotic cells suspended within the anterior chamber were visible. Feline iris melanoma is discussed in Chapter 15.

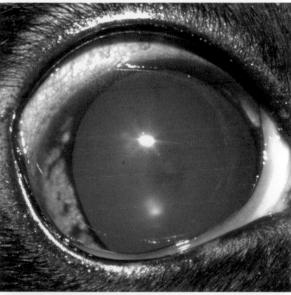

Figure 6.26 This dog was referred for evaluation and removal of a slow-growing, pigmented iridal mass in the left eye. The mass is flat, brown to black, and located within the peripheral iris from approximately 1 to 3 o'clock. Histopathology confirmed anterior uveal melanocytoma. Canine iris melanocytoma is further discussed in Chapter 15.

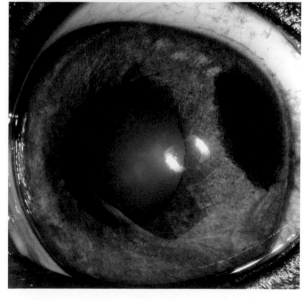

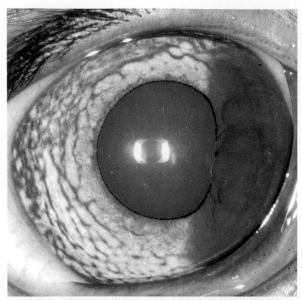

Figure 6.27 Rapidly progressing iridal hyperpigmentation in the right eye of a 7-month-old, spayed female retriever cross. The bulk of the mass is visible within the medial iris. The affected iris is thickened and raised with impaired muscle function (dyscoria is visible, due to incomplete dilation of the medial pupil). Enucleation was performed. Histopathology confirmed iridal melanocytoma. Canine iris melanocytoma is further discussed in Chapter 15.

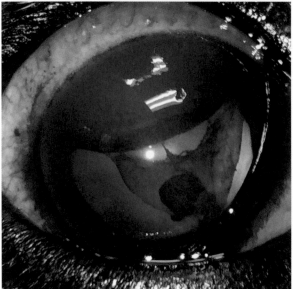

Figure 6.28 Right eye of a geriatric boxer. This patient presented for recent onset of ocular discomfort and redness. Ophthalmic examination revealed a mass in the dorsal iris as well as secondary glaucoma (the IOP was 30 mm Hg at the time of the photograph). The pupil is crescent-shaped because the mass prevents pupillary dilation in the affected areas of iris. The green tapetal reflection is visible but attenuated as a result of inflammatory debris in the anterior chamber. Also shown in this photograph are episcleral hyperemia and corneal edema (most notable in the dorsal cornea, where the mass is contacting the cornea). This patient was lost to follow-up. Iridal neoplasia is discussed in Chapter 15.

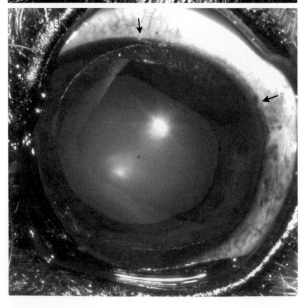

Figure 6.29 Left eye of an 11-year-old spayed female poodle mix. An iris mass was diagnosed incidentally on ophthalmic examination. It extends from approximately 12 o'clock to 3 o'clock (between the arrows). The mass is raised and more pigmented when compared to the surrounding iris. White opacities overlying the mass are flash artifact. This patient did not show signs of discomfort. Ophthalmic examination did not show signs of uveitis, and the IOP was 19 mm Hg. Monitoring was elected. Iridal neoplasia is discussed in Chapter 15.

Figure 6.30 Iridociliary adenoma. The mass is pink because it contains little melanin and is vascular. It is located in the ventromedial posterior chamber of the left eye. The eye appeared comfortable and visual, but enucleation was recommended due to enlargement of the mass noted on serial visits. This condition is discussed in Chapter 15.

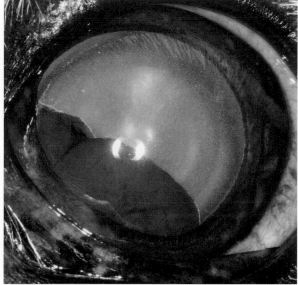

Figure 6.31 Right eye of a 7-year-old, spayed female border collie. There is a mass near the ventromedial pupillary margin that is presumed to be an iridociliary adenoma. Similar to the mass in Figure 6.30, this mass is pink. Because it arises from the ciliary body, ophthalmic examination shows that the mass arises from behind (posterior to) the iris. Iridociliary neoplasia is discussed in Chapter 15.

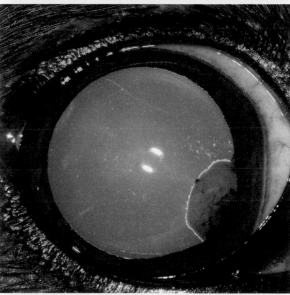

Figure 6.32 Anterior uveitis in the right eye of a dog. Chemosis and episcleral congestion are present, as well as deep corneal vasculature (visible at the lateral limbus) and marked corneal edema. The pupil was miotic. Anterior uveitis is discussed in Chapter 15.

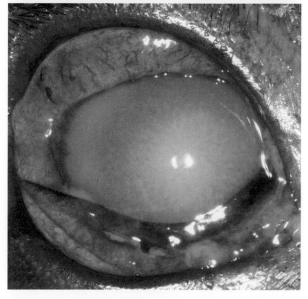

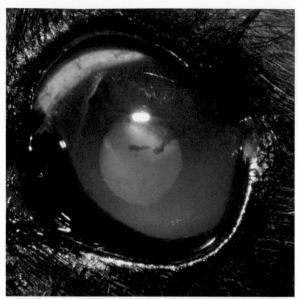

Figure 6.33 Left eye of a miniature schnauzer. This patient was diabetic and had lipemic serum. Episcleral hyperemia and lipemic aqueous are signs of anterior uveitis. This patient has a complete cataract that is secondary to diabetes mellitus and the likely cause of the uveitis. Corneal melanosis was also present without an obvious cause. Uveitis is discussed in Chapter 15.

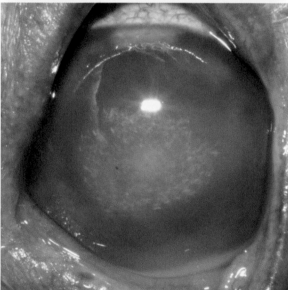

Figure 6.34 Left eye of a mixed breed dog. This patient was diabetic and had previously undergone phacoemulsification. Episcleral hyperemia, corneal edema, and hypopyon are present and consistent with anterior uveitis. Note the settling of the white blood cells in the ventral anterior chamber (hypopyon). Also shown in this photograph are corneal fibrosis (at the dorsal limbus, due to phacoemulsification surgery), a superficial corneal ulcer centrally (appearing green due to fluorescein uptake), and corneal lipid deposition surrounding the ulcer. Uveitis is discussed in Chapter 15.

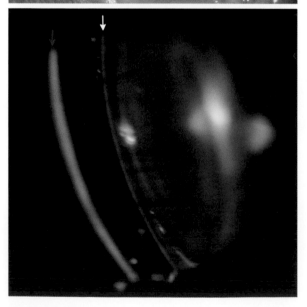

Figure 6.35 In a normal, uninflamed eye, the examiner's light is reflected off the cornea (red arrow) and anterior lens capsule (white arrow), and the two reflections are separated by a dark space, the anterior chamber. The reason the anterior chamber appears black is because normal aqueous humor is devoid of particulate matter that can scatter light. The iris is minimally visible in this photograph because the pupil is dilated. The visible iris, which is brown in this individual, is seen at the bottom on the photograph, at the termination of the reflection off the anterior lens capsule. Please compare and contrast this normal eye with the inflamed eye in Figure 6.36. The anterior uvea is discussed in Chapter 15.

Figure 6.36 Photograph of an eye with anterior segment inflammation (anterior uveitis). In the presence of inflammation, anterior chamber debris (inflammatory cells and proteins) reflects light that traverses the anterior chamber. The result is a white band of light visible between the corneal reflection (red arrow) and the anterior lens capsule (white arrow). This white band of light is referred to as aqueous flare and is indicative of anterior uveitis. The patient in this photograph had a blue iris and the pupil was miotic. Anterior uveitis is discussed in Chapter 15.

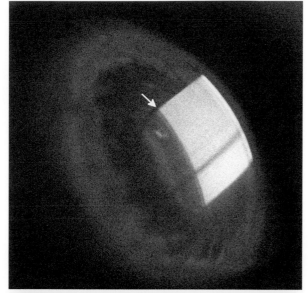

Figure 6.37 Multiple bright, white corneal opacities are visible in the ventral one-fourth of the cornea in this photograph. These are keratic precipitates, which are clusters of white cells and inflammatory debris adhered to the corneal endothelium. The presence of keratic precipitates indicates a past episode of anterior uveitis or current anterior uveitis. Anterior uveitis is discussed in Chapter 15.

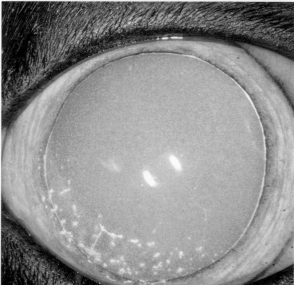

Figure 6.38 Chronic, ulcerative, stromal keratitis and anterior uveitis in a 9-year-old, spayed female miniature poodle. Concurrent diseases included diabetes mellitus and KCS. This photograph depicts episcleral congestion, deep corneal vascularization, corneal stromal loss (black arrow), corneal fluorescein retention, and corneal edema. White blood cells have settled in the ventral anterior chamber (hypopyon). The multiple round, white opacities visible within the medial cornea (red arrowhead) are keratic precipitates. The ovoid, white opacity medial to the fluorescein uptake is the pupil (the black arrowhead indicates the dorsal pupillary margin). Both miosis and dyscoria are present. Anterior uveitis is discussed in Chapter 15. Corneal ulcers are discussed in Chapter 14.

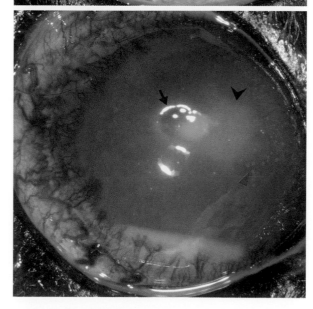

CHAPTER 6

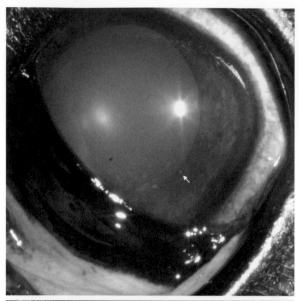

Figure 6.39 Left eye of 10-year-old, spayed female Labrador retriever mix that presented for evaluation of red eyes. The photograph shows episcleral hyperemia, diffuse corneal edema, and keratic precipitates (arrow). Similar lesions were found in the right eye. The lesions were consistent with anterior uveitis. An underlying cause for the uveitis was not found. Anterior uveitis is discussed in Chapter 15.

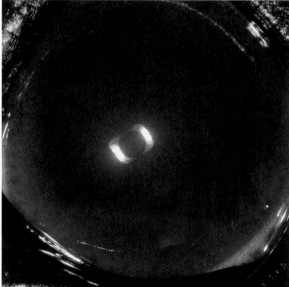

Figure 6.40 Hyphema in the left eye of a dog. Blood is present throughout the anterior chamber, but has settled ventrally as a result of gravity. Also visible in this photograph are deep corneal vessels (most noticeable along the ventral and medial limbus) and mild corneal edema (bluish-white discoloration most noticeable near the limbus). Anterior uveitis is discussed in Chapter 15.

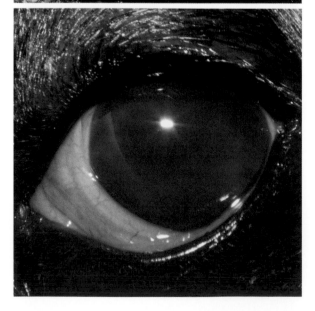

Figure 6.41 The same patient as in Figure 4.9. Hyphema is still present after approximately 2 weeks of steroid therapy. Red blood cells are suspended throughout the anterior chamber. The hyphema, which occurred as a result of trauma, never fully resolved and the eye remained blind and in need of chronic anti-inflammatory therapy. Hyphema is discussed in Chapter 15.

Figure 6.42 Right eye of a 22-year-old, spayed female snowshoe cat. This patient had a chronic history of systemic hypertension and hypertensive chorioretinopathy. At the time of this photograph, she had experienced a recent episode of uncontrolled hypertension. The hyphema in this photograph was attributed to the high blood pressure. Additional findings include dyscoria, due to posterior synechiae, and iris bombé. Iris bombé occurs when the iris is adhered to the lens (posterior synechiae) for the entire pupillary circumference, trapping aqueous humor posterior to the iris. The buildup of aqueous humor behind the iris causes the iris collarette to billow forward. Hyphema is discussed in Chapter 15. Hypertensive chorioretinopathy is discussed in Chapter 17.

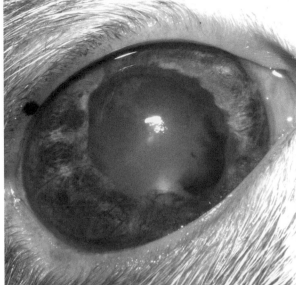

Figure 6.43 Left eye of the same patient as in Figure 6.42. The hyphema in this eye is much more severe than in the right eye. The entire anterior chamber is filled with blood such that examination of intraocular structures was not possible. Hyphema is discussed in Chapter 15. Hypertensive chorioretinopathy is discussed in Chapter 17.

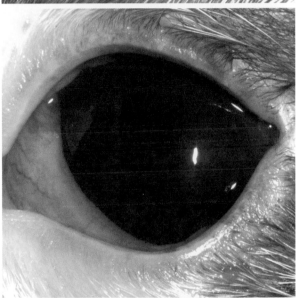

Figure 6.44 Rubeosis iridis is increased redness of the iris due to inflammation. The color change is secondary to vascular engorgement and formation of new blood vessels. Also visible in this photo are deposits of inflammatory debris and red blood cells on the anterior lens capsule (seen within the dorsolateral pupil and paracentral pupil). Anterior uveitis is discussed in Chapter 15.

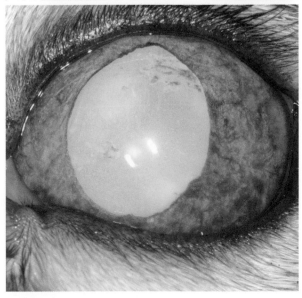

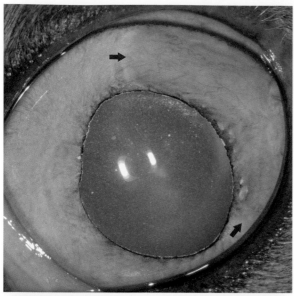

Figure 6.45 Focal rubeosis iridis and iris thickening in the left eye of a DSH with suspected spinal cord lymphoma. The lateral iris between the two arrows is raised, thickened, and more pink than normal. Dyscoria is also present. Anterior uveitis is discussed in Chapter 15.

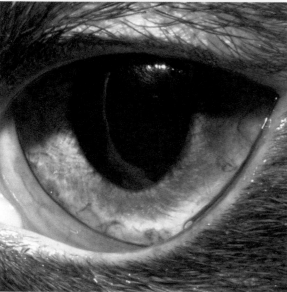

Figure 6.46 Left eye of a 13-year-old, castrated male Himalayan mix who presented for color change to the left eye. Examination revealed engorgement of iridal vessels peripherally and ventrally, consistent with iridal inflammation. Contrast the appearance of the inflammatory changes in this patient with the normal appearance of blood vessels within a blue iris in Figure 6.1. Diagnostic testing did not reveal an obvious underlying systemic disease in this patient. Treatment with an ophthalmic NSAID was associated with regression of the vessels. Rubeosis iridis and anterior uveitis are discussed in Chapter 15.

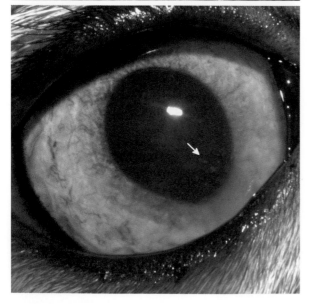

Figure 6.47 Diffuse rubeosis iridis in the right eye of a 6-year-old, castrated male DSH. The owners reported mydriasis and cloudiness of the right eye for 2 years prior to presentation. This patient's irides were green. However, iris inflammation and engorgement of iris vessels has changed the color of the right iris. In addition to rubeosis iridis, there are keratic precipitates (arrow). These have caused the ventral cornea to be translucent; as a result, visualization of the ventral iris is slightly blurred. These changes are indicative of anterior uveitis. Diagnostic testing did not reveal an obvious underlying cause for the inflammation. This patient also had secondary glaucoma; at the time of this photograph, the IOP was 31 mm Hg. The patient was treated with prednisolone acetate and dorzolamide. Anterior uveitis is discussed in Chapter 15.

Figure 6.48 Left eye of a 1-year-old, castrated male DSH presenting for evaluation of color change to the eye. The third eyelid was elevated, consistent with ocular pain. Centrally, the view of intraocular structures is blurry due to keratic precipitates and anterior chamber fibrin. There is rubeosis iridis and dyscoria. These changes are consistent with anterior uveitis. The suspected underlying cause for the uveitis was FIP, because of abnormalities seen on labwork. These included positive coronavirus titers, decreased hemoglobin, decreased hematocrit, and elevated globulins. Anterior uveitis is discussed in Chapter 15.

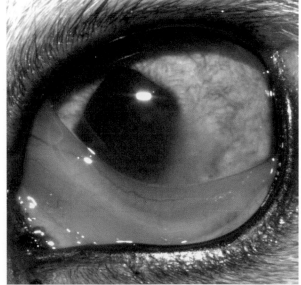

Figure 6.49 Left eye of a young Siberian husky who presented for "spots in eyes" that had been present for a few days. Multiple areas of iridal hemorrhage are visible. Similar changes were documented in the right eye. Physical examination revealed gingival petechiae. Labwork showed severe thrombocytopenia; this patient was later diagnosed with immune-mediated thrombocytopenia. Anterior uveal diseases are discussed in Chapter 15.

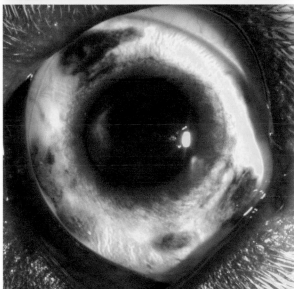

Figure 6.50 Left eye of a mixed breed kitten. Arrows indicate the dorsal and lateral pupillary margins. There are broad adhesions (anterior synechiae) between the medial and ventral pupil margins and the cornea. The central cornea, where the iridal tissue attaches, is fibrotic. These changes were suspected to be due to a previous globe perforation. Contrast the appearance of these adhesions with the appearance of the iris-to-cornea PPMs earlier in this chapter (Figures 6.3 and 6.4). The PPMs are much thinner than these synechiae and arise from the iris collarette, rather than the pupillary zone. Anterior synechiae and PPMs are discussed in Chapter 15.

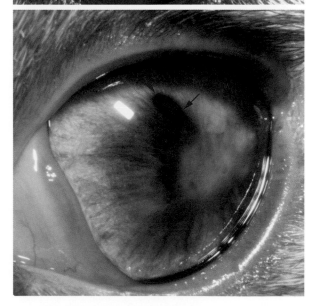

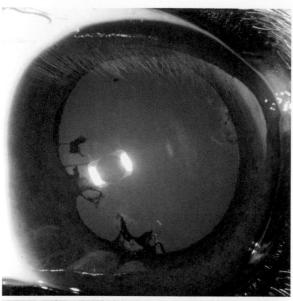

Figure 6.51 Posterior synechiae. The synechiae arise from the pupillary margin from 6 to 9 o'clock and are adherent to the anterior lens capsule. Where present, these adhesions prevent complete dilation of the pupil, and mild dyscoria has resulted. Linear white opacities in the dorsal cornea are reflections and not true changes. Anterior uveitis is discussed in Chapter 15.

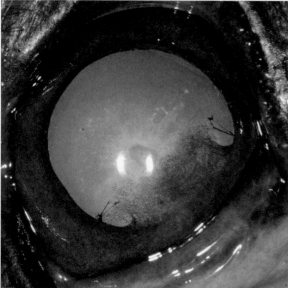

Figure 6.52 Posterior synechiae. Two thin adhesions are visible, extending from the pupillary margin to the anterior lens capsule at 3 and 7 o'clock. A broader adhesion is also present, arising from the pupillary margin from 3 to 6 o'clock. As a result of the adhesions, the ventromedial pupil is unable to completely dilate. An incipient cataract is also present in the central lens. Anterior uveitis is discussed in Chapter 15.

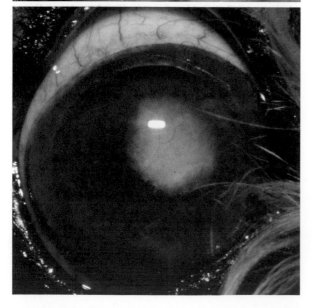

Figure 6.53 Right eye of a 10-year-old, castrated male miniature schnauzer. This patient was a poorly-controlled diabetic. There is dyscoria as a result of posterior synechiae involving the entire circumference of the pupil. The adhesions are also the reason the pupillary margin is irregular. Note the blood vessels visible within the pupil; this is within a fibrovascular membrane that has formed in the presence of chronic uveitis. Also shown in this photograph are episcleral hyperemia and a complete cataract. Anterior uveitis is discussed in Chapter 15.

Figure 6.54 Iris bombé following traumatic uveitis. Note the mild episcleral hyperemia and miotic pupil (due to uveitis). The pupillary and peripheral zones of the iris are located posterior relative to the iris collarette, which is billowing anteriorly. The small amount of visible lens is completely opaque (complete cataract), with a sparkly appearance indicating resorption. The crescent-shaped, white opacity near the limbus from 6 to 9 o'clock is a reflection. Uveitis is discussed in Chapter 15.

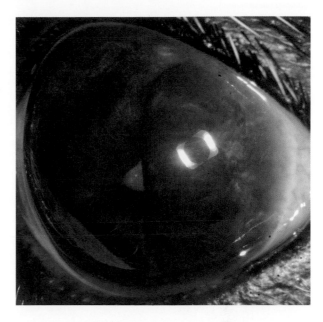

7 Lens

Please see Chapter 16 for more information about diseases, diagnostic testing, and treatment plans related to the lens.

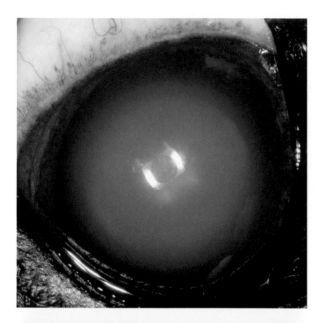

Figure 7.1 Nuclear sclerosis in the right eye of a 12-year-old, castrated male Gordon setter. Due to the angle of light, the sclerotic nucleus appears opaque. However, changes to the angle of viewing and the angle of light will reveal a clear, unobstructed tapetal reflection similar to that in Figures 7.3 and 7.4. Nuclear sclerosis is discussed in Chapter 16.

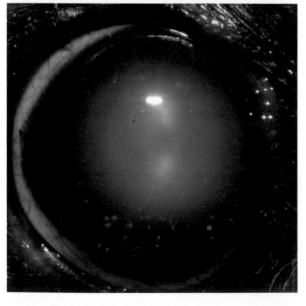

Figure 7.2 Right eye of an elderly miniature poodle. The characteristic appearance of nuclear sclerosis is a gray circle in the central pupil. Peripheral to this, the lens is less dense so in this photo the peripheral pupil appears black. Pinpoint opacities are visible in the ventral peripheral pupil; these are asteroid hyalosis. Nuclear sclerosis is discussed in Chapter 16.

Small Animal Ophthalmic Atlas and Guide, Second Edition. Christine C. Lim.
© 2023 John Wiley & Sons, Inc. Published 2023 by John Wiley & Sons, Inc.
Companion website: www.wiley.com/go/lim/atlas

Figure 7.3 Nuclear sclerosis in the left eye of a 10-year-old, spayed female miniature schnauzer. The nuclear density is circular and central within the pupil. Outer edges of the nucleus are marked with arrows. Colors are visible near the outer nucleus (also indicated by arrows) due to differences in refraction of various wavelengths of light. The appearance of these colors is also typical of the appearance of nuclear sclerosis. Nuclear sclerosis is discussed in Chapter 16.

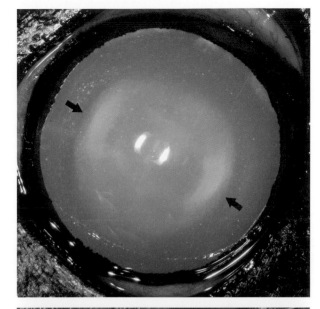

Figure 7.4 Typical retroilluminated appearance of nuclear sclerosis. The outer edges of the nucleus are indicated by arrows. Colors are more visible in these areas due to differences in refraction of various wavelengths of light. Nuclear sclerosis is discussed in Chapter 16.

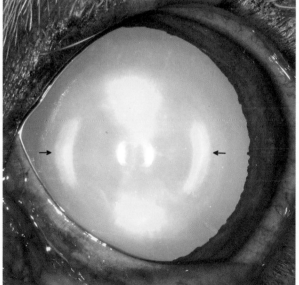

Figure 7.5 Incipient cataract. The cataract, visible in the central pupil, appears bright yellow due to the reflection of light from the light source. Signs of visual compromise were absent. Routine monitoring was recommended. Cataracts are discussed in Chapter 16.

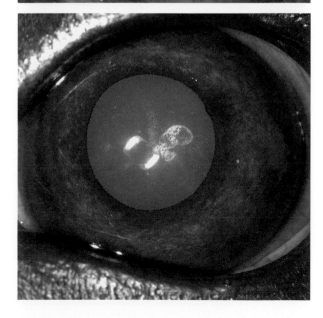

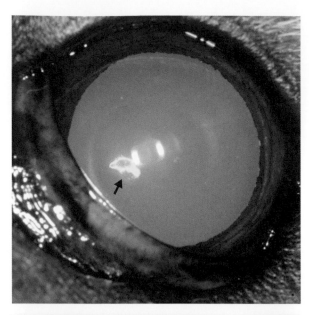

Figure 7.6 Incipient cataract (arrow). Note the bright appearance of the cataract, resulting from scattering of light from the light source. The patient did not show any signs of vision compromise. No treatment was instituted but monitoring was recommended. Cataracts are discussed in Chapter 16.

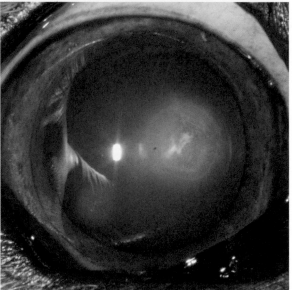

Figure 7.7a Incipient cataract in the right eye of an elderly great Dane. In this photograph, the cataract appears round and white, and is slightly off-center within the pupil, closer to the medial pupillary margin. Adjacent opacities are reflections. Cataracts are discussed in Chapter 16.

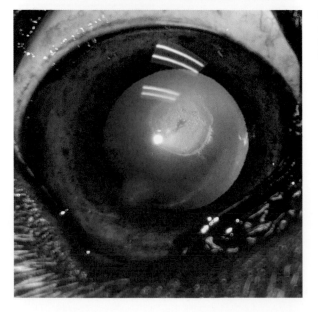

Figure 7.7b Retroilluminated view of the same eye as in Figure 7.7a The tapetal reflection is visible. Because the cataract is backlit by the tapetal reflection, it has a slightly different appearance when compared to the previous photograph. Cataracts are discussed in Chapter 16.

Figure 7.8 Incomplete cataract in the right eye of a DSH. No change in vision was noticed by the owners. The tapetal reflection (green to yellow color) is partially blocked by the white cataract, which is densest in the dorsal one-third of the lens, but which also affects the lens more ventrally. Melanin is adhered to the dorsal anterior lens capsule, a result of contact between the iris and lens. Topical anti-inflammatory medications were started, and routine monitoring was advised. Cataracts are discussed in Chapter 16.

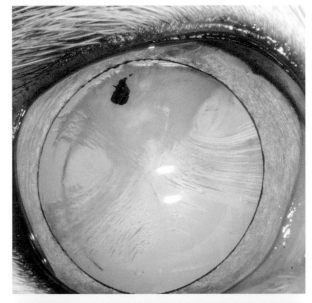

Figure 7.9 Unilateral incomplete cataract. This dog was still able to navigate around the home because the other eye was unaffected. The tapetal reflection (red) is visible throughout the lens, but is less bright in areas where the cataract is more dense. This owner elected topical anti-inflammatory therapy and periodic monitoring. Cataracts are discussed in Chapter 16.

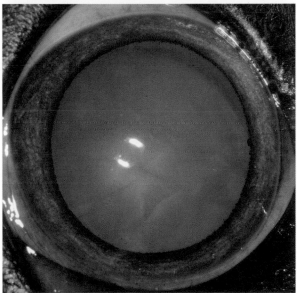

Figure 7.10 In this photograph, the lens appears diffusely opaque, with only a small amount of tapetal reflection visible (faint yellow visible in portions of the lens). Because some tapetal reflection is still visible, the cataract is classified as incomplete. This dog was bilaterally affected and severely visually impaired. Topical anti-inflammatory medications were initiated, and phacoemulsification with intraocular lens implantation was performed. Cataracts are discussed in Chapter 16.

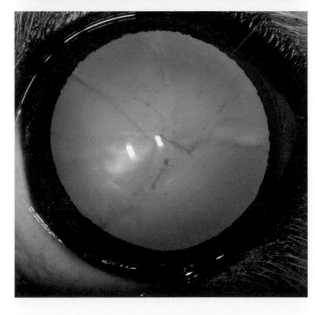

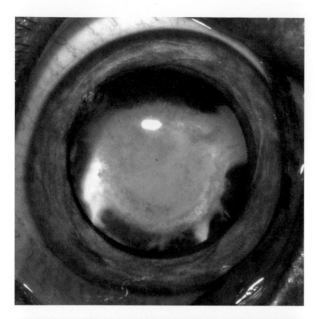

Figure 7.11 Incomplete cataract in the right eye of a young pit bull. The affected lens is white, while the unaffected, clear lens appears black in this photograph. Cataracts are discussed in Chapter 16.

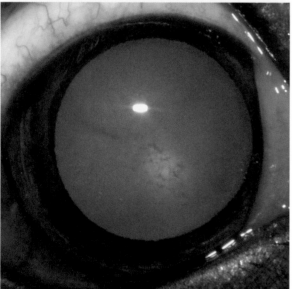

Figure 7.12 Incomplete cataract in the right eye of an Australian shepherd. The orange tapetal reflection is still visible through the cataractous lens. The tapetal reflection is attenuated by the cataract, and varies in brightness due to variability in the cataract density throughout the lens. Cataracts are discussed in Chapter 16.

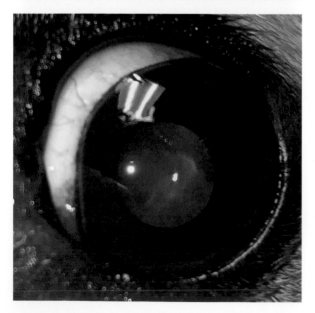

Figure 7.13a Incomplete cataract in the left eye of a young Jack Russell terrier mix. In this photograph, the eye is viewed with diffuse illumination and the pupil appears gray. Compare this photograph to Figure 7.13b. Cataracts are discussed in Chapter 16.

Figure 7.13b Retroilluminated view of the same eye as in Figure 7.13a. In this photograph, the green tapetal reflection is visible because retroillumination is employed. The tapetal reflection is attenuated because of the cataract and is brighter in areas where the cataract is less dense. Cataracts are discussed in Chapter 16.

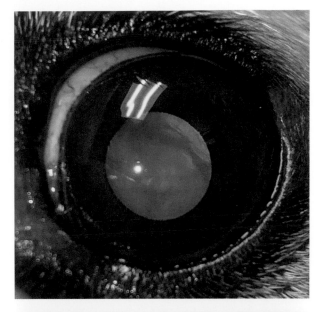

Figure 7.14a Incomplete cataract in the right eye of a miniature pinscher mix. This patient was referred for altered appearance of the right eye. The linear and curvilinear white streaks in the pupil are the cataract. In this photograph, the cataract is viewed with direct illumination and the cataract appears white. Where the lens is unaffected, the pupil is black. Compare this photograph to Figure 7.14b. Cataracts are discussed in Chapter 16.

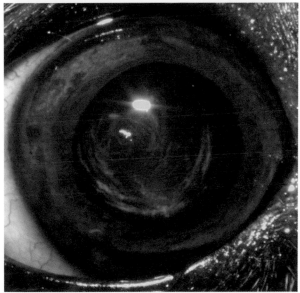

Figure 7.14b Retroilluminated view of the same eye as in Figure 7.14a. Although attenuated by the cataract, the tapetal reflection is visible. Because the cataract is backlit in this photograph, it appears slightly differently than in the previous photograph. This emphasizes the importance of looking at an eye from different angles during the ophthalmic examination. Cataracts are discussed in Chapter 16.

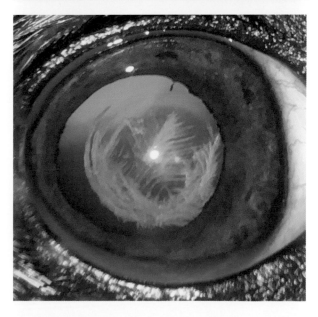

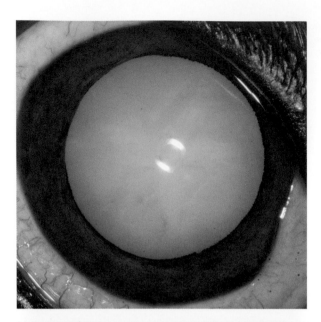

Figure 7.15 Complete diabetic cataracts. Both eyes were similarly affected. This dog was blind. The cataracts are considered complete because no tapetal reflection is visible. Note the conjunctival and episcleral hyperemia, resulting from LIU. Topical anti-inflammatories were started, and phacoemulsification with intraocular lens implantation was performed. Cataracts are discussed in Chapter 16.

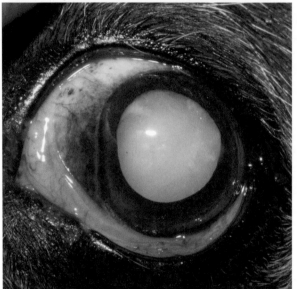

Figure 7.16 Complete cataract in a patient previously diagnosed with PRA. The tapetal reflection is not visible because of the cataract. This patient was treated with topical anti-inflammatory medications to control LIU. Cataracts are discussed in Chapter 16.

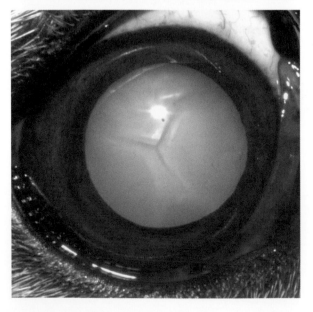

Figure 7.17 Complete, intumescent cataracts in a diabetic Labrador retriever. Note the Y sutures visible in the center of the lens. The cataracts were bilaterally symmetrical and blinding. As is typical for diabetic dogs, the cataracts developed rapidly. They were first noticed less than 2 weeks prior to this photograph. In addition to topical anti-inflammatories for control of LIU, this patient was treated with phacoemulsification and intraocular lens implantation. Cataracts are discussed in Chapter 16.

Figure 7.18 This is a left eye viewed from the left side of the dog, highlighting the contours of the anterior lens capsule. Note the uneven, wrinkled surface of the anterior lens capsule, which occurs with leakage of lens protein from the lens. The tapetal reflection is not visible. The cataract was therefore classified as complete and resorbing. Cataracts are discussed in Chapter 16.

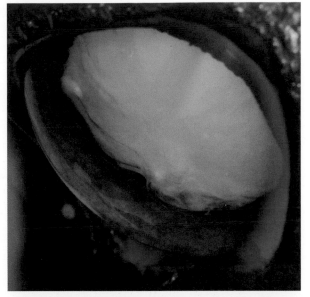

Figure 7.19 Incomplete, resorbing cataract. In this photograph, chronicity is indicated by the sparkly appearance to the lens. Ophthalmic examination also detected wrinkling of the lens capsule. The tapetal reflection is yellow and can be seen in the peripheral lens, particularly ventrolaterally. Mild episcleral hyperemia is a reflection of LIU. Superficial corneal vascularization and corneal melanosis are visible, extending from the 9 o'clock limbus into the cornea. Cataracts are discussed in Chapter 16.

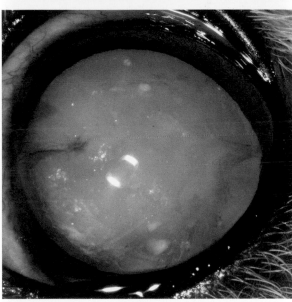

Figure 7.20 Hypermature cataract in a 13.5-year-old, spayed female miniature poodle. This cataract had been present for at least 2 years. The lens cortex is resorbing and beginning to clear, but the lens nucleus remains dense. The cataract is incomplete because when the lens is retroilluminated, tapetal reflection can be seen through the resorbing portion of the lens. The sparkly appearance throughout the lens indicates mineralization. This and the yellowing of the lens (brunescence) are indicators of cataract chronicity. Note the melanin deposit on the anterior lens capsule near the dorsal pupillary margin, which is a result of contact between the iris and lens. Secondary glaucoma was also diagnosed; the IOP at the time of the photograph was 33 mm Hg. Cataracts are discussed in Chapter 16.

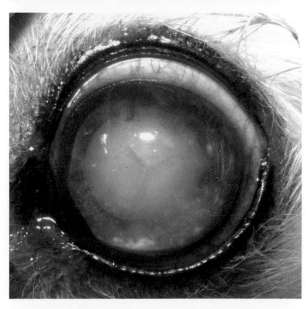

CHAPTER 7

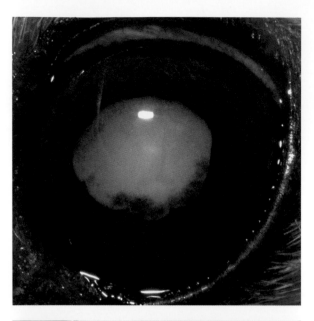

Figure 7.21 Complete, hypermature cataract in a diabetic Pomeranian. There is mineralization within the cataract, seen as pinpoint sparkly areas. There is dyscoria as a result of posterior synechia. Cataracts are discussed in Chapter 16.

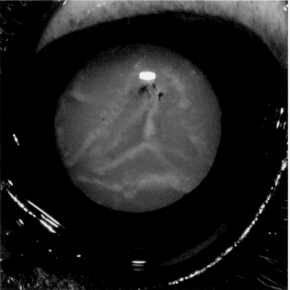

Figure 7.22 Complete, hypermature cataract in a diabetic terrier mix. The varying degrees of opacity within the lens are due to variations in the density of the cataract. Pinpoint sparkly deposits visible dorsally within the lens are areas of mineralization. Note the melanin deposit on the anterior lens capsule, which is a result of contact between the iris and lens. Cataracts are discussed in Chapter 16.

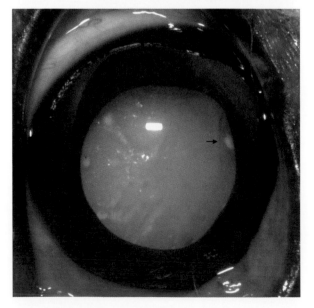

Figure 7.23 Complete, hypermature cataract in an elderly diabetic poodle mix. Pinpoint, sparkly deposits visible laterally within the lens represent areas of mineralization. Resorption of lens proteins has reduced lens volume, causing wrinkling of the lens capsule (arrow). Cataracts are discussed in Chapter 16.

Figure 7.24 Complete, hypermature cataract in a 3-year-old poodle. Mineralization, which appears sparkly, is visible throughout the lens. Cataracts are discussed in Chapter 16.

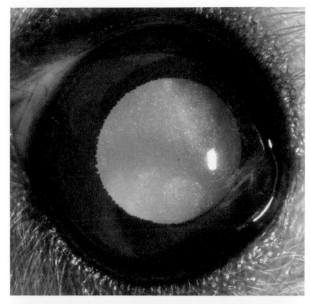

Figure 7.25 Lens subluxation, incipient cataracts (arrowheads), and nuclear sclerosis. The equator of the lens is indicated by the arrow. The aphakic crescent is the space between the lens equator and the pupillary margin, in this case extending from approximately 8 to 12 o'clock. At the tapered edges of the crescent, zonules extend radially across the aphakic cresent (from lens equator to the ciliary body). Nuclear sclerosis is the clear, circular shape within the central lens. Lens subluxation is discussed in Chapter 16.

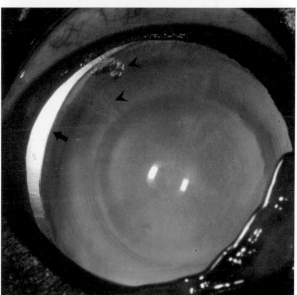

Figure 7.26 Nuclear sclerosis, incipient cataracts, and lens subluxation in the right eye of a 14-year-old, castrated male Chihuahua. The aphakic crescent is between the medial lens equator and pupillary margin from approximately 12 to 5 o'clock. The nuclear sclerosis is the cloudy circle within the central lens, and the incipient cataracts are the gray streaks within the ventrolateral nucleus. Iris atrophy is also visible in the medial iris. Lens subluxation is discussed in Chapter 16.

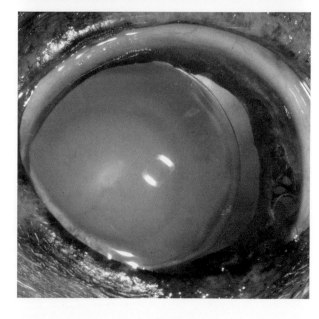

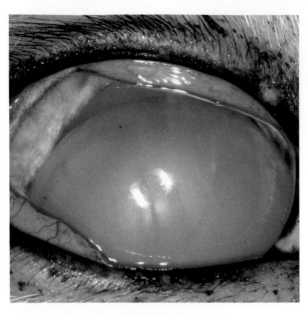

Figure 7.27 Complete cataract and anterior lens luxation in the right eye of a cat. The opaque lens prevents complete visualization of the iris. Green tapetal reflection is visible through the aphakic crescent (between the dorsal pupillary margin and the lens). Anterior uveitis and IOP elevation were also present. Note the chemosis, conjunctival and episcleral hyperemia, and superficial corneal vascularization (dorsolateral limbus). Lens luxation is discussed in Chapter 16.

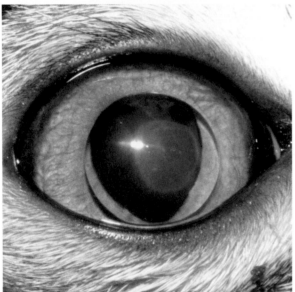

Figure 7.28 Right eye of a young kitten. The right lens is microphakic and luxated into the anterior chamber. Fibrosis is present in the central cornea, where the lens and cornea make contact. Anterior lens luxation is discussed in Chapter 16.

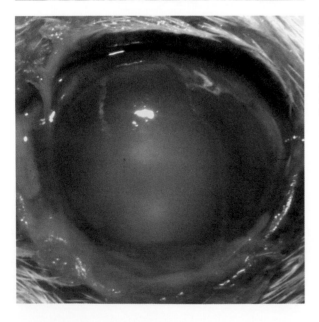

Figure 7.29 Left eye of an 8-year-old Chihuahua. The lens has luxated anteriorly into the anterior chamber. Red arrows indicate the lens equator. Corneal edema makes it somewhat difficult to visualize the luxated lens; this is often the case in clinical patients. The IOP was 54 mm Hg, consistent with glaucoma. The mucopurulent discharge is characteristic of KCS, which was also diagnosed at presentation because the STT was 8 mm/min. Keratoconjunctivitis sicca is discussed in Chapter 14. Anterior lens luxation is discussed in Chapter 16. Glaucoma is discussed in Chapter 18.

Figure 7.30 Right eye of a 9-year-old poodle mix. The lens has luxated anteriorly into the anterior chamber. Because the lens is now in front of the iris, it prevents complete visualization of the iris. Also shown in this photograph are episcleral hyperemia and mild, central corneal edema. Anterior lens luxation is discussed in Chapter 16.

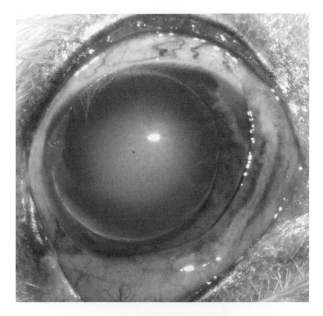

Figure 7.31 Right eye of a shiba inu. The lens is completely cataractous and is luxated posteriorly into the vitreous cavity. Because of gravity, it is located ventrally within the vitreous. The dorsal lens equator (arrows) is visible. Lens luxation is discussed in Chapter 16.

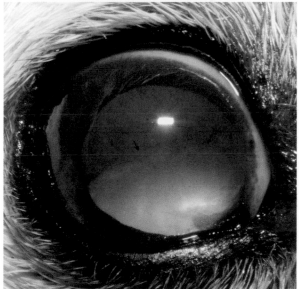

Figure 7.32 Left eye of an elderly shih tzu. The lens, which is completely cataractous, is luxated posteriorly into the vitreous cavity. Black arrows indicate the lens equator. Also present in this photo is episcleral hyperemia. Lens luxation is discussed in Chapter 16.

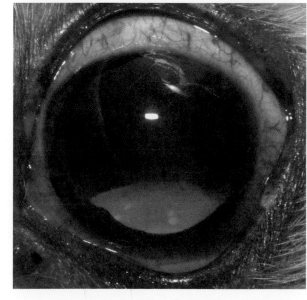

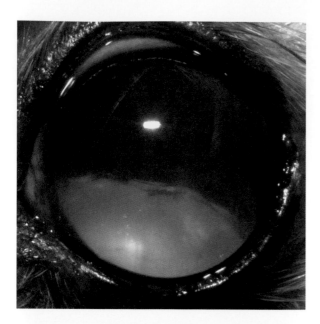

Figure 7.33 Left eye of an elderly Yorkshire terrier. The lens is completely cataractous and is luxated posteriorly into the vitreous cavity. Wrinkling of the lens capsule is visible at the equator (arrows), indicating chronicity of the cataract (hypermature/resorbing). Lens luxation and cataract are discussed in Chapter 16.

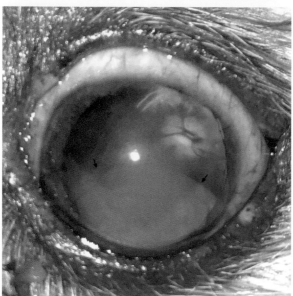

Figure 7.34 Left eye of a shih tzu mix. Black arrows indicate the equator of the lens, which is cataractous and luxated posteriorly into the vitreous cavity. The optic nerve, which is not normally visible with casual illumination of the eye, can be seen in the aphakic crescent because of the lack of lens. Lens luxation is discussed in Chapter 16.

8 Posterior segment

Please see Chapter 17 for more information about diseases, diagnostic testing, and treatment plans related to the posterior segment.

Figure 8.1 Normal appearance of the canine fundus. The canine tapetum is usually yellow, green, or orange. The canine optic nerve is white, due to myelin, and is usually round to triangular in shape. It is located near the tapetal–nontapetal junction near the central fundus. Three to four larger vessels cross the optic nerve head and extend into the peripheral fundus. Of these, the dorsal retinal venule is most visible; the others are more difficult to see against the brown nontapetal fundus. The normal fundus is discussed in Chapter 17.

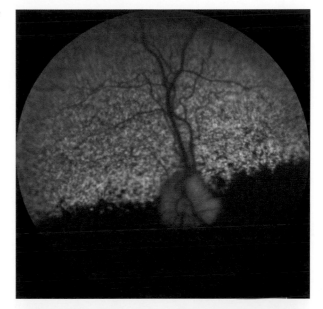

Figure 8.2 More magnified photograph of the normal canine fundus. For orientation purposes, please note that dorsal is the upper, left-hand corner of this photograph (i.e., the photo is slightly tilted). In this dog, the tapetal fundus is orange whereas the nontapetal fundus is brown. The transition from tapetal to nontapetal fundus can be smooth, but is often irregular, as in this photo. The optic nerve is white, and vessels can be seen crossing the optic nerve head. The vessels extend to the periphery of the fundus. The normal fundus is discussed in Chapter 17.

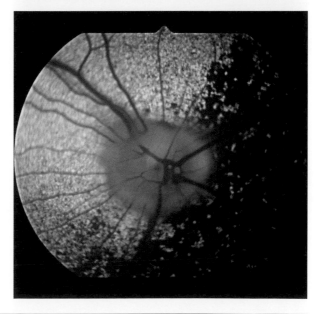

Small Animal Ophthalmic Atlas and Guide, Second Edition. Christine C. Lim.
© 2023 John Wiley & Sons, Inc. Published 2023 by John Wiley & Sons, Inc.
Companion website: www.wiley.com/go/lim/atlas

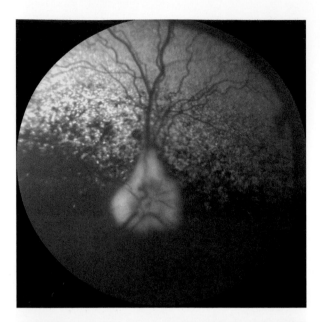

Figure 8.3 Photograph of a normal canine fundus. The tapetum is orange. The transition from tapetal to nontapetal fundus can be smooth, but is often irregular, as in this photo. The optic nerve is white, and vessels can be seen crossing the optic nerve head. The vessels extend to the periphery of the fundus. The normal fundus is discussed in Chapter 17.

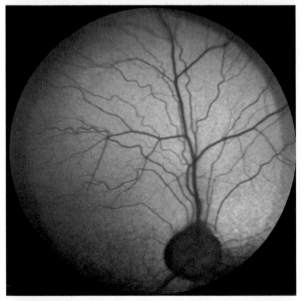

Figure 8.4 Normal canine fundus. Only the tapetal fundus is shown. The optic nerve is myelinated. Blood vessels can be seen crossing the optic nerve head, then extending to the peripheral tapetal fundus, which is yellow and green. The normal fundus is discussed in Chapter 17.

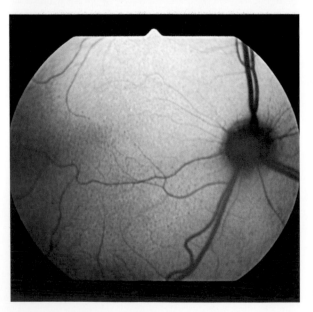

Figure 8.5 Normal appearance of the feline tapetal fundus. The ventral, nontapetal fundus is not pictured. The feline tapetum is usually green or yellow. The nontapetum is usually brown. The optic nerve is round and is gray due to the lack of myelin. Typically, three to four larger vessels extend from the periphery of the optic nerve to the peripheral fundus. The vessels do not cross the anterior surface of the optic nerve. Smaller retinal vessels are also present. The normal fundus is discussed in Chapter 17.

Figure 8.6 Normal appearance of the feline tapetal fundus. The junction between the tapetal and nontapetal fundus is at the bottom of the photograph. Three larger blood vessels extend from the optic nerve to the periphery of the fundus. The optic nerve is small, round, and gray. The normal fundus is discussed in Chapter 17.

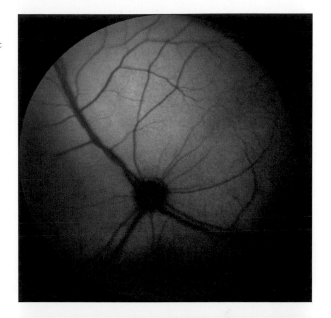

Figure 8.7 Normal appearance of the feline tapetal fundus. The optic nerve is small, round, and gray. Three larger blood vessels extend from the optic nerve to the periphery of the fundus. The normal fundus is discussed in Chapter 17.

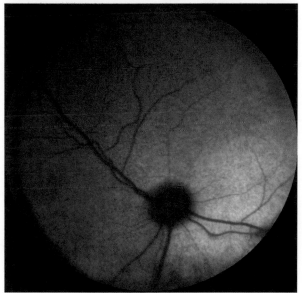

Figure 8.8 Subalbinotic, atapetal canine fundus. This is a normal variant. Instead of the typically brown nontapetal fundus, choroidal vessels are visible in the subalbinotic fundus. In contrast to retinal vessels, choroidal vessels do not arise from the optic nerve, tend to be wider than retinal vessels, and are arranged parallel to one another. The lack of tapetum is a common finding in subalbinotic fundi. The normal fundus is discussed in Chapter 17.

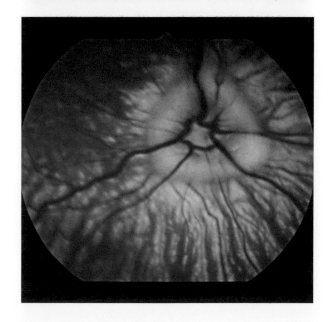

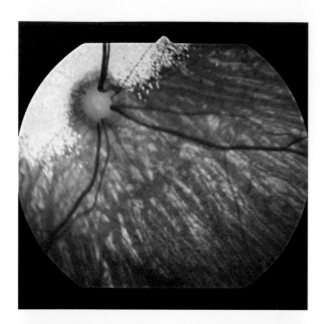

Figure 8.9 Normal appearance of a subalbinotic feline fundus. For orientation purposes, please note that dorsal is the upper, left-hand corner of this photograph (i.e., the photo is slightly tilted). The tapetum is present in this cat. Because the RPE in the nontapetal fundus contains little melanin, choroidal vessels are visible throughout the nontapetal fundus. Choroidal vessels are wider than retinal vessels, do not extend from the optic nerve, and appear parallel to each other. The normal fundus is discussed in Chapter 17.

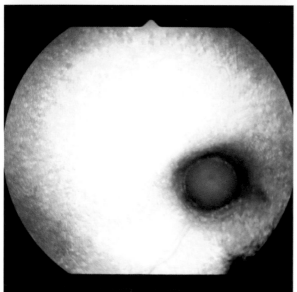

Figure 8.10 Diffuse tapetal hyperreflectivity and marked retinal vascular attenuation in a 1-year-old, castrated male Bengal. The changes were bilaterally symmetrical. This kitten had always been quieter and clumsier than his littermates and 3 months prior to presentation stopped chasing his toys and could no longer navigate the house without bumping into furniture. This patient was diagnosed with PRA, which is discussed in Chapter 17.

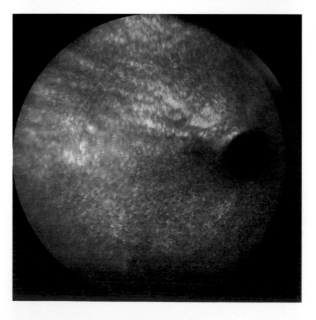

Figure 8.11 Right fundus of a 10-year-old DSH that presented for evaluation of vision loss. There is diffuse tapetal hyperreflectivity, retinal vessel attenuation, and optic nerve atrophy. Because there was no history of fluoroquinolone use and the patient was fed a commercial feline diet, PRA was the presumed cause of the retinal degeneration. PRA is discussed in Chapter 17.

Figure 8.12 Left fundus of the same patient as in Figure 8.11. As in the right eye, the left fundus is diffusely hyperreflective with marked vascular attenuation. The optic nerve, which is atrophied, is only partially visible as a dark circle at the bottom edge of the photograph. This patient was presumed to have retinal degeneration secondary to PRA, which is discussed in Chapter 17.

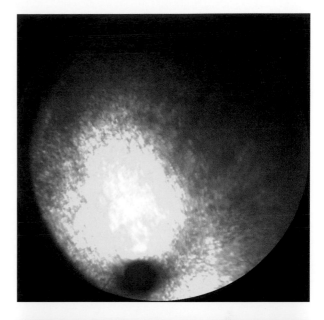

Figure 8.13 Diffuse tapetal hyperreflectivity and marked retinal vascular attenuation in a 4-year-old, castrated male mixed breed dog. The patient experienced progressive vision loss over a 6-month period and exhibited severe visual deficits at presentation. The changes were present bilaterally. This patient was diagnosed with PRA, which is discussed in Chapter 17.

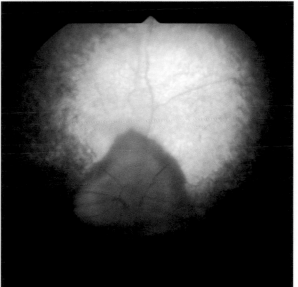

Figure 8.14 Left eye of a 3-year-old, intact male pitbull that presented for evaluation of gradually declining vision. This photograph shows tapetal hyperreflectivity (which is diffuse, but most noticeable dorsolateral to the optic nerve due to the flash) and retinal vessel attenuation. Note how the vessels are not visible beyond the immediate peripapillary region. The optic nerve is also smaller and paler than normal (compare to earlier figures of normal fundi). The changes were bilateral and symmetrical. Due to the history and clinical findings, PRA was suspected. PRA is discussed in Chapter 17.

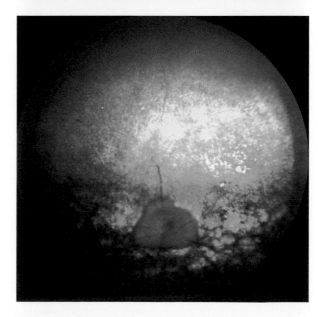

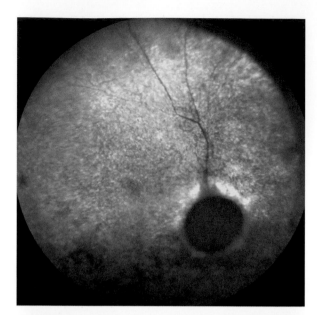

Figure 8.15 Left fundus of a 4-year-old Australian shepherd. He presented for an abnormal appearance to the right eye, but his owner did not report compromised vision. There is diffuse tapetal hyperreflectivity, retinal vessel attenuation, and optic nerve atrophy. Although the vessels extend to the edge of this photograph, they do not extend to the peripheral fundus, which is consistent with attenuation. Another feature of attenuation is narrowing of the vessels (compare to earlier figures of normal fundi). The atrophied nerve is smaller and darker when compared to normal. Incipient cataracts were present in the lens of this eye. The right fundus was not visible due to the presence of an incomplete cataract. Due to the association between PRA and cataract, the age of the patient, and the breed, the retinal degeneration was suspected to be bilateral and due to PRA. PRA is discussed in Chapter 17.

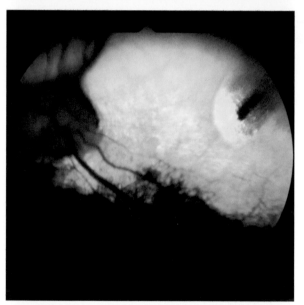

Figure 8.16 Typical appearance of a chorioretinal scar/focal retinal degeneration (far right edge of photo). The peripheral portion of the oval lesion is hyperreflective (seen as bright yellow to orange), and the center of the lesion is dark. Hyperreflectivity is due to thinning of the degenerate retina, and the hyperpigmentation is due to melanin clumping. Retinal degeneration of causes other than PRA and SARDS is discussed in Chapter 17.

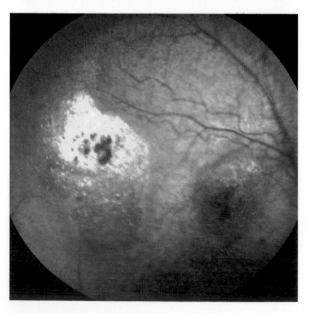

Figure 8.17 Two foci of retinal degeneration, which were incidental findings during ophthalmic examination. These areas, also referred to as chorioretinal scars, are flat, round, and hyperreflective (orange to yellow in the photograph) with black centers. For orientation, please note that the optic nerve, outside of the photo, is to the lower right-hand side of this photo. Retinal degeneration of causes other than PRA and SARDS is discussed in Chapter 17.

Figure 8.18 Right eye of an 8-year-old, castrated male beagle mix. The fundic changes were found incidentally on ophthalmic examination. For orientation purposes, please note that the optic nerve is located at the bottom of this photograph. There is an ovoid chorioretinal scar dorsal to the optic nerve, through which the dorsal retinal venule passes. Areas within the center of the scar are melanotic, while the periphery of the scar is hyperreflective. There is a second area of tapetal hyperreflectivity at the left-hand side of this photograph that is out of focus. Retinal degeneration of causes other than PRA and SARDS is discussed in Chapter 17.

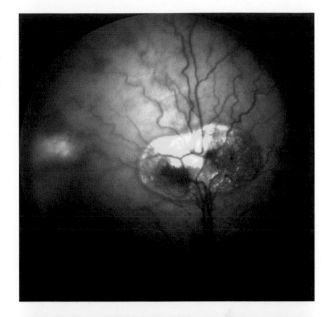

Figure 8.19 Multifocal tapetal hyporeflectivity in a 12-year-old, spayed female DSH with a blood pressure measurement of 220 mm Hg. For orientation, please note that the optic nerve, outside of the photo, is to the lower right-hand side of this photo. The normal areas of the tapetal fundus are yellow, while the hyporeflective areas are green to gray. The hyporeflectivity is due to retinal edema and fluid in the subretinal space, resulting from systemic hypertension. The central, circular lesion is retina that has detached as a result of fluid in the subretinal space. Hypertensive chorioretinopathy is discussed in Chapter 17.

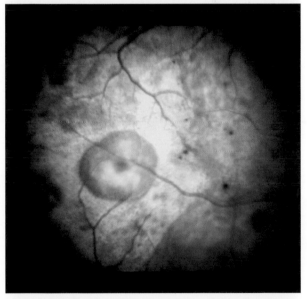

Figure 8.20 Multiple serous retinal detachments in the left eye of a 20-year-old castrated male DSH. The detached areas are hyporeflective, appearing round and dark in the photograph. The most prominent area of detachment is dorsolateral to the optic nerve and approximately 1 optic disc in diameter (arrow). The systolic blood pressure at the time of the photograph was 190 mm Hg. Hypertensive chorioretinopathy is discussed in Chapter 17.

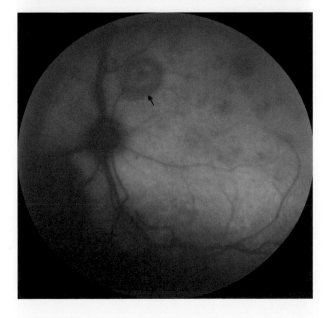

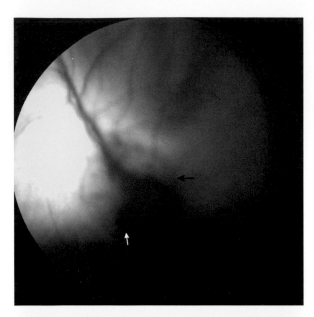

Figure 8.21 Left fundus of an 11-year-old spayed female DSH. There is a hyporeflective, gray lesion (red arrow) dorsal to the optic nerve and lateral to the dorsal retinal venule that was suspected to be a retrobulbar mass pressing on the globe. The peripapillary retina is also hyporeflective (black arrow). This area also appeared more blurry than surrounding fundus, suggestive of chorioretinitis. A white arrow indicates hemorrhage adjacent to the optic nerve. Ophthalmic examination revealed additional lesions, such as external ophthalmoplegia and internal ophthalmoplegia. Neoplasia was suspected. Fundic lesions are discussed in Chapter 17.

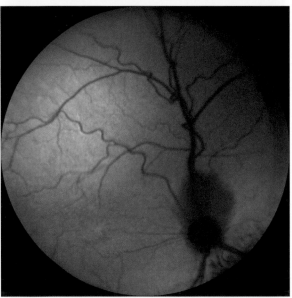

Figure 8.22 Right fundus of a young DSH that was positive for FIV. He presented for evaluation of bilateral mydriasis, vision loss, and periocular dermatitis. Ophthalmic examination revealed periocular excoriations, hyperesthesia, external ophthalmoplegia, internal ophthalmoplegia, and focal peripapillary hyporeflectivity. The appearance of the lesion was suggestive of cellular infiltrate. Due to the location of the lesion and neurologic abnormalities, more extensive neurologic disease was suspected. Diagnostic testing was not pursued and this patient was lost to follow-up. Tapetal hyporeflectivity is discussed in Chapter 17.

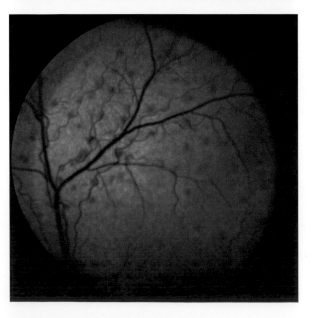

Figure 8.23 Multifocal tapetal hyporeflectivity in a 4-month-old, female mixed breed dog. For orientation, please note that the optic nerve is immediately outside of the frame at the bottom, left-hand corner of the photograph. This patient had many congenital ocular abnormalities in both eyes, including cataract, lens subluxation, and retinal detachment. The hyporeflective areas are pinpoint and gray, and were presumed to be areas of dysplastic retina. Tapetal hyporeflectivity is discussed in Chapter 17.

Figure 8.24 Right eye of a 10-year-old castrated male flat-coated retriever. For orientation purposes, the optic nerve is located immediately outside of the frame of this photograph, at the lower right corner. The dorsal retinal venule leads to an ovoid, hyporeflective, black lesion in the dorsal tapetal fundus. This lesion was found incidentally on ophthalmic examination and was presumed to be a choroidal melanoma. Tapetal hyporeflectivity is discussed in Chapter 17.

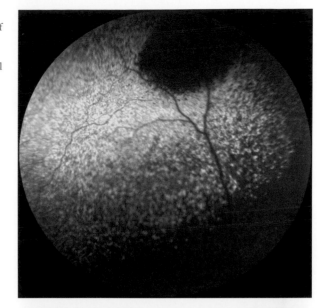

Figure 8.25 Left eye of a young Pekingese with systemic blastomycosis. There are multiple areas of tapetal hyporeflectivity immediately dorsal to the tapetal–nontapetal junction. The area immediately dorsal to the optic nerve is slightly blurry, suggesting focal inflammation and likely a low-lying retinal detachment as well. Chorioretinitis is discussed in Chapter 17.

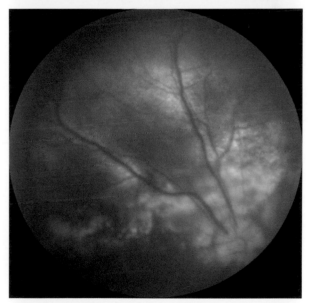

Figure 8.26 Left fundus of a golden retriever diagnosed with blastomycosis and chorioretinitis. The optic nerve is at the lower right-hand corner of the photograph and is not clearly visible. There are two round areas of tapetal hyporeflectivity, one larger than the other, dorsal and medial to the optic disc. They are both gray compared with the surrounding yellow–green tapetum. Both of these areas were presumed to be infiltrates of *Blastomyces* organisms and white blood cells. Tapetal hyporeflectivity is discussed in Chapter 17.

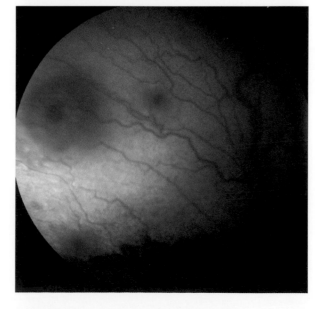

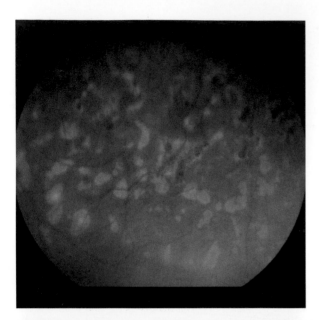

Figure 8.27 Multifocal areas of increased pigmentation and decreased pigmentation in the nontapetal fundus. The patient was a 6-year-old, castrated male Labrador retriever that was diagnosed with a brain tumor. The darker areas were thought to be clumps of melanin, while the whiter areas were thought to be accumulations of fluid and cells. Decreased pigmentation in the nontapetal fundus is discussed in Chapter 17.

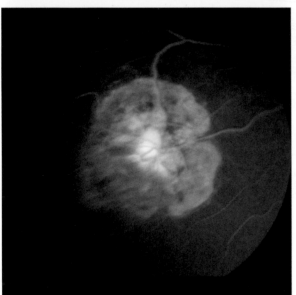

Figure 8.28 Decreased pigmentation of the nontapetal fundus in a 2-year-old, castrated male Doberman pinscher. This dog had undergone months of treatment for blastomycosis. The center of the white lesion is a thicker, creamier white than the periphery. The center of the lesion was due to white cell infiltrate, while the white areas at the periphery of the lesion were due to post-inflammatory thinning and depigmentation of the RPE and choroid. Decreased pigmentation in the nontapetal fundus is discussed in Chapter 17.

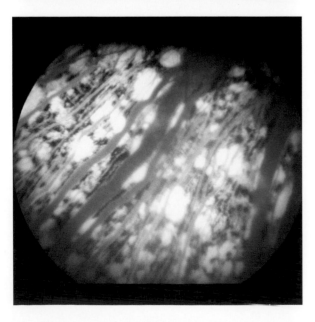

Figure 8.29 Multifocal areas of retinal degeneration in a 2-year-old, castrated male Bernese mountain dog. The area shown is in the nontapetal fundus. The blood vessels that are visible in this photograph are choroidal vessels. The degenerate areas appear white and are the result of previous chorioretinitis. Retinal degeneration is discussed in Chapter 17.

Figure 8.30 Pinpoint retinal hemorrhage (arrow) in the left fundus of a 10-year-old, castrated male shih tzu. This patient presented for evaluation of keratitis, and the hemorrhage was an incidental finding. Blood pressure was within normal limits on the day this photograph was taken. Retinal hemorrhage is discussed in Chapter 17.

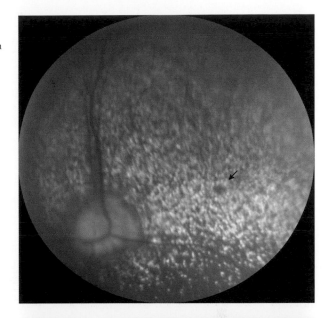

Figure 8.31 Preretinal hemorrhage in the ventral, nontapetal fundus. The keel shape indicates that the hemorrhage is anterior to the retina. The preretinal location is also known because the hemorrhage obscures visualization of the RPE. Retinal hemorrhage is discussed in Chapter 17.

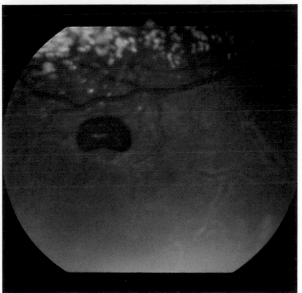

Figure 8.32 Multiple red, ovoid lesions consistent with intraretinal hemorrhage in a 5-year-old, castrated male cocker spaniel. This patient was diagnosed with optic neuritis and chorioretinitis, but a diagnostic workup was declined. Retinal hemorrhage is discussed in Chapter 17.

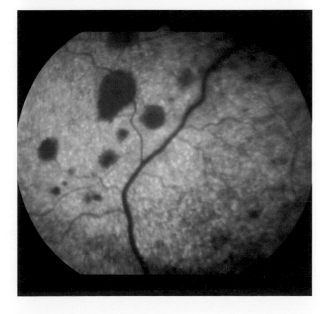

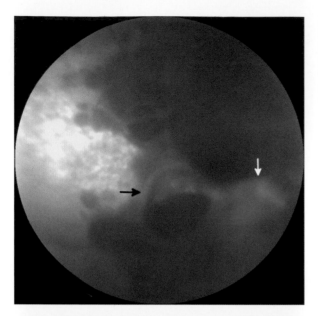

Figure 8.33 Left fundus of an 8-year-old, spayed female shih tzu with a long history of immune-mediated thrombocytopenia. She became acutely blind 2 days before presentation. For orientation, a white arrow indicates the optic nerve. Some yellow tapetum is visible on the left side of this photograph, but the remaining tapetal and nontapetal fundus are obscured by multiple areas of vitreous and retinal hemorrhage. The black arrow shows a white, curvilinear lesion that is an edge of torn retina. Retinal hemorrhage is discussed in Chapter 17.

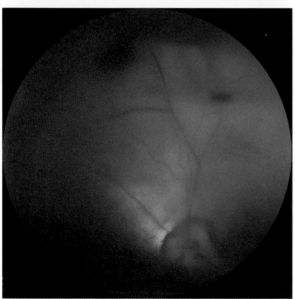

Figure 8.34 Left eye of an 11-year-old castrated male border collie cross. There is vitreous and retinal hemorrhage. Some retinal vessels are in focus while others are not, consistent with retinal detachment. There is tapetal hyporeflectivity as a result of the hemorrhage. This patient was later diagnosed with hemangiosarcoma. Retinal hemorrhage is discussed in Chapter 17.

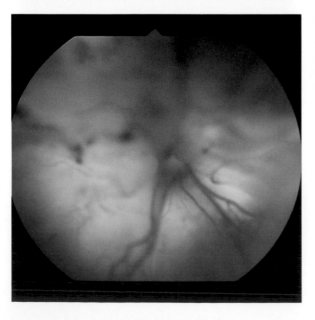

Figure 8.35 Complete, serous retinal detachment and hemorrhage in a 16-year-old, castrated male DSH diagnosed with systemic hypertension. Detachment is recognized by multiple planes of focus in this image and an obscured view of the optic nerve (due to retina suspended anterior to the nerve). On the day of this photograph, the blood pressure was 180 mm Hg. Hypertensive chorioretinopathy is discussed in Chapter 17.

CHAPTER 8

Figure 8.36 Left fundus of an elderly Himalayan. At the time this photograph was taken, the systolic blood pressure was 196 mm Hg, which was improved from >300 mm Hg at her initial ophthalmic examination. Multiple retinal and vitreous hemorrhages are present. There is attenuation of the retinal vasculature. The vessels immediately dorsal to the optic disc are blurry, suggestive of fluid infiltrate in this area. Hypertensive chorioretinopathy is discussed in Chapter 17.

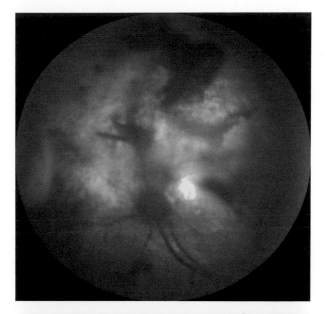

Figure 8.37 Left eye of an elderly retriever mix with complete retinal detachment. The only areas of retinal attachment are at the ciliary body and optic nerve. When a significant portion of the retina is detached, the retina is usually visible on external ophthalmic examination. The cream-colored retina and its vessels are visible in the pupillary space. The linear black structure (arrow) is a fold within the detached retina. Retinal detachment is discussed in Chapter 17.

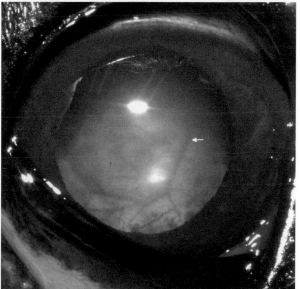

Figure 8.38 Left eye of a young rescue dog with unknown history. Both eyes were blind as a result of retinal detachments, suspected to be related to congenital ocular abnormalities. This photograph shows detached retina (gray to pink, at central and medial pupil) and hemorrhage (red) adhered to the posterior lens capsule. Retinal detachment is discussed in Chapter 17.

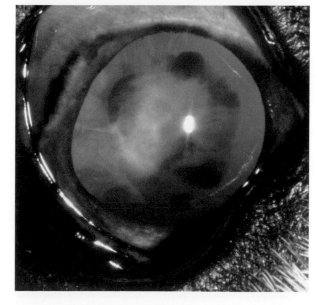

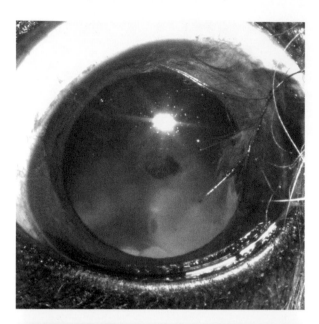

Figure 8.39 Right eye of the same patient as in Figure 8.33. The detached retina is the white to gray opacity in the ventral pupil. Intraretinal hemorrhage can be seen in addition to a vitreous blood clot in the central pupil. Retinal detachment is discussed in Chapter 17.

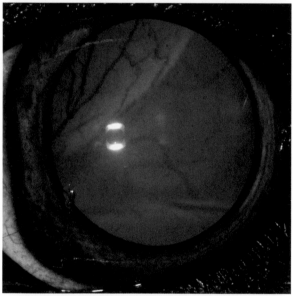

Figure 8.40a Complete, serous retinal detachment of unknown cause in a 4-year-old, castrated male German shepherd. The only areas of retinal attachment are at the ciliary body and optic nerve. When a significant portion of the retina is detached, the retina is usually visible on gross, external ophthalmic examination. The detached retina is visible within the pupil and looks like a gray to white membrane containing blood vessels. Folds within the detached retina are usually visible, as in this patient. The detachments in this dog resolved with systemic steroid therapy. Retinal detachment is discussed in Chapter 17.

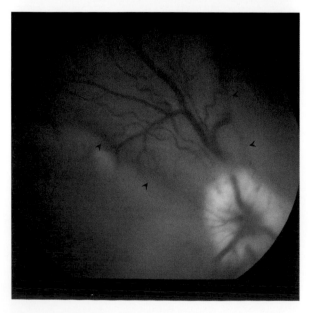

Figure 8.40b Fundic photograph of the same eye as in Figure 8.40a. Note that the dorsal retina is in focus, while the remainder of the retina and the optic nerve are out of focus, indicating that these structures are at different planes. The folds that were visible on external examination are also visible in this photograph (arrowheads). Retinal detachment is discussed in Chapter 17.

Figure 8.41 Right fundus of a young Labrador retriever with systemic blastomycosis. There is tapetal hyporeflectivity due to cellular infiltrates, most prominent dorsally. The lower half of the photo is out of focus because the retina is detached and is closer to the camera when compared to the upper half of the photo. Chorioretinitis is discussed in Chapter 17.

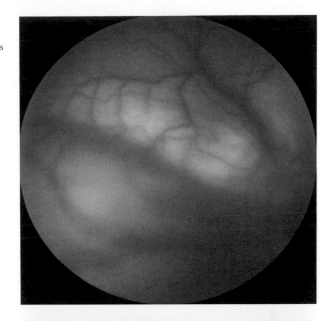

Figure 8.42 Rhegmatogenous retinal detachment. The optic nerve is at 12 o'clock in the photograph. The optic nerve cannot be seen clearly because the retina has torn dorsally along its attachments to the ciliary body, allowing it to fall ventrally and anterior to the optic nerve. The appearance of the retina resembles a white veil. Two retinal blood vessels are visible within the detached retina. Retinal detachment is discussed in Chapter 17.

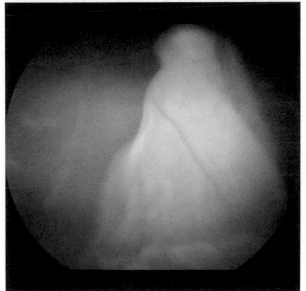

Figure 8.43 Left eye of a 2-year-old Chihuahua mix with multiple congenital abnormalities. It is difficult to visualize the optic nerve (black arrow) because the dorsal retina has fallen anterior to the nerve. In order for the retina to be anterior to the optic nerve, there must be a tear located dorsally, likely at the ciliary body. A white arrow shows one edge of the detached retina. Retinal detachment is discussed in Chapter 17.

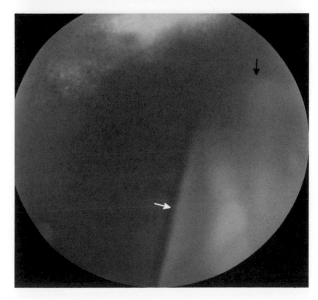

CHAPTER 8

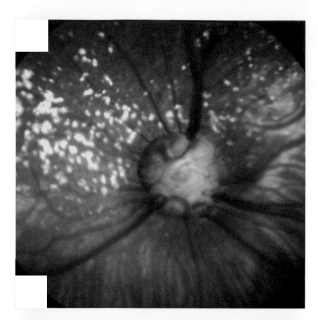

Figure 8.44 Optic nerve atrophy in a subalbinotic canine fundus. This atrophied nerve has less myelin than a normal nerve and is therefore smaller and darker than a normal nerve (see earlier figures for examples of normal). Loss of myelin is particularly noticeable from 6 to 11 o'clock, where the edge of the nerve appears black. The blood vessels do not form a robust vascular ring on the optic nerve head in contrast to the normal nerve. Careful examination shows subtle bending of the vessels at the nerve edge and darker retina immediately around the optic nerve. These changes at the edge of the nerve occur because the optic nerve head is recessed (more posterior to the retina) and reflect the transition of planes between the retina and the atrophied optic nerve. Pathologic changes to the optic nerve are discussed in Chapter 17.

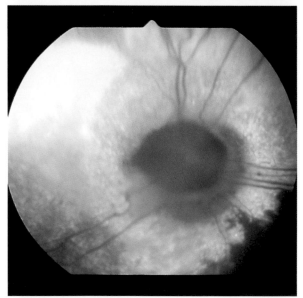

Figure 8.45 Optic nerve atrophy and retinal degeneration as a sequela to severe chorioretinitis. The degeneration is more severe in this photograph than in Figure 8.44. This optic nerve is small and dark due to demyelination. In addition, the vessels no longer cross over the optic nerve head, reaching only the nerve periphery. The tapetum immediately around the optic nerve is hyperreflective (seen as yellow in this photograph), indicating retinal degeneration. Retinal degeneration discussed in Chapter 17.

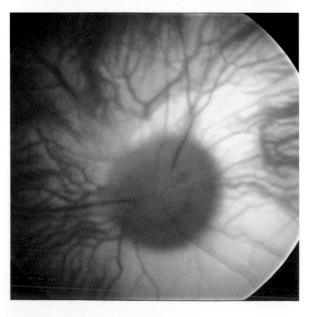

Figure 8.46 Optic disc cupping in a subalbinotic canine fundus. This is the result of chronic glaucoma. The retina immediately around the optic nerve appears darker than normal. Retinal blood vessels reach the edge of the optic nerve, but do not cross over the optic nerve head. It is difficult to distinguish the edges of the nerve from surrounding retina because both tissues are dark. Glaucoma is discussed in Chapter 18.

Figure 8.47 Typical appearance of a cupped optic nerve. When compared with a normal optic nerve (see earlier figures for examples of normal), the edges of the cupped nerve are dark, the cupped nerve is misshapen, the retinal vessels only reach its edge (rather than crossing over the nerve head), and the nerve is located more posteriorly than normal. Near the nerve head, there is subtle bending of the retinal vessels because they must change planes when transitioning between the retina and the more posteriorly located optic nerve. The peripapillary tapetum is also darker than in the normal dog. Glaucoma is discussed in Chapter 18.

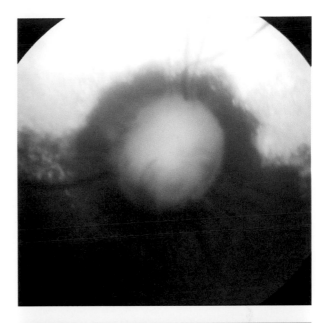

Figure 8.48 Canine optic neuritis. The edges of the optic nerve are indistinct. Because it is in focus while the remainder of the fundus is out of focus, it must be in a different plane than the retina. This is due to the severe swelling of the nerve and protrusion into the vitreous. Optic neuritis is discussed in Chapter 17.

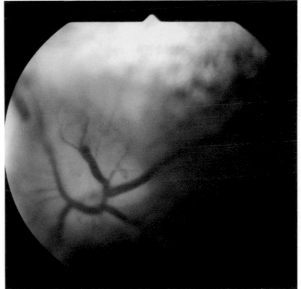

Figure 8.49 Optic neuritis and retinal hemorrhage in a cat suspected of having FIP. Inflammation of the optic nerve is inferred by its swelling and indistinct borders. Focal hemorrhage is present around the optic nerve as well. Optic neuritis is discussed in Chapter 17.

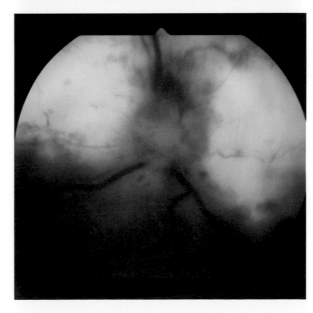

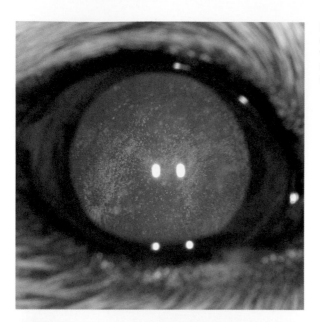

Figure 8.50 The typical appearance of asteroid hyalosis is multiple small, refractile objects suspended throughout the vitreous. Because of their location, they will be visible anterior to the retina and optic nerve on funduscopy but rarely interfere significantly with visualization of the fundus. Asteroid hyalosis is discussed in Chapter 17.

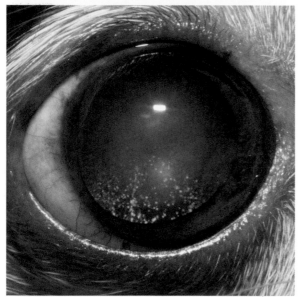

Figure 8.51 Asteroid hyalosis in a 12-year-old Chihuahua. Asteroid hyalosis describes calcium and phospholipid particles suspended within the vitreous. Due to the location of the camera flash, this photograph shows asteroid hyalosis only within the ventral region of the pupil. Because these particles are located throughout the vitreous, they would be visible within the entire pupillary space with retroillumination, as is the case in Figure 8.50. Asteroid hyalosis is discussed in Chapter 17.

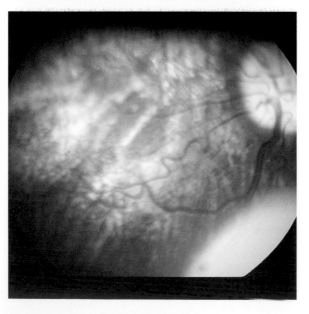

Figure 8.52 Choroidal hypoplasia in the right eye of a collie dog. The choroid lateral to the optic nerve is less pigmented than normal, and its vessel pattern is disorganized. Normal choroid, which is seen ventral to the area of hypoplasia, is more melanotic and the vessels are arranged relatively parallel to one another. The round, white object in the bottom right-hand corner of the photograph is a flash artifact. Collie eye anomaly is discussed in Chapter 17.

Figure 8.53 Choroidal hypoplasia and optic nerve coloboma in the left eye of a collie dog. The lateral aspect of the optic head, which appears gray and is devoid of blood vessels, is colobomatous and depressed. The hypoplastic choroid is lateral to the optic nerve; it is the less pigmented tissue to the right of the nerve in the photograph. Choroidal vessels are present within the area of choroidal hypoplasia, but they are not arranged in a regular, linear pattern. Collie eye anomaly is discussed in Chapter 17.

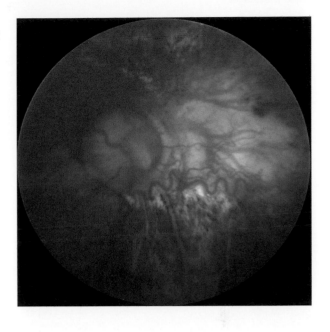

9 Glaucoma

Please see Chapter 18 for more information about diseases, diagnostic testing, and treatment plans related to glaucoma.

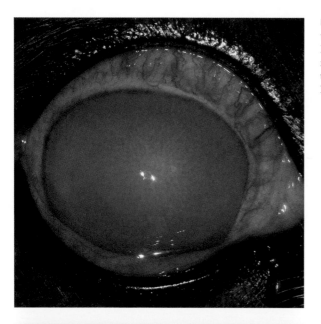

Figure 9.1 The typical presentation of primary glaucoma is acute onset of unilateral marked episcleral congestion, diffuse corneal edema, and mydriasis. Because this photograph was taken following administration of latanoprost, mydriasis is not present in this photograph. This patient, a 3-year-old male Boston terrier, also has deep corneal vessels because he presented 6 days after the acute IOP spike. Glaucoma is discussed in Chapter 18.

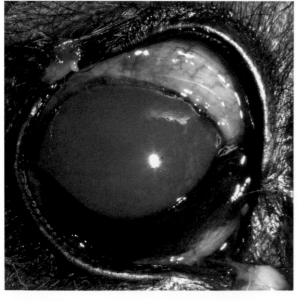

Figure 9.2 Right eye of a 5-year-old, spayed female standard poodle. She presented for a 1-day history of redness and clouding of the right eye. At the time this photograph was taken, the IOP was 74 mm Hg. The IOP changed minimally after emergency and maintenance therapy for glaucoma. Therefore, this eye was enucleated. Histopathology confirmed primary glaucoma. Glaucoma is discussed in Chapter 18.

Small Animal Ophthalmic Atlas and Guide, Second Edition. Christine C. Lim.
© 2023 John Wiley & Sons, Inc. Published 2023 by John Wiley & Sons, Inc.
Companion website: www.wiley.com/go/lim/atlas

Figure 9.3 Left-sided buphthalmos as a result of chronic, primary glaucoma in a basset hound. The left lens has luxated posteriorly as a result of buphthalmos. At the time this photo was taken, the left IOP was 46 mm Hg. The left eye was enucleated. Glaucoma is discussed in Chapter 18.

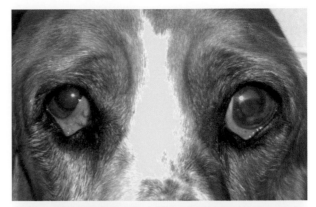

Figure 9.4 Left-sided buphthalmos in a shih tzu with chronic glaucoma. The IOP was 51 mm Hg prior to this photo being taken. Other abnormalities of the left globe include episcleral hyperemia, corneal edema, and corneal melanosis. The corneal melanosis is likely secondary to exposure, which increases when an eye is enlarged and the eyelids can no longer adequately blink over the ocular surface (lagophthalmos). This eye was enucleated. Glaucoma is discussed in Chapter 18.

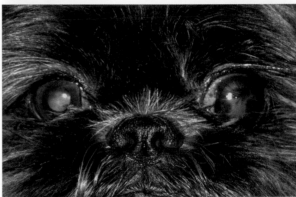

Figure 9.5 Haab's striae (arrowheads) are curvilinear corneal opacities seen with chronic glaucoma. They are breaks within Descemet's membrane that occur as the eye stretches. Glaucoma is discussed in Chapter 18.

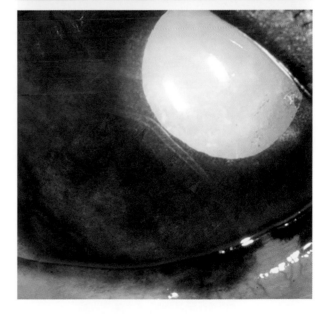

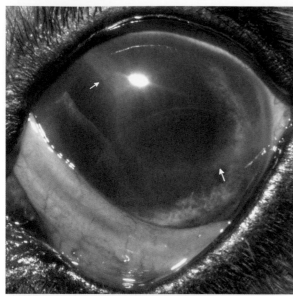

Figure 9.6 Close-up photograph of the left eye shown in Figure 9.3. The IOP was 46 mm Hg. Two Haab's striae (white arrows) cross the cornea. The red arrow indicates the lens equator, which is visible because the lens has luxated posteriorly into the vitreous cavity. Glaucoma is discussed in Chapter 18.

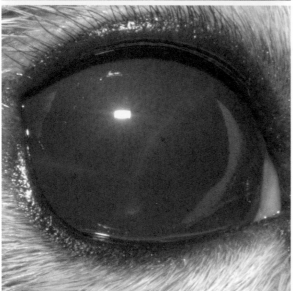

Figure 9.7 Right eye of a 5-year-old, castrated male American shorthair. The IOP was 71 mm Hg. There is diffuse corneal edema. Two Haab's striae (red arrows) are visible as curvilinear white lesions within the edematous cornea. The iris is not visible in the photograph because the pupil was widely dilated as a result of glaucoma. The fellow eye was similarly affected. This patient had a previous diagnosis of FIV. Histopathology of both eyes revealed chronic, lymphoplasmacytic endophthalmitis and optic neuritis, which is often seen with FIV-related uveitis, and which is the presumed cause of the secondary glaucoma in this patient. Glaucoma is discussed in Chapter 18.

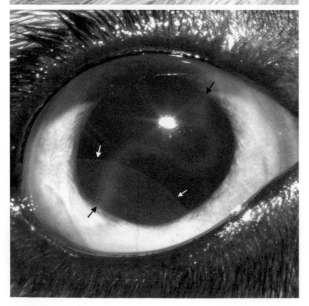

Figure 9.8 Right eye of a 1-year-old mixed breed spayed female dog. This eye was buphthalmic, consistent with chronic glaucoma. Changes seen in this photograph include Haab's striae (between the black arrows) and posterior lens luxation (white arrows indicate the lens equator). This eye was enucleated. Histopathology confirmed primary glaucoma. Glaucoma is discussed in Chapter 18.

Figure 9.9 Posterior lens luxation secondary to glaucoma. The IOP was 38 mm Hg. Buphthalmos led to zonular breakdown and luxation of the lens into the vitreous cavity. Note the episcleral congestion and mydriasis, also consistent with a diagnosis of glaucoma. Lens dislocation is discussed in Chapter 16. Glaucoma is discussed in Chapter 18.

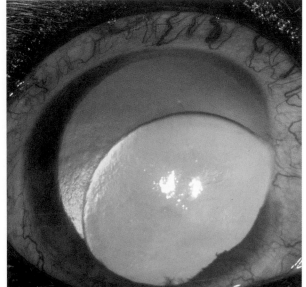

Figure 9.10 Left eye of an elderly mixed breed dog. The IOP was 72 mm Hg at presentation. The lens is cataractous and luxated into the anterior chamber. Arrows indicate the lens equator. In addition to anterior lens luxation, this photograph shows episcleral hyperemia, deep corneal vascularization, and diffuse corneal edema. Histopathology confirmed chronic uveitis causing secondary glaucoma, and supported chronic lens-induced uveitis as the cause of the lens luxation. Anterior lens luxation is discussed in Chapter 16. Glaucoma is discussed in Chapter 18.

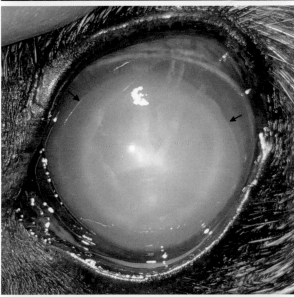

Figure 9.11 Right eye of a 10-year-old, spayed female Labradoodle. At the time of this photograph, this patient was being treated with dorzolamide and the IOP was 35 mm Hg. The optic nerve is small and dark as a result of chronically elevated IOP (optic nerve cupping). Because the eye was blind and the IOP uncontrolled, enucleation was performed. Histopathology showed goniodysgenesis, consistent with primary glaucoma. Changes to the optic nerve are discussed in Chapter 17. Glaucoma is discussed in Chapter 18.

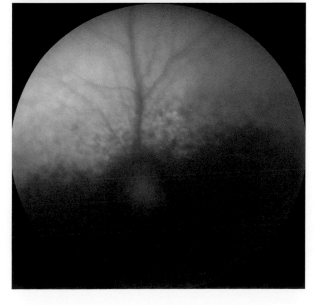

SECTION II

Guide

10 Orbit

Please see Chapter 1 for images of the orbit.

The bony orbit is a relatively enclosed space. In addition to the globe, the orbit contains the following:
- Extraocular muscles
  - Dorsal, medial, ventral, and lateral rectus muscles
  - Dorsal and ventral oblique muscles
  - Retractor bulbi muscle
- Third eyelid
- Glands
  - Orbital lacrimal gland
  - Gland of the third eyelid
- External ophthalmic artery and its branches
- An ophthalmic venous plexus and branches of the external ophthalmic vein
- Cranial nerves II through VI
- Orbital fat pad
- Conjunctiva
- Lymphatics
- Connective tissue

The walls of the orbit are composed of the following:
- Lateral aspect
  - Orbital ligament
  - Temporal muscle
- Dorsal aspect
  - Frontal bone
- Medial aspect
  - Frontal bone
- Ventral floor
  - Sphenoid bone
  - Palatine bone
  - Medial pterygoid muscle
  - Zygomatic salivary gland
- Apex
  - Presphenoid bone
- Ventral orbital rim
  - Lacrimal bone
  - Frontal bone
  - Maxillary bone
  - Zygomatic bone

Structures adjacent to the orbit include the following:
- Frontal sinus (dorsomedial to orbit)
- Maxillary sinus (anteroventral to orbit)
- Nasal cavity (ventromedial to orbit)
- Roots of the fourth maxillary premolars and maxillary molars
- Ramus of the mandible
- Masticatory muscles

Diseases of any structures within or adjacent to the orbit tend to cause a space-occupying effect and displacement of the orbital structures. This predominantly occurs through the path of least resistance, meaning anteriorly through the palpebral fissure. Therefore, orbital structures tend to become more visible in the presence of orbital disease. General and common signs of orbital disease include the following:
- *Exophthalmos* (Figures 1.1, 1.2a, 1.2b, 1.3)
  - That is, the eye is pushed anteriorly and is more prominent than normal.
  - Subtle exophthalmos can be missed if the eyes are not viewed from above the head and from the side of the head (in addition to the examination conducted while facing the patient).
  - Do not confuse exophthalmos with buphthalmos.
    - The latter is an enlargement of the eye, which also gives it a more prominent appearance.
    - Exophthalmos can be differentiated from buphthalmos by measurement of the horizontal corneal diameter.
    - The horizontal corneal diameter of the buphthalmic eye is greater than the measurement for the fellow eye, whereas diameters are equal if an eye is exophthalmic.
- *Third eyelid elevation* (Figures 1.1, 1.3, 1.5, 1.11, 1.12a, 1.12b, 1.13a, 1.13b)
- Chemosis (Figures 4.3, 4.4)
- Conjunctival and episcleral vascular engorgement
- Periocular tissue swelling (Figures 1.2a, 1.2b, 1.3)
- *Decreased retropulsion of the globe*

The aforementioned clinical signs are almost always present in orbital cellulitis/abscess and orbital neoplasia.

Enophthalmos (Figures 1.4, 1.6, 1.11, 1.13a) can also indicate orbital disease, although this is less common than exophthalmos.

Small Animal Ophthalmic Atlas and Guide, Second Edition. Christine C. Lim.
© 2023 John Wiley & Sons, Inc. Published 2023 by John Wiley & Sons, Inc.
Companion website: www.wiley.com/go/lim/atlas

It is seen with Horner's syndrome, in some cases of orbital neoplasia, in association with facial fractures, as a sequela to severe orbital inflammation, and in diseases where orbital volume decreases (e.g., atrophy of the orbital fat pad, which accompanies weight loss).

Diseases of the orbit

Brachycephalic ocular syndrome

What it is
- Brachycephalic ocular syndrome refers to a set of conformational abnormalities affecting the eyelids and the orbit.
- This syndrome is usually accompanied by chronic surface ocular irritation and trauma occurring secondary to the conformational abnormalities.

Predisposed individuals
- The syndrome occurs most often in brachycephalic dogs and cats, but some nonbrachycephalic dogs also exhibit the same orbit and eyelid abnormalities.
- Commonly affected dog breeds include the pug, shih tzu, lhasa apso, and Pekingese. Affected cat breeds include the Persian, Himalayan, and Burmese.

Defining characteristics
Affected individuals exhibit the following facial characteristics:
1. Bilateral exophthalmos (Figures 1.7, 1.8)
   - Due to bony orbits that are shallower than those of mesocephalic and dolichocephalic individuals.
   - The result of exophthalmos is increased ocular exposure. The exposure in turn makes the eyes more susceptible to trauma.
2. Enlarged palpebral fissures (Figures 1.7, 1.8, 1.9)
   - Excessively large eyelid openings.
   - Also referred to as macropalpebral fissure.
   - Contributes to lagophthalmos and corneal exposure, leading to chronic corneal drying and irritation.
3. Medial trichiasis (Figures 1.9, 1.10)
   - Ventromedial entropion of varying severity is present. Epiphora is a common secondary effect; the entropion can misalign nasolacrimal puncta and prevent tears from entering the nasolacrimal drainage system.
   - Often, hair follicles are present within the medial canthus. The hairs usually are directed onto the cornea.
   - In breeds with prominent nasal folds, the folds may lie against the cornea.
   - Constant corneal contact with hairs results in chronic irritation to the medial cornea.

Clinical significance
- The aforementioned abnormalities chronically irritate the cornea and allow the ocular surface to become exposed and dry.

- The exposure and dryness are irritating.
- This exposure predisposes to keratitis and corneal ulceration, especially of the medial and central cornea.
   - Therefore, pathologic changes to the cornea are predominantly visible in the medial and central portions of the cornea.
- In addition to chronic ocular surface inflammation, the abnormalities associated with brachycephalic ocular syndrome impair or even prevent healing of corneal ulcers.
- In dogs, pigmentary keratitis (see Chapter 14) is a common consequence of brachycephalic ocular syndrome.
   - This condition causes vision impairment and, if progressive, even blindness.
- In cats, corneal sequestra (see Chapter 14) commonly develop as a result of brachycephalic ocular syndrome.
   - This condition is painful and predisposes the cornea to infection.

Diagnosis
Diagnosis of brachycephalic ocular syndrome is made by observation of the conformational abnormalities.

Treatment
- The goals of treatment are to
   - reduce surface ocular irritation and
   - prevent development of corneal changes or, if changes are already present, slow progression of corneal lesions.
- Treatment may be limited to medical management, may include surgery, or may be a combination of medications and surgery.
- For eyes that have not yet developed keratitis, and when the severity of conformational abnormalities is mild, ophthalmic lubrication alone may be sufficient to prevent development of surface ocular inflammation.
- However, for eyes with mild keratitis, addition of an ophthalmic anti-inflammatory medication is likely needed.
- When keratitis is present, or when conformational abnormalities are pronounced, medications should be started and the patient referred for potential surgery.
1. Medical management of brachycephalic ocular syndrome
   - Tear film replacements (ophthalmic lubricating solutions or ointments)
      - These are prescribed to reduce exposure and drying of the central cornea.
      - Apply two to four times daily, or more often, if needed.
      - Preservative-free preparations are preferred when application is frequent, since ophthalmic preservatives themselves can irritate the ocular surface.
   - Ophthalmic anti-inflammatory medications (corticosteroids, CsA, or both in combination)
      - These are used to decrease corneal inflammation (i.e., to treat keratitis), often concurrently with tear film replacements.
      - Degree of improvement with medications can be variable.

- Corticosteroids
  - Prednisolone acetate ophthalmic 1% suspension or dexamethasone 0.1% ophthalmic solution.
  - Frequently prescribed for dogs with keratitis.
  - Not recommended to treat feline keratitis due to the relationship between feline corneal disease and FHV-1 infection.
  - Because inflamed corneas and individuals with brachycephalic ocular syndrome are at higher risk of corneal ulceration, patients should be monitored closely while being treated with corticosteroids.
  - Do not use in presence of corneal ulceration because corticosteroids reduce healing and may potentiate infections.
  - Initial dosing may be as high as one drop of suspension applied to the affected eyes three to four times daily, especially for severe, nonulcerative keratitis.
  - As the level of keratitis improves (i.e., as the inflammation decreases), the dose should gradually be tapered to no more than one to two times daily if used long term.
  - Corticosteroids can be used concurrently with CsA.
  - Improvement in the severity of keratitis usually starts to become noticeable within 3–4 weeks.
- CsA
  - CsA 0.2% ophthalmic ointment (Optimmune®).
  - This is frequently prescribed to both dogs and cats with keratitis.
  - The dose is 1/4″ strip applied to the affected eyes q12h.
  - CsA can be used concurrently with corticosteroids.
  - Improvement in the severity of keratitis usually starts to become noticeable within 6–8 weeks.
  - CsA is preferred over corticosteroids for long-term use. This is because of the predisposition of brachycephalics to corneal ulceration (for which corticosteroids are contraindicated) and potential for steroids to induce keratopathy.
- The first recheck examination is recommended for within 4–6 weeks of beginning medical therapy.
  - The purpose of the recheck is to document any changes to the corneal health.
  - If improvement is lacking, the patient should be referred for surgery.
  - Further recheck intervals are determined by the progress of the patient (i.e., degree of improvement of corneal lesions and time course for improvement to be visible).
2 Surgical management
  - Medical management may be sufficient as the only form of therapy if conformational abnormalities and keratitis are mild.
  - However, referral for medial canthoplasty is recommended in most cases, especially for individuals with severe or progressive keratitis or recurrent corneal ulceration.

- Medial canthoplasty
  - Shortens the length of the palpebral fissures.
  - The shortened palpebral fissures increase eyelid coverage of the corneas and improve corneal protection by the eyelids.
  - Because the surgery is performed at the medial canthus, it eliminates the ventromedial entropion.
  - During surgery, the hair follicles within the medial canthus are excised, thereby eliminating these hairs as a source of irritation.
- Nasal fold resection
  - Performed in dogs with nasal folds that rest against the cornea, especially if medial canthoplasty does not eliminate contact between cornea and nasal fold.

Prognosis

- Some degree of corneal opacification will persist in the long term and the goal is to slow/limit progression of corneal opacities rather than achieving significant regression.
- If therapy is instituted prior to development of significant corneal disease, the prognosis is good for minimizing progression of corneal lesions (corneal vascularization, melanosis, and fibrosis).
- Therapy starting after development of more significant keratitis usually results in only a modest reduction of surface ocular changes (corneal vascularization, melanosis, and fibrosis).

Additional information

- Affected pets often sleep with their eyelids partially open.
  - This exposes the cornea to prolonged periods of exposure and dryness.
  - To reduce the exposure, apply an ophthalmic ointment lubricant to the exposed corneas before sleep.
  - An ointment is used instead of a solution because it will stay on the corneal surface for a prolonged period of time when compared with a solution.
- Corneal sensitivity in brachycephalic individuals is reduced when compared with nonbrachycephalic individuals (Barrett et al., 1991; Blocker & van der Woert, 2001).
  - This means that overt signs of ocular pain (blepharospasm, epiphora, and raised third eyelid) may not be visible even in the presence of keratitis or corneal ulceration, and significant corneal pathology can be present by the time patients are presented for evaluation.

Horner's syndrome

What it is

- Horner's syndrome occurs when there is loss of sympathetic innervation to the eye.
- The lesions can occur anywhere along the sympathetic pathway to the eye. Regions at which the lesions occur are roughly divided into (1) central neurons, (2) preganglionic neurons,

and (3) postganglionic neurons. A brief review of the course of sympathetic neurons is included here for background:

1 Central neurons
   - Sympathetic innervation to the eye originates from the hypothalamus and travels along the spinal cord to the first (T1) through third (T3) thoracic spinal cord segments, where synapse with preganglionic neurons occurs.
2 Preganglionic neurons
   - Cell bodies of the preganglionic neurons reside between T1 and T3.
   - Axons of the preganglionic neurons exit the spinal cord between T1 and T3, then travel to the head through the chest and the neck, along the thoracic and cervical sympathetic trunks.
   - When they reach the cranial cervical ganglion, the preganglionic neurons then synapse with the postganglionic neurons.
   - The location of the cranial cervical ganglion is ventromedial to the tympanic bulla.
3 Postganglionic neurons
   - The cell bodies of the postganglionic neurons reside in the cranial cervical ganglion.
   - Axons of the postganglionic neurons pass through the middle ear and then run toward the orbit.

Predisposed individuals
- Dogs and cats of any age, gender, or breed can be affected with Horner's syndrome.

Defining characteristics
- Affected animals show the following ocular abnormalities (Figures 1.11, 1.12a, 1.12b, 1.13a, 1.13b)

1 Ptosis
   - This is drooping of the upper eyelid.
   - This results from the loss of sympathetic innervation to Mueller's muscle.
   - Because Mueller's muscle assists with elevation of the upper eyelid, the upper eyelid cannot be completely raised.
      - Occasionally, some individuals will show "reverse ptosis," which is drooping of the lower eyelid instead of the upper eyelid.
2 Enophthalmos
   - This results from the loss of sympathetic tone to the orbitalis muscle.
      - This muscle, found in the connective tissue of the orbit, wraps around the cone of extraocular muscles that are located posterior to the eye.
   - The contraction of the orbitalis muscle around the extraocular muscle cone pushes the eye anteriorly and keeps it in its normal position within the orbit.
   - With loss of orbitalis muscle tone, it no longer holds the eye in position and instead the eye moves posteriorly.

3 Third eyelid elevation
   - This occurs passively when the enophthalmic globe displaces the third eyelid from the orbit.
4 Miosis
   - When sympathetic innervation to the iris dilator muscle is lost, the pupillary constrictor muscle is unopposed.

Clinical significance
- Ocular abnormalities resulting from Horner's syndrome are not harmful and do not cause pain.
- However, the raised third eyelid may cause varying degrees of visual impairment in the affected eye, depending on how much of the visual axis is obscured.
- The significance of Horner's syndrome relates to its underlying cause.
- The underlying cause of the neurologic lesion may be idiopathic, may have only a minor effect on overall health and be easily treatable, or could be fatal.

Potential causes of Horner's syndrome:

1 Lesions of the central neuron
   - These are rare and are usually accompanied by obvious neurologic abnormalities.
   - Intracranial and spinal neoplasia (Kern et al., 1989; Luttgen et al., 1980; van den Broek, 1987).
   - Intervertebral disc disease (de Lahunta et al., 2021).
   - Ischemic myelopathy (de Lahunta et al., 2021).
2 Lesions of the preganglionic neuron
   - Lesions at the spinal cord
      - Ischemic myelopathy (de Lahunta & Alexander, 1976)
   - Lesions along the thoracic sympathetic trunk
      - Thoracic neoplasia, for example, lymphoma (Kern et al., 1989)
      - Thoracic trauma following car accident (common, especially when brachial plexus avulsion is present) (Kern et al., 1989)
   - Lesions along the cervical sympathetic trunk
      - Neoplasia, for example, thyroid adenocarcinoma (Melian et al., 1996)
      - Traumas such as bite wound to the neck, choke collar injury, and venipuncture (de Lahunta et al., 2021)
3 Lesions of the postganglionic neuron
   - Diseases of the ear
      - Otitis media or otitis interna (van den Broek, 1987)
      - Nasopharyngeal polyps (Anders et al., 2008)
      - Ear cleaning (Morgan & Zanotti, 1989)
      - Surgery to the middle or inner ear (Spivack et al., 2013)
      - Neoplasia (Wainberg et al., 2019)
   - Orbital disease
      - Orbital cellulitis or orbital abscess (de Lahunta et al., 2021)
      - Orbital neoplasia (de Lahunta et al., 2021)
4 Idiopathic
   - This is the most common cause of Horner's syndrome in dogs and cats and accounts for about half of cases (Kern et al., 1989; Morgan & Zanotti, 1989).

○ This is a diagnosis of exclusion.

○ Idiopathic Horner's syndrome is usually determined to be postganglionic when pharmacologic testing is performed.

○ Idiopathic Horner's syndrome disproportionately affects golden retrievers (Boydell, 2000).

○ Horner's syndrome is more likely to be idiopathic than due to underlying disease when it occurs in an individual without other clinical signs of disease (Lockhart *et al.*, 2021).

Diagnosis

The diagnostic process for Horner's syndrome consists of three parts: (1) confirming Horner's syndrome, (2) localizing the lesion, and (3) determining the underlying cause of the lesion.

1 Confirming Horner's syndrome

○ Cocaine testing has been used to confirm Horner's syndrome, but this medication is difficult to obtain.

○ Therefore, the diagnosis of Horner's syndrome is made by ophthalmic examination when the clinical signs as mentioned in "Defining characteristics" are seen.

○ Because other ophthalmic conditions (e.g., anterior uveitis) can mimic the signs of Horner's syndrome, diagnosis of Horner's syndrome requires careful ophthalmic examination.

2 Lesion localization via pharmacologic testing

○ In practice, direct sympathomimetic drugs are used almost exclusively.

○ Approximately 0.1 ml of 0.001% epinephrine (Bistner *et al.*, 1970) or 1% phenylephrine ophthalmic solution (Ramsay, 1986) is applied to both eyes.

▪ A positive response is indicated by a decrease in severity of clinical signs, with improvement of miosis and third eyelid elevation the most obvious and reliable changes (Figures 1.12a, 1.12b, 1.13a, 1.13b).

▪ There will be little to no change in the pupil of the unaffected eye.

▪ If a response does not occur until 30–40 minutes after application of medications, this is consistent with a preganglionic lesion.

▪ If a response occurs within 20 minutes of application of medications, this is consistent with a postganglionic lesion.

□ The rapid response is due to denervation hypersensitivity, which is an upregulation of receptors for the neurotransmitter that occurs with postganglionic lesions.

3 Determining the underlying cause of Horner's syndrome

○ Although idiopathic is the most common "cause" of Horner's syndrome, it is a diagnosis of exclusion.

○ Other causes of Horner's syndrome should be ruled out before concluding that the cause is idiopathic.

○ The choice of diagnostic tests (performed in addition to the physical examination) is determined by the location of the lesion (as determined by pharmacologic testing).

▪ Diagnostic testing for central Horner's syndrome should include the following:

□ Neurological examination

□ CBC, serum biochemical profile, and urinalysis

□ Infectious disease titers as appropriate for geographic location

□ MRI or CT scan of the brain and/or spinal cord

□ Collection of cerebrospinal fluid for cytology, culture and sensitivity, or infectious disease titers

▪ Diagnostic testing for preganglionic Horner's syndrome should include the following:

□ CBC, serum biochemical profile, and urinalysis

□ Infectious disease titers as appropriate for geographic location

□ Thoracic radiographs or CT scan

▪ Diagnostic testing for postganglionic Horner's syndrome should include the following:

□ CBC, serum biochemical profile, and urinalysis

□ Infectious disease titers as appropriate for geographic location

□ Otic examination

□ Skull radiographs, MRI, or CT scan focusing on tympanic bulla and orbit

Treatment

• Idiopathic Horner's syndrome is not treated.

• For Horner's syndrome of identifiable, treatable causes, the goal of treatment is to resolve the underlying disease, that is, direct specific treatment toward the underlying cause.

• The ocular abnormalities themselves are rarely treated since they do not cause harm.

○ However, occasionally there is visual impairment as a result of third eyelid elevation.

○ If vision is noticeably impaired, phenylephrine (2.5 or 10%) ophthalmic solution can be applied to the affected eye as infrequently as needed to lower the third eyelid.

▪ This medication can induce cardiovascular side effects; therefore, use caution. Avoid use in cats and small dogs, and do not use in patients with preexisting cardiovascular disease.

Prognosis

• Prognosis depends on the underlying cause of Horner's syndrome.

○ If the underlying cause (and therefore the neurologic lesion) can be treated, then it is possible for the ocular changes to resolve.

○ In general, the prognosis for postganglionic lesions is usually better than that for preganglionic or central lesions due to the types of diseases that cause lesions in these locations.

• The prognosis for idiopathic Horner's syndrome is good.

○ Most cases spontaneously resolve 6 weeks to 6 months following diagnosis (Boydell, 2000).

Orbital cellulitis and abscess

What it is
- Orbital cellulitis refers to inflammation of the extraocular soft tissues of the orbit.
- Orbital abscess refers to accumulation of white blood cells and inflammatory debris (pus) within the orbit.

Predisposed individuals
- Dogs and cats of any age, gender, or breed can be affected.
- The average affected individual is less than 10 years old.

Defining characteristics
Ophthalmic abnormalities develop acutely and occur as a result of physical displacement of orbital structures by the swollen, inflamed tissues. Clinical signs include the following (Figures 1.2a, 1.2b, 1.3):
- *Exophthalmos*
- *Third eyelid elevation*
- Chemosis
- *Conjunctival and episcleral vascular engorgement*
- Serous or mucoid ocular discharge
- Periocular tissue swelling
- *Decreased retropulsion of the eye*
- *Extreme pain when the mouth is opened*
  Physical examination may be unremarkable or may show the following abnormalities:
- Signs of general malaise, such as lethargy and inappetence
- Pyrexia or enlargement of the ipsilateral submandibular lymph node
- Sensitivity to periocular palpation of the affected side

Clinical significance
- Orbital inflammation is extremely painful.
  - Patients usually react violently to attempts at opening the mouth.
- Bacterial infection is usually present and must be treated.
  - The definitive source of the bacteria is often not identified.
- Fungal infection may also occur (Baron *et al.*, 2011; Barrs *et al.*, 2012).
- Some other potential causes of orbital inflammation include the following:
  - Orbital trauma
    - Iatrogenic penetration of the orbit during a dental procedure such as an extraction
    - Bite wound to the orbit
    - Foreign body migration to the orbit
  - Extension of inflammation from adjacent structures
    - Dental disease
    - Nasal disease
    - Frontal or maxillary sinusitis
    - Osteomyelitis
- Exophthalmos causes lagophthalmos and corneal exposure. This in turn can lead to surface ocular diseases such as keratitis and corneal ulceration.

- Complications following orbital inflammation are common and can include KCS, corneal disease, strabismus, and optic nerve atrophy (Fischer *et al.*, 2018).

Diagnosis
Although acute development of the aforementioned clinical signs is highly suggestive of inflammatory orbital disease, diagnostics are warranted to (i) confirm inflammatory disease and (ii) determine the underlying etiology of the inflammation. Recommended diagnostics include the following:
- CBC, serum biochemical profile, and urinalysis
  - Neutrophilic leukocytosis, when present, is highly suggestive of an inflammatory process.
- Oral examination
  - If swelling is visible caudal to the most caudal ipsilateral maxillary molar, this is suggestive of an abscess.
    - Obtaining purulent material from this swelling (see treatment discussed later) supports abscessation.
- Dental radiographs
  - Identification of tooth root lesions is not possible with oral examination alone.
  - Lack of overt oral lesions on gross oral examination does not rule out subgingival lesions.
  - Dental radiographs are required to rule out subgingival lesions.
- Orbital ultrasound
  - Can sometimes be used to identify orbital abscess, neoplasia, or foreign body, but is also often nondiagnostic (Mason *et al.*, 2001).
  - Ultrasound is less sensitive than MRI and CT for the identification of orbital lesions.
- Skull radiographs
  - Poor soft-tissue visualization limits the usefulness of this diagnostic test.
- MRI or CT
  - Advanced imaging is sometimes required to rule out orbital neoplasia, nasal disease, or foreign body.

Treatment
- Goals are to clear the bacterial infection and eliminate inflammation so that the eye can return to normal position, and the patient can return to comfort.
- Treatment consists of systemically administered, broad-spectrum antibiotics and anti-inflammatory therapy.
- When an abscess is present, its contents must be drained.
1 Abscess drainage (performed under general anesthesia)
  - Using a #15 scalpel blade, superficially incise the gingival swelling caudal to the last maxillary molar.
    - Use caution due to the proximity of the branches of the external ophthalmic artery.
  - Gently insert tips of closed hemostats into the orbit through this incision.
    - Gently open hemostats during insertion.

- Do not close the hemostats because of the risk of crushing vital arteries, veins, or the optic nerve.
  - If an abscess is present, purulent material will be liberated.
    - Massage side of face to encourage drainage of the purulent material.
    - If pus is not obtained, cellulitis is more likely than abscess.
      - Do not continue to look for pus by continuously probing the orbit with the hemostat because this will cause further trauma to the orbital structures.
    - Collect samples of the discharge for cytology and culture and sensitivity.
    - Gently flush orbit with sterile saline to maximize removal of the purulent material.
    - Allow the gingival incision to heal by second intention.
2 Antibiotic therapy
  - Culture and sensitivity ultimately determines the antibiotic of choice.
    - Isolates are usually a mixture of aerobic and anaerobic bacteria.
    - Antibiotics should be started at the time of diagnosis, prior to availability of culture and sensitivity results.
      - Some reasonable empirical choices include potentiated penicillins (e.g., amoxicillin/clavulanic acid) and cephalosporins.
    - Due to the high probability of bacterial infection, antibiotics should be prescribed even if culture and sensitivity yields no growth.
  - At least 3–4 weeks of antibiotic therapy is recommended.
3 Anti-inflammatory therapy
  - Systemically administered anti-inflammatory therapy is recommended for 7–14 days to reduce pain and swelling.
  - Use veterinary-labeled NSAIDs at labeled doses.
    - Use caution; patients usually exhibit an overall malaise and may have decreased food and water intake.
      - These patients may be more susceptible to the adverse effects of NSAIDs.
    - Avoid corticosteroids due to the potential for immunosuppression in the face of an infectious process.
- The first recheck examination should be within 1–2 weeks of the initial examination.
- Further recheck intervals are determined by patient progress (i.e., reduction of orbital abnormalities and return to normal behavior).

Prognosis

- The prognosis is good for resolution of inflammation, provided any underlying causes (e.g., tooth root abscess) have been addressed and antibiotic therapy is not discontinued prematurely.
- Patients with severe or prolonged orbital inflammation are at risk of developing complications such as KCS, optic nerve atrophy, or enophthalmos secondary to atrophy of orbital tissues.
  - These patients may experience these sequelae even if orbital inflammation is ultimately controlled; therefore, continued follow-up after resolution of inflammation is recommended.

Additional information

- Assess oral pain after completion of the ophthalmic examination because the pain response is extreme.
  - The patient may not allow further handling after the assessment of pain.
- Exophthalmos caused by the inflammation is often pronounced enough to cause lagophthalmos and exposure keratitis.
  - At minimum, begin therapy with ophthalmic lubricants to minimize development/progression of keratitis or corneal ulceration.
  - Often, a partial, temporary tarsorrhaphy is required to provide corneal coverage until the exophthalmos subsides.
- Injectable therapy may initially be required because the severity of oral pain may preclude oral administration of medications.
- Feed soft foods until patients become less painful.

Orbital neoplasia

What it is

- Neoplasia involving the orbit or structures within the orbit.
- Includes neoplasms that arise within the orbit as well as neoplasms that extend to the orbit from adjacent structures.

Predisposed individuals

- Dogs and cats of either gender are affected.
- Individuals over 10 years of age are overrepresented.

Defining characteristics

The onset of clinical signs tends to be slower than that for orbital cellulitis and abscess (Figures 1.1, 1.4, 1.5).

- *Exophthalmos* or *enophthalmos*
- Strabismus
- *Medial, lateral, dorsal, or ventral displacement of the globe*
- Restricted eye movement
- *Third eyelid elevation*
- Chemosis
- *Conjunctival and episcleral vascular engorgement*
- Serous or mucoid ocular discharge
- Periocular tissue swelling
- Distortion of the palpebral fissure
- Decreased or absent PLRs
- Anisocoria
- *Decreased retropulsion of the eye*
- Blindness
- Retinal detachment

- Signs of pain upon opening the mouth are typically minimal to absent.

Physical examination
- Physical examination may be unremarkable.
- If the neoplasm originated from a structure adjacent to the orbit, physical examination may reveal abnormalities of these structures.
  - For example, altered airflow ipsilateral to the affected orbit or sneezing is often found when a primary nasal tumor is affecting the orbit.

Clinical significance
- Most orbital neoplasms are malignant.
- Neoplasms can arise from within the orbit or from structures adjacent to the orbit (e.g., nasal cavity).
- Numerous tumor types have been documented in the orbit. Some examples are squamous cell carcinoma, lymphoma, fibrosarcoma, melanoma, rhabdomyosarcoma, and meningioma.

Diagnosis
Diagnostic testing is aimed at identifying the tumor type and determining the extent of the tumor.
- CBC, serum biochemical profile, and urinalysis
  - Often unremarkable
- Oral examination
  - Little to no pain response when mouth is opened
- Orbital ultrasound
  - Retrobulbar masses are sometimes visualized but results are often nondiagnostic.
- Skull radiographs
  - Soft-tissue changes can be difficult to interpret; therefore, the usefulness of this test is limited.
  - Evidence of bone destruction can support a neoplastic process.
- MRI or CT
  - Confirms the presence of a mass.
  - Determines the extent of neoplasm.
- Fine-needle aspirate and cytology or biopsy of neoplasm
  - Often via ultrasound guidance after completion of MRI or CT.
- Also consider ruling out metastatic disease (e.g., thoracic radiographs or CT, abdominal ultrasound or CT, and lymph node aspirates).

Treatment
- Goals of treatment depend on the type of tumor.
- Treatment ranges from attempting to achieve cancer remission to palliative therapy.
- The type of treatment employed depends on the specific tumor type.
  - For some neoplasms, tumor size can be reduced with chemotherapy or radiation therapy.
  - Surgical debulking or resection can be the sole treatment or can be combined with chemotherapy or radiation therapy.
    - To achieve surgical margins, enucleation is often required at the time of tumor debulking or resection.

Prognosis
- Regardless of tumor type, the majority of orbital neoplasms are advanced at the time of diagnosis and the prognosis is therefore poor.
- Patients usually die or are euthanatized within weeks to months of diagnosis.

Additional information
- Because the onset of clinical signs tends to be slow, overt abnormalities are often not noticed by pet owners until they are pronounced.
  - This means that patients often do not present for evaluation until late in the course of disease.
- In younger animals, orbital neoplasms tend to behave more aggressively and progress more rapidly than those occurring in older animals.
- Exophthalmos often results in lagophthalmos and exposure keratitis.
  - At minimum, treat with ophthalmic lubricants to minimize development or progression of keratitis or corneal ulceration.
  - Partial, temporary tarsorrhaphy may be required to protect the cornea.

Proptosis

What it is
- Sudden, anterior displacement of the eye from the orbit, secondary to trauma.

Predisposed individuals
- Dogs and cats of any gender or age can develop proptosis following trauma.
- Due to shallow orbits, less trauma is required to cause proptosis in a brachycephalic dog than in a nonbrachycephalic dog or a cat.
- Male dogs are affected more often than female dogs (Gilger et al., 1995).
- Intact male dogs are affected more often than neutered male dogs (Gilger et al., 1995; Pe'er et al., 2020).

Defining characteristics
- The eye is anterior to the orbit (Figures 1.14, 1.15).
- The eye is usually also anterior to the eyelids at the time of presentation.
- Eyelid margins are almost always trapped posterior to the globe and are therefore not visible on initial facial examination.
- Excessive sclera is visible because of the position of the eye.

- Some degree of conjunctival hemorrhage is usually present.
- Corneal abrasions, globe lacerations, or hyphema may also be present.

Clinical significance

- Because proptosis is caused by trauma (e.g., car accident and dog fight), life-threatening injuries may be present.
- Proptosis is painful.
- Prompt treatment may improve the potential of retaining ocular function.
- Proptosis frequently results in blindness.

Diagnosis

- The diagnosis is based on clinical appearance.

Treatment

- The goals of treatment are to (i) ensure that the patient is systemically stable, (ii) replace the eye into the orbit and maintain it within the orbit, (iii) prevent bacterial infection, and (iv) treat periocular inflammation.
- While replacement of the globe should be performed as soon as possible, the priority at presentation is to identify and stabilize nonocular injuries, as these can be life-threatening.
  - A lubricant (e.g., ophthalmic lubricants and sterile lubricating jelly) should be applied to the eye in order to keep it moist.
- Proptosis should be addressed only after the patient has been deemed systemically stable.
- For the eye, the main treatment goal is to retain a comfortable eye in the long term, with or without vision.

Treatment of proptosis is either replacement of the globe or enucleation. Unless it is obviously ruptured or collapsed, eye replacement is acceptable; enucleation can always be performed at a later date, if necessary. The technique for eye replacement involves bringing the eyelid margins anterior to the globe, then placing a temporary tarsorrhaphy to keep the eyelids in front of the eye. This should only be performed after the patient has been stabilized and deemed safe for general anesthesia.

Technique for replacement of the globe

- Gently and copiously lavage the globe with a dilute (5%) povidone–iodine solution, sterile eyewash, sterile saline, or lactated Ringer's solution to cleanse the ocular surface and to remove any debris.
- Carefully place stay sutures within the dorsal and ventral eyelids.
- Use the stay sutures to pull the eyelids anteriorly while a lubricated, gloved finger applies gentle pressure to the eye, directing it into the orbit (posteriorly).
  - The eye is unlikely to return to its original position due to extensive swelling and bleeding within the orbit.
  - If swelling is severe, a lateral canthotomy may be necessary to allow the eyelids to move anteriorly and the eye to move posteriorly.

- Once the eyelids are anterior to the eye, remove the stay sutures.
- Place a temporary tarsorrhaphy using 5-0 to 3-0 nonabsorbable sutures in a horizontal mattress pattern.
  - Use of stents will decrease the amount of skin trauma caused by sutures.
  - To prevent contact between the suture and the cornea, place sutures partial thickness (*not* full thickness) within the eyelid, and ensure that the needle and suture enter/exit in the hairless eyelid margin anterior to the Meibomian gland openings.
  - Do not close the entire length of the eyelids. Leave approximately one-fourth to one-third of the palpebral fissure open to allow drainage of ocular discharge and application of ophthalmic medications onto the ocular surface.
  - Sutures should remain in place for a minimum of 2–3 weeks.
    - Over time, sutures will require adjustment because they will become looser as tissue swelling resolves.
    - Loose sutures should be adjusted because they can rub on the cornea and induce corneal ulceration.

Following eye replacement, the following therapy should be prescribed:

1 Broad-spectrum, oral antibiotics
  - For example, cephalosporins or amoxicillin/clavulanic acid (Clavamox®) is usually chosen empirically.
  - Treat for 7–10 days.
2 Broad-spectrum, ophthalmic antibiotic
  - For example, triple antibiotic (neomycin/polymyxin B/bacitracin ophthalmic ointment or neomycin/polymyxin B/gramicidin ophthalmic solution), erythromycin ophthalmic ointment, and oxytetracycline/polymyxin B (Terramycin®) ophthalmic ointment.
  - Use of ophthalmic solution may result in less periocular crusting and medication accumulation within periocular hairs than ophthalmic ointment.
  - Treat for 7–10 days; longer if corneal ulceration is present and persists.
3 Oral anti-inflammatory medications
  - Corticosteroids (anti-inflammatory doses) or veterinary NSAIDs at labeled doses.
  - Do not use corticosteroids and NSAIDs concurrently.
4 Ophthalmic lubricants
  - Proptosed eyes often have decreased tear production.
5 Placement of an Elizabethan collar.
  - To prevent self-trauma or suture removal.

Recheck

- The patient should be rechecked within 1 week of eye replacement and tarsorrhaphy.
- Adjustments to the tarsorrhaphy can be made at this time, if necessary.
- Further rechecks are determined by patient progress and reduction of periocular swelling.

- Removal of tarsorrhaphy sutures should not occur until at least 2–3 weeks after replacement of the eye.
  - Development of scar tissue will help maintain the eye within the orbit after the sutures are removed.

Prognosis

- The prognosis for return of vision is poor.
- The majority of dogs and virtually all cats will remain blind in the proptosed eye.
- The prognosis for retaining the globe depends on the extent of the initial globe displacement (i.e., globes with shorter distance of proptosis are more likely to remain within the orbit after repair than globes that displaced further).
- The prognosis for maintaining ocular comfort is fair.
  - Due to development of sequelae (see below)

Positive prognostic indicators

- Short duration of proptosis
- Short distance of proptosis
- Brachycephalic dog (Gilger *et al.*, 1995)
  - Because less force is required to proptose the globe and it does not travel as far to proptose.
- Positive direct and consensual PLRs (Gilger *et al.*, 1995; Pe'er *et al.*, 2020)
  - Direct PLR: the pupil of the affected eye constricts in response to light directed at it.
  - Consensual PLR: the pupil of the fellow eye constricts when light is shone into the proptosed eye.

Negative prognostic indicators

- Prolonged duration of proptosis
- Increased distance of globe displacement
  - Avulsed extraocular muscles or the optic nerve may be seen.
- Corneal or scleral ruptures or lacerations
- Hyphema (Gilger *et al.*, 1995)
- Optic nerve damage
- Facial fractures (Gilger *et al.*, 1995)
- Feline or nonbrachycephalic canine patient (Gilger *et al.*, 1995)

Proptosed eyes are also susceptible to development of complications following removal of tarsorrhaphy sutures.

- The majority of eyes will be blind (Gilger *et al.*, 1995; Pe'er *et al.*, 2020).
- Strabismus (Gilger *et al.*, 1995)
  - Lateral strabismus is most common, as the insertion of the medial rectus muscle often breaks during proptosis.
- Lagophthalmos leading to chronic keratitis or corneal ulceration (Gilger *et al.*, 1995)
  - This is because the final globe position, while within the orbit, is often more anterior than its original (pre-proptosis) position.
- KCS
- Recurrent proptosis
  - Due to more anterior position of the eye and the weakened attachments maintaining it within the orbit.

Additional information

- When pet owners call prior to presentation, advise them to lubricate the eye with items found in the home during transportation to the veterinary clinic, such as ophthalmic lubricants, eyewash, personal lubricant, and petroleum jelly.
- Because significant trauma is needed to proptose a feline globe, severe bodily injuries and skull fractures are often present at presentation.
  - These must be addressed before concentrating on the eye.
- Brachycephalic dogs may require only minor trauma for proptosis to occur.
  - For example, restraint in the veterinary clinic can cause ocular proptosis.

Further reading

Horner's syndrome
Zwueste, DM & Grahn, BH. 2019. A review of Horner's syndrome in small animals. *Canadian Veterinary Journal.* 60(1):81–88.

Orbital cellulitis and abscess
Betbeze, C. 2015. Management of orbital diseases. *Topics in Companion Animal Medicine.* 30(3):107–117.

References

Anders, BB, *et al.* 2008. Analysis of auditory and neurologic effects associated with ventral bulla osteotomy for removal of inflammatory polyps or nasopharyngeal masses in cats. *Journal of the American Veterinary Medical Association.* 233(4):580–585.

Baron, ML, *et al.* 2011. Intracranial extension of retrobulbar blastomycosis (Blastomyces dermatitidis) in a dog. *Veterinary Ophthalmology.* 14(2):137–141.

Barrett, PM, *et al.* 1991. Absolute corneal sensitivity and corneal trigeminal nerve anatomy in normal dogs. *Progress in Veterinary & Comparative Ophthalmology.* 1(4):245–254.

Barrs, VR, *et al.* 2012. Sinonasal and sino-orbital aspergillosis in 23 cats: aetiology, clinicopathological features and treatment outcomes. *The Veterinary Journal.* 191(1):58–64.

Bistner, SI, *et al.* 1970. Pharmacologic diagnosis of Horner's syndrome in the dog. *Journal of the American Veterinary Medical Association.* 157(9):1220–1224.

Blocker, T & van der Woert, A. 2001. A comparison of corneal sensitivity between brachycephalic and domestic short-haired cats. *Veterinary Ophthalmology.* 4(2):127–130.

Boydell, P. 2000. Idiopathic Horner syndrome in the golden retriever. *Journal of Neuro-ophthalmology.* 20(4):288–290.

de Lahunta, A & Alexander, JW. 1976. Ischemic myelopathy secondary to presumed fibrocartilaginous embolism in nine dogs. *Journal of the American Animal Hospital Association.* 12(1):37–48.

de Lahunta, A, *et al.* 2021. Lower motor neuron: general visceral efferent system. In: Veterinary Neuroanatomy and Clinical Neurology, 5th edn, pp. 203–229. Elsevier, Philadelphia, PA.

Fischer, MC, *et al.* 2018. Retrobulbar cellulitis and abscessation: focus on short- and long-term concurrent ophthalmic diseases in 41 dogs. *Journal of Small Animal Practice.* 59(12):763–768.

Gilger, BC, *et al.* 1995. Traumatic ocular proptoses in dogs and cats: 84 cases (1980–1993). *Journal of the American Veterinary Medical Association.* 206(8):1186–1190.

Kern, TJ, *et al.* 1989. Horner's syndrome in dogs and cats: 100 cases (1975–1985). *Journal of the American Veterinary Medical Association.* 195(3):369–373.

Lockhart, RL, *et al.* 2021. The diagnostic yield of advanced imaging in dogs with Horner's syndrome presenting with and without additional clinical signs: a retrospective study of 120 cases (2000–2018). *Veterinary Ophthalmology.* doi:10.1111/vop.12918.

Luttgen, PJ, *et al.* 1980. A retrospective of twenty-nine spinal tumors in the dog and cat. *Journal of Small Animal Practice.* 21(4): 213–226.

Mason, DR, *et al.* 2001. Ultrasonographic findings in 50 dogs with retrobulbar disease. *Journal of the American Animal Hospital Association.* 37(6):557–562.

Mclian, C, *et al.* 1996. Horner's syndrome associated with a functional thyroid carcinoma in a dog. *Journal of Small Animal Practice.* 37(12):591–593.

Morgan, RV & Zanotti, SW. 1989. Horner's syndrome in dogs and cats: 49 cases (1980–1986). *Journal of the American Veterinary Medical Association.* 194(8):1096–1099.

Pe'er, O, *et al.* 2020. Prognostic indicators and outcome in dogs undergoing temporary tarsorrhaphy following traumatic proptosis. *Veterinary Ophthalmology.* 23(2):245–251.

Ramsay, DA. 1986. Dilute solutions of phenylephrine and pilocarpine in the diagnosis of disordered autonomic innervation of the iris. Observations in normal subjects, and in the syndromes of Horner and Holmes-Adie. *Journal of the Neurological Sciences.* 73(1):125–134.

Spivack, RE, *et al.* 2013. Postoperative complications following TECA-LBO in the dog and cat. *Journal of the American Animal Hospital Association.* 49(3):160–168.

van den Broek, AHM. 1987. Horner's syndrome in cats and dogs: a review. *Journal of Small Animal Practice.* 28(10):929–940.

Wainberg, SH, *et al.* 2019. Comparison of complications and outcome following unilateral, staged bilateral, and single-stage bilateral ventral bulla osteotomy in cats. *Journal of the American Veterinary Medical Association.* 255(7):828–836.

11 Eyelids

Please see Chapter 2 for images of the eyelids.

The main function of the eyelids is to protect the eyes. One way they achieve this is through direct physical protection of the eyes from the external environment. The eyelids also protect the eyes by ensuring that the corneas remain moist; adequate moisture is crucial for maintaining surface ocular health. With each blink, the eyelids distribute fresh tears across the ocular surface, remove wastes and debris from the ocular surface, and push older tears into the nasolacrimal drainage system for disposal. The eyelids also contribute to formation of the precorneal tear film. Specifically, the Meibomian glands within the eyelid tissue form the lipid portion of the precorneal tear film. While eyelids are very similar to haired skin elsewhere (with associated muscle, fat, connective tissue, nerves, blood supply, and glandular tissue), certain modifications allow the eyelids to serve their specialized functions.

1 Periocular hairs
- Cilia
    - These are hairs along the external edge of the upper eyelid margin.
    - Cilia provide physical protection for the eye.
- Vibrissae
    - These are also hairs, but are longer than cilia.
    - Vibrissae are located above the medial canthus.
    - Vibrissae have a sensory function similar to those of whiskers.
2 Hairless eyelid margin
- By having a "buffer zone" between the haired skin and the eye itself, potential for contact between hairs and the ocular surface (and therefore irritation) is minimized.
3 Puncta (Figures 2.1, 2.2)
- These are small openings in the eyelid conjunctiva.
- Puncta are located in both the upper and the lower eyelids of cats and dogs, within the palpebral conjunctiva adjacent to the eyelid margin, approximately 2 mm lateral to the medial canthus.
- Puncta are the entry into the nasolacrimal duct.

4 Muscles
- Muscles that control movement of the eyelids, specifically eyelid opening and closing.
- The upper eyelid is more mobile in cats and dogs than the lower eyelid is.
- Orbicularis oculi muscle
    - The muscle fibers run circumferentially around the palpebral fissure so that contraction closes eyelids.
        - Action is similar to a sphincter muscle.
    - This muscle is innervated by the facial nerve.
- Levator palpebrae superioris muscle
    - This muscle is found in the upper eyelid but not the lower eyelid.
    - The muscle fibers run dorsally and are perpendicular to the eyelid margin so that contraction elevates the upper eyelid.
    - This muscle is innervated by the oculomotor nerve.
- Mueller's muscle
    - This muscle is found in the upper eyelid but not the lower eyelid.
    - Similar to the levator palpebrae superioris muscle, Mueller's muscle runs perpendicular to the eyelid margin so that contraction elevates the upper eyelid.
    - This muscle receives sympathetic innervation.
5 Tarsal plate
- This is fibrous connective tissue within the eyelid.
- This provides eyelids with a slightly rigid structure.
6 Glands
- Meibomian glands
    - These are also referred to as tarsal glands.
    - These produce the lipid portion of the tear film.
    - Multiple glands are present along the eyelid margin, located approximately 3 mm proximal to the eyelid margin.
    - Ducts of the Meibomian glands open onto the eyelid margin.

Small Animal Ophthalmic Atlas and Guide, Second Edition. Christine C. Lim.
© 2023 John Wiley & Sons, Inc. Published 2023 by John Wiley & Sons, Inc.
Companion website: www.wiley.com/go/lim/atlas

- The openings of the ducts are visible along the eyelid margin as a series of depressions (20–40 per eyelid) referred to as the gray line (Figures 2.2, 2.3).
7 Conjunctiva (discussed in Chapter 13)
  - The bulbar surface of the eyelids is lined with conjunctiva, referred to as palpebral conjunctiva.
  - This allows the eyelids to move smoothly over the ocular surface.
8 Rich vascular supply
  - Improves recovery from injuries.

Because of eyelids' role in the protection and nourishment of the eye, diseases of the eyelids can have a significant impact on corneal and conjunctival health. For example, eyelid disease can

- Impair Meibomian gland function, and therefore formation of the lipid portion of the precorneal tear film.
- Hinder distribution of tears across the ocular surface, causing the eye to dry out.
- Impair removal of debris and wastes within the tear film from the ocular surface.
- Result in failure to protect the eye, if blinking is compromised.
- Directly irritate the eye. For example, eyelid masses and margin irregularities are sources of frictional irritation.

Clinical effects of eyelid disease can range from mild to marked surface ocular irritation and inflammation (superficial keratitis, conjunctivitis, or keratoconjunctivitis) (see Chapters 13 and 14) and even lead to the development of corneal ulceration (Chapter 14).

Diseases of the eyelid

Distichiasis

What it is

- Distichiae are hairs that arise from the Meibomian glands and emerge from the openings of the Meibomian glands.

Predisposed individuals

- Distichiasis mainly affects dogs.
- Commonly affected breeds include the cocker spaniel, English bulldog, golden retriever, Labrador retriever, and shih tzu.
- Distichiasis rarely affects cats.

Defining characteristics

- A single hair (distichia) or multiple hairs (distichiae) emerging from the Meibomian gland openings along the eyelid margins (Figures 2.5, 2.6, 2.7, 2.8, 2.9).
- The following clinical signs may be present:
  - Blepharospasm
  - Epiphora
  - Tear staining
  - Conjunctival hyperemia
  - Corneal fibrosis
  - Corneal edema

- Superficial corneal vascularization
- Corneal ulceration

Clinical significance

- A single fine distichia or small numbers of very fine distichiae may not cause any outward signs of discomfort or ocular surface irritation, and may therefore be clinically insignificant.
- Large numbers of distichiae or coarse distichiae usually irritate the ocular surface to varying degrees.

Diagnosis

- Distichiasis is diagnosed when hairs are seen emerging from the Meibomian gland openings.

Treatment

- In the absence of clinical signs and surface ocular inflammation, treatment is not necessary.
- Treatment is indicated if clinical signs and/or evidence of keratoconjunctivitis are present.
- The goal of treatment is to eliminate ocular irritation and corneal damage by removal of the hairs.
- Common definitive treatment options include cryoepilation, transconjunctival thermal cautery, and follicle resection.
  - Electrolysis is sometimes used, but may be associated with a higher rate of hair regrowth and is less suitable for treating large numbers of hairs.
  - Until definitive treatment, application of topical ophthalmic lubricants may reduce ocular surface irritation.
1 Cryoepilation
  - Epilation alone is not recommended because the hairs will likely regrow.
  - Cryoepilation is the preferred technique when distichiae are numerous.
  - Using a cryoprobe, two fast-freeze, slow-thaw cycles at −80°C are applied to palpebral conjunctiva overlying the affected Meibomian glands (~3 mm from the eyelid margin).
    - The duration of each freeze is approximately 25 seconds.
    - After the conjunctiva has thawed from the second freeze, the hairs are manually epilated.
  - Potential adverse effects:
    - Eyelid inflammation occurs following cryotherapy.
    - Depigmentation occurs at cryotherapy sites.
      - This may be a transient or a permanent depigmentation.
      - If transient, several weeks will pass before pigmentation starts to return to the eyelids.
    - With excessive freezing, eyelid structure may become distorted, or skin may necrose and slough.
    - Hairs may occasionally regrow despite appropriate application of cryotherapy.
2 Follicle resection
  - In this procedure, the hair follicle and the overlying palpebral conjunctiva are excised.
  - Referral to a veterinary ophthalmologist is advised.

- While this technique can be employed for numerous distichiae, resection is more suitable for small numbers of hairs.
- Potential adverse effects:
  - Persistent hemorrhage necessitating surgical closure of the defect.
  - Postoperative scarring that alters eyelid conformation and predisposes to formation of cicatricial entropion.
  - Incomplete excision of the follicle, which can result in regrowth of the hairs.

3 Thermal cautery
  - In this procedure, heat is applied to the hair follicle and overlying palpebral conjunctiva.
  - Referral to a veterinary ophthalmologist is advised.
  - While this technique can be employed for numerous hairs, it may be more suitable when few distichiae are present.
  - Potential adverse effects (Zimmerman & Reinstein, 2019):
    - Transient eyelid depigmentation
    - Inflammation of the eyelids
    - Distortion of the eyelid structure and potential entropion
    - Regrowth of distichiae

Prognosis

- The prognosis is very good for elimination of distichiae and improvement of patient comfort.
- Although regrowth of the hairs is possible, it can be managed with the previously mentioned techniques.
- Also, if hair regrowth occurs, the number of hairs is usually less than the number of hairs present prior to removal.

Additional information

- Cryotherapy, applied with a cryoprobe, is easily performed in general veterinary practice.
  - However, use of cryogen sprays for removal of aberrant hairs on the eyelids is not recommended.
    - This is because the direction of the spray cannot be accurately controlled and there is a risk of inadvertent freezing of adjacent structures such as the eye itself.
  - Referral to a veterinary ophthalmologist is advised if a cryoprobe is not available.

Ectopic cilia

What it is

- Ectopic cilia are hairs that arise from the Meibomian glands and exit through the palpebral conjunctiva (Figures 2.3, 2.4, 2.10).

Predisposed individuals

- Ectopic cilia rarely occur in cats.
- This condition mainly affects younger dogs.

Defining characteristics

- Single (cilium) or multiple (cilia) hairs protruding through the palpebral conjunctiva, approximately 3 mm from the eyelid margin.

- Ectopic cilia occur most often in the central upper eyelid, but can be found in other locations.
- The length of the hairs varies.
- Hairs may be extremely short, minimally protruding from the conjunctival surface (similar to day-old beard stubble), and therefore difficult to see (Figures 2.3, 2.4).
- Hairs can also protrude several millimeters from the conjunctival surface (with an appearance similar to eyelashes) (Figure 2.10).
  - Longer ectopic cilia are usually seen in breeds such as shih tzu and lhasa apso.
- Clinical signs of pain are usually pronounced.
  - The exception is in breeds of dog with brachycephalic ocular syndrome, where clinical signs of pain can be minimal.
- The following clinical signs may be seen:
  - *Blepharospasm*
  - *Epiphora*
  - Conjunctival hyperemia
  - Superficial corneal vascularization
  - Corneal fibrosis
  - Corneal ulceration

Clinical significance

- Because the hairs are in direct contact with the ocular surface, ectopic cilia cause ocular pain.
- Ectopic cilia are associated with development of keratitis.
- Ectopic cilia predispose to development of corneal ulceration.

Diagnosis

- An ectopic cilium is diagnosed when a hair is seen emerging from the palpebral conjunctiva, usually centrally within the upper eyelid.

Treatment

- The goal of treatment is similar to that for distichiasis: to eliminate ocular irritation by removal of the hairs.
- This is achieved in a similar manner as for distichiasis: cryoepilation, transconjunctival thermal cautery, or follicle resection.
  - See the earlier section on distichiasis for details of treatment and the potential complications of treatment.

Prognosis

- The prognosis is very good for permanent removal of the offending hairs.
- Regrowth is possible, but the original treatments can be repeated.
  - Multiple recurrences of ectopic cilia are highly unlikely.

Additional information

- Visualizing an ectopic cilium can be challenging, especially if the hair is light in color or if the hair is very short.
- Magnification greatly increases the chances of detecting ectopic cilia.

- Plastic head loupes are inexpensive options that provide a reasonable amount of magnification.
- Otoscopes also provide a reasonable amount of magnification.
- Slit lamp attachments designed for use with regular transilluminator handles are slightly more expensive than head loupes and otoscopes but are excellent light sources with built-in magnification.
- Corneal ulcers caused by ectopic cilia are usually located dorsal to the central cornea.
  - The position of the corneal ulcer correlates with the location of the hair.
  - These ulcers also tend to be chronic or recurrent due to the continued presence of the ectopic cilium.
- Corneal ulcers associated with ectopic cilia tend to be very painful.
  - Signs of ocular pain do not improve during treatment.
  - Signs of pain tend to persist even after the ulcer has re-epithelialized (after a negative fluorescein stain).

Trichiasis

What it is

- Trichiasis refers to hairs that arise from a normal location but contact the ocular surface.
- Examples include the following:
  - Medial canthal trichiasis
    - Hairs arising from follicles within the medial canthus.
  - Nasal fold trichiasis
    - In some brachycephalic individuals, the nasal fold rests directly on the corneal surface.
  - Trichiasis due to entropion (Figures 2.12, 2.13, 2.14, 2.15, 2.16)
  - Trichiasis from periocular facial hairs
    - For example, long periocular hairs such as those found in the shih tzu, lhasa apso, and miniature poodle (Figure 2.11).
    - For example, as a consequence of eyelid defects or injuries that direct hair toward the eye (Figures 2.20, 2.22).

Predisposed individuals

- Medial canthal trichiasis, nasal fold trichiasis, and trichiasis due to ventromedial entropion occur to varying degrees in individuals with brachycephalic ocular syndrome.
- Dogs with prominent nasal folds are also at higher risk of trichiasis.
  - Even if the folds do not rest against the ocular surface, long hairs from the nasal folds can reach to the cornea.
- Trichiasis affects many cats with eyelid agenesis.
- Previous eyelid injury or eyelid surgery without careful repair of eyelid margins predisposes to trichiasis.
  - For example, second-intention healing of an eyelid laceration may alter anatomy and redirect eyelid hairs toward the cornea.

Defining characteristics

- Hairs arise from a normal location on the face but are in contact with the ocular surface.
- Clinical signs are similar to those for distichiasis and ectopic cilia and may include the following:
  - Blepharospasm
  - *Epiphora*
  - Tear staining
  - Conjunctival hyperemia
  - *Superficial corneal vascularization*
  - Corneal fibrosis
  - *Corneal melanosis*
  - Corneal ulceration

Clinical significance

- Mild or intermittent trichiasis can be asymptomatic.
- However, trichiasis is often irritating and causes keratitis.
- Trichiasis associated with keratitis is very common in brachycephalic dogs. See "Pigmentary keratitis" in Chapter 14.
  - Chronically, trichiasis may predispose to corneal ulceration and can impair ulcer healing.

Diagnosis

- Trichiasis is diagnosed when hairs arising from a normal location (see "What it is" for examples) are seen to be in contact with the ocular surface.

Treatment

- In the absence of clinical signs or evidence of keratitis, trichiasis may not require treatment.
  - Monitor periodically for development of keratitis, then institute treatment if keratitis develops.
- If long periocular hairs are the source of trichiasis, these should be kept trimmed to a length that prevents contact with the eyes.
- When blepharospasm and/or epiphora is reported, or when keratitis is present, trichiasis should be treated.
  - The goal is to eliminate ocular irritation; this is achieved by eliminating or reducing contact between hairs and the ocular surface.
  - Application of topical ophthalmic lubricants may decrease, but not eliminate, ocular irritation until definitive treatment.
- Medial canthal trichiasis is usually treated by cryoepilation (see Treatment section under "Distichiasis").
  - Due to close proximity to the eye, referral to a veterinary ophthalmologist is advised.
  - If medial canthal trichiasis occurs in conjunction with brachycephalic ocular syndrome, then medial canthoplasty may be performed instead of cryotherapy.
- Nasal fold trichiasis is treated by resection of the nasal fold.
- Surgical correction of entropion will also correct associated trichiasis.

- Trichiasis resulting from other eyelid defects is treated by addressing the specific eyelid defect.
  - For example, surgical repair of eyelid agenesis, surgical repair of cicatricial entropion, and so on.

Prognosis

- The prognosis is very good for removal of hairs and improvement of ocular discomfort.
- As with distichiasis and ectopic cilia, the offending hairs can regrow.
  - In many cases, regrowth involves fewer hairs than in the original problem.
  - It is therefore possible that regrowth can be clinically insignificant.
  - If the hairs that regrow are seen to be in contact with the eyes, or if they are accompanied by signs of ocular irritation or progression of keratitis, retreatment is warranted.

Additional information

- Trichiasis is very common in patients with breed-related exophthalmos (e.g., dogs with brachycephalic ocular syndrome). Therefore, these patients should be carefully examined for trichiasis and associated corneal changes.
- When performing eyelid surgery (e.g., laceration repair, mass removal, or similar procedures), taking care to ensure accurate apposition of the eyelid margins is crucial for preventing development of trichiasis after injury and eyelid surgery.

Eyelid agenesis

What it is

- Eyelid agenesis refers to the congenital absence of a portion of the eyelid.
- Also referred to as eyelid coloboma.

Predisposed individuals

- Eyelid agenesis affects cats.

Defining characteristics

- A portion of the upper eyelid is absent (Figures 2.20, 2.21a, 2.21b, 2.22).
- The length of missing eyelid varies; the defect can range from barely perceptible to the entire length of the upper eyelid.
- The defect preferentially affects the lateral aspect of the eyelid.
- The dorsal conjunctival fornix adjacent to the defect is usually shallow or absent.
  - Haired eyelid skin often directly transitions to the ocular surface.
- The defect is usually bilateral and symmetrical.
- Clinical signs may include the following:
  - Blepharospasm
  - *Ocular discharge*
  - *Superficial corneal vascularization*
  - Corneal edema
  - *Corneal fibrosis*
  - Corneal ulceration
  - Conjunctival hyperemia
  - Chemosis
  - Trichiasis

Clinical significance

- Clinical significance varies with severity of tissue defect; that is, a larger defect means there is less eyelid coverage to the ocular surface, increased corneal exposure, and decreased distribution of the precorneal tear film.
  - The size of the eyelid defect therefore correlates directly with the severity of ocular damage and clinical signs.
  - The corneal exposure is due to a gap between the upper and the lower eyelid that persists even when the eyelids are closed (Figure 2.21b).

Diagnosis

- The diagnosis is made when ophthalmic examination reveals the absence of some or all of the upper eyelid margins in a cat.
- The diagnosis is usually made when cats are under 1 year of age.
  - However, the diagnosis is usually not made before 2–3 months of age, likely because the small size of the eyes means the eyelid defects are not yet noticed.

Treatment

- The goal is to provide adequate corneal coverage and protection, thereby reducing ocular surface disease.
- This can be achieved in several ways; the specific treatment chosen will depend on the magnitude of the tissue defect and clinical signs.
- In very mild cases where the gap between the eyelids is minimal but trichiasis is present, cryoepilation (see Treatment section under Distichiasis) and regular application of ophthalmic lubricant may be sufficient.
  - The eyes should be monitored periodically for progression of surface ocular inflammation.
- Larger eyelid defects should be referred for surgical treatment.
  - These will have large areas of corneal exposure that must be corrected.
  - These defects are treated by surgical skin grafts that replace the missing eyelid tissue with tissue from elsewhere on the face.
  - Various techniques exist (e.g., lip-to-lid graft and Roberts and Bistner graft) and are published elsewhere.

Prognosis

- For very minor eyelid defects with minimal keratitis, the prognosis is good for reducing or eliminating ocular surface damage, if medical and/or surgical management of ocular surface exposure is pursued.

- For larger defects, the prognosis is fair to good for improving eyelid coverage to the corneas and reducing keratoconjunctivitis, as long as medical management and surgical correction are pursued.
  - Keratitis, of lesser degree than presurgically, can persist after surgical correction.
  - Corneal opacities present prior to surgery are likely to persist.

Additional information

- Eyelid agenesis is sometimes mistaken for entropion; careful ophthalmic examination will prevent this misdiagnosis.
- With large eyelid defects, severe keratitis and corneal ulceration often accompany eyelid agenesis.
  - In young kittens, this is often attributed only to severe FHV-1 infection, and the underlying eyelid defect is missed.
  - Careful ophthalmic examination to rule out eyelid defects is crucial to avoid missing this diagnosis.
- Eyelid agenesis can be accompanied by other congenital ocular defects such as microphthalmos, PPMs, or cataract.
  - Careful ophthalmic examination is warranted.
- In addition to being inflamed, the exposed corneal surface can be ulcerated.
  - For these cases, treatment for corneal ulceration, as discussed in the cornea chapter, is also indicated.

Entropion

What it is

- Inward rolling of the eyelids allowing haired eyelid skin to rub the ocular surface (Figures 2.12, 2.13, 2.14, 2.15, 2.16).
- Entropion is categorized according to its cause as follows:
  - Conformational entropion
    - Inward rolling of the eyelids as a result of excessive eyelid and facial skin present in some breeds.
  - Cicatricial entropion
    - Acquired inward rolling of the eyelids that occurs after eyelid inflammation or injury.
    - Scar tissue contraction results in distortion of the eyelid.
  - Spastic entropion
    - Also referred to as blepharospastic entropion.
    - This occurs in the presence of a painful ocular condition, most commonly, corneal ulceration.
    - The ocular pain incites blepharospasm.
    - With severe blepharospasm, the eyelids roll inward.
    - This causes trichiasis, which then creates further ocular discomfort, perpetuating the ocular pain and blepharospasm.
  - Entropion secondary to enophthalmos.
    - The normal position of the eyelids is partially maintained by the eye itself.

- When the eye moves deeper into the orbit, it no longer holds the eyelids in position and the eyelids fall posteriorly as well.
- Since the eyelids are not completely rigid, the result is inward rolling of the eyelids.

Predisposed individuals

- Entropion occurs frequently in dogs and less frequently in cats.
- Conformational entropion is common in dogs. Some predisposed breeds include the following:
  - Shar Pei
  - Bloodhound
  - Basset hound
  - Labrador retriever
  - Golden retriever
  - German shorthaired pointer
  - English bulldog
  - Chow chow
- Feline entropion may occur secondary to conformation, but is more often cicatricial (as a result of severe FHV-1–induced keratoconjunctivitis) or due to enophthalmos (secondary to age-related loss of orbital fat).

Defining characteristics

- The eyelid margin is not visible in the area of the entropion.
- Instead, haired eyelid skin is seen to be in direct contact with the ocular surface (Figures 2.12, 2.13, 2.14, 2.15, 2.16).
- The hairs near the eyelid margin are wet or tear-stained.
- Keratitis (see Chapter 14) is often present at a site corresponding to the location of entropion.
- Conformational entropion in dogs is usually bilateral and tends to affect the lateral lower eyelids and lateral canthi.
- Clinical signs can include the following:
  - *Blepharospasm*
  - *Epiphora*
  - Tear staining
  - Ocular discharge
  - *Conjunctival hyperemia*
  - Chemosis
  - *Superficial corneal vascularization*
  - Corneal edema
  - Corneal fibrosis
  - Corneal ulceration

Clinical significance

- Contact between the haired skin and the cornea is uncomfortable, causes keratoconjunctivitis, predisposes to corneal ulceration, and impairs healing of corneal ulcers.

Diagnosis

- Entropion should be suspected when the lateral portions of the eyelid margins are wet or tear-stained.
- Entropion is diagnosed when inward rolling of the eyelid is seen when the individual is at rest.

Treatment

- The goal is to return the eyelid margin to its proper alignment against the ocular surface.
  - This eliminates contact between the eye and the eyelid hairs and therefore also relieves ocular irritation.
- This is achieved with either temporary (nonsurgical) or permanent (surgical) corrections.
  - Whether temporary or permanent procedures are chosen depends on the type of entropion and the age of the affected individual.
  - For example, conformational entropion in young dogs is expected to persist in the long term, but the degree of eyelid rolling may change with growth of the individual.
  - For example, blepharospastic entropion is a temporary condition that will resolve once the underlying painful ocular condition resolves.
1. Temporary eyelid tacking (Figure 2.17)
   - Recommended for conformational entropion in growing dogs.
     - Permanent surgical correction is often delayed until adult size is reached because the degree of entropion, and therefore the extent of the repair needed, changes as the head grows to adult size.
   - Also recommended for spastic entropion.
     - A permanent surgical correction is not recommended because resolution of ocular pain (by treatment of the underlying condition) alone will correct entropion.
   - With this technique, nonabsorbable sutures are placed into the eyelids and used to evert the eyelids.
     - Suture size ranges from 2-0 to 4-0, depending on the size of the dog.
   - Technique:
     - Under sedation or general anesthesia, inject a small amount of 2% lidocaine subcutaneously at the site of suture placement.
     - Approximately 2 mm from the eyelid margin, place one partial-thickness bite into the eyelid skin, directed perpendicular to the eyelid margin.
       - That is, to treat upper eyelid entropion, start this bite 2 mm dorsal to the margin and direct suture dorsally.
       - That is, to treat lower eyelid entropion, start this bite 2 mm ventral to the margin and direct suture ventrally.
       - That is, to treat the lateral canthus, start this bite 2 mm lateral to the canthus and direct suture laterally.
     - Do not tie any knots in the suture yet.
     - To place the second, partial-thickness bite, move the needle to a position farther away from the eyelid margin but in line with the first bite.
       - That is, for the upper eyelid, move directly dorsal to the first bite before placing the second bite.
       - That is, for the lower eyelid, move directly ventral to the first bite before placing the second bite.

- That is, for the lateral canthus, move directly lateral to the first bite before placing the second bite.
- The distance between bites is equal to the amount of unrolling needed to correct the entropion.
- The sutures are then tied.
- The eyelid will unroll as the suture is tightened.
- As an example, where the lower eyelid must be unrolled by 5 mm to correct ventral entropion, the following procedure can be followed:
  - The first bite is placed 2 mm ventral to the eyelid margin and is directed ventrally. The needle is moved 5 mm ventral to the point from which the needle just exited the skin, and a second bite is placed (also directed ventrally). The suture ends are then tied.
- The total number of sutures placed depends on the length of the eyelid affected by entropion.
  - Only place as many sutures as are required to repair the length of entropion.
- Use an Elizabethan collar to prevent early suture removal.
- Sutures remain in place until resolution of the painful eye disease (for spastic entropion) or until the patient has reached adult size (for conformational entropion in a young dog).
- Active dogs can remove sutures in spite of consistent placement of an Elizabethan collar.
  - Replacement of missing sutures may be needed over time.
2. Subdermal injection of hyaluronic acid (McDonald & Knollinger, 2019)
   - Can be used in many types of entropion.
     - Is often used to correct entropion secondary to enophthalmos in geriatric individuals and conformational entropion in young dogs that are still physically maturing.
   - Placement of the hyaluronic acid filler into the subdermal space corrects entropion.
   - After injection, the filler is slowly resorbed by the body.
   - Corrective effects can last for several months or longer, meaning the correction is permanent for some individuals, while others may require repeat injection or subsequent permanent surgical correction.
   - This procedure is performed under local anesthetic, with or without sedation.
   - Referral to a veterinary ophthalmologist is recommended.
3. Permanent surgical repair
   - This is recommended for repair of conformational and cicatricial entropion in fully grown individuals.
   - Surgical techniques for correction of entropion are published elsewhere.
     - The most common techniques, which are appropriate for uncomplicated entropion, include the Hotz-Celsus, wedge resection, and arrowhead. All of these techniques evert the eyelids by removing tissue from the eyelids.
     - For dogs with many facial folds (e.g., Shar Pei and bloodhound), referral to a veterinary ophthalmologist for more complex procedures such as coronal rhytidectomy

or brow suspension may be required because simple eversion of the eyelids will not be sufficient to correct entropion.

- When entropion is secondary to enophthalmos, entropion can resolve with correction of underlying disease and restoration of normal eye position.
  - However, if return to normal globe position is not possible, permanent surgical correction should be pursued.

Following permanent surgical repair, a recheck examination should be performed in 10–14 days, at the same time as suture removal. A second recheck is recommended 1–2 months later, to monitor for any postoperative changes to eyelid position.

Prognosis

- The prognosis for correction of entropion is very good.
  - Multiple surgeries are sometimes required for optimal correction, even in dogs that have finished growing.
- If substantial keratitis was present prior to correction of entropion, corneal scarring may persist in the long term after entropion repair.

Additional information

- Allow patients a few minutes to relax before assessing the degree of entropion.
  - When a patient is excited, increased eyelid muscle tone and palpebral fissure width can make the degree of entropion seem less than it truly is at rest.
- During examination, avoid excessive manipulation of the head to prevent distortion of eyelid position and inaccurate assessment of entropion.
- Determine the amount of correction required while the patient is awake.
  - General anesthesia alters muscle tone and the appearance of entropion.
- Prior to assessing entropion, a topical anesthetic (e.g., proparacaine hydrochloride 0.5% ophthalmic solution) should be applied to both eyes.
  - This eliminates any ocular pain, and therefore eliminates any blepharospasm that may be present.
  - This is a necessary step because spastic entropion exacerbates preexisting entropion of a separate cause, making entropion seem worse than it truly is.
  - For example, a dog with conformational entropion develops a corneal ulcer. The pain from the corneal disease then incites a spastic entropion. Without application of a topical anesthetic, initial assessment would overestimate the amount of entropion because it would reflect both temporary, spastic entropion as well as conformational entropion. Surgical correction based on this initial assessment would therefore be excessive, and could result in ectropion.
- If the exact amount of surgical correction required is not completely clear, err on the side of undercorrection.
  - It is much easier to perform a second surgery to remove more tissue than it is to correct ectropion.

Ectropion

What it is

- Ectropion refers to eversion, or outward rolling, of the eyelids.
- As with entropion, consider ectropion in the context of the cause:
  - Conformational ectropion
    - Excess length of the eyelid can result in ectropion.
    - This often affects the central, lower eyelid.
    - Concurrent entropion of the lateral lower eyelid and lateral canthus is common.
  - Cicatricial ectropion
    - Contraction of scar tissue following injury or inflammation can result in eyelid eversion.
  - Ectropion secondary to previous entropion surgery
    - Ectropion results when the amount of tissue removed during entropion surgery is disproportionate to the degree of entropion.

Predisposed individuals

- Ectropion, especially conformational, mainly affects dogs.
- Dog with excessive eyelid and facial skin are predisposed to conformational ectropion. Some breeds include the following:
  - St. Bernard
  - Newfoundland
  - Mastiff
  - Bloodhound
- Ectropion is uncommon in cats.
  - When present, it is likely cicatricial.

Defining characteristics

- Eversion of the ventral eyelid, usually midway between the medial and the lateral canthi (Figures 2.18, 2.19).
- Variable amounts of the palpebral and ventral fornicial conjunctivae will be exposed.
- Clinical changes include the following:
  - Chronic epiphora or ocular discharge
  - *Conjunctival hyperemia*
  - Chemosis

Clinical significance

- Mild ectropion may not be associated with any secondary clinical changes and can therefore be clinically insignificant.
- However, more pronounced eyelid eversion will be associated with clinical signs due to the exposure of the conjunctiva and ocular surface.
- Most dogs with conformational ectropion have some degree of conjunctivitis, the severity of which varies with the degree of ectropion.
- Dogs with concurrent entropion tend to be visibly irritated and usually have keratitis affecting the lateral cornea.

Diagnosis

- The diagnosis is made when eversion of the eyelid is seen.

Treatment

- Because conformational ectropion is desired in some breeds, treatment is often not requested.
- Mild conjunctivitis associated with mild eyelid eversion can be treated with tear film replacements or ophthalmic anti-inflammatory medications. See Chapter 13 for conjunctivitis treatment.
- Moderate to marked ectropion should be treated surgically because these are associated with higher levels of keratoconjunctivitis.
  - For eyes undergoing surgical therapy, the goal is to return the eyelids to correct apposition against the ocular surface, thereby reducing keratoconjunctivitis.
  - Surgical techniques are published elsewhere and include wedge resection (very useful for ectropion that is due solely to excessive eyelid length), Kuhnt Szymanowski, and V to Y plasty.

Prognosis

- The prognosis is good for achieving comfort.
- More than one surgical procedure may be required to achieve optimal eyelid position.

Eyelid neoplasia

What it is

- For this discussion, eyelid neoplasia refers to neoplasms arising from the eyelids.

Predisposed individuals

- Dogs and cats of any age or gender can develop eyelid neoplasia, but it is more common in older individuals.
- Squamous cell carcinoma disproportionately affects white and lightly pigmented cats.

Defining characteristics

- Most eyelid neoplasms are distinct masses arising from the eyelid skin, margin, or conjunctiva (Figures 2.23, 2.24, 2.25, 2.26, 2.27, 2.28, 2.29).
- Eyelid neoplasia can also diffusely thicken the eyelid (Figure 2.30).
- Eyelid neoplasia can also sometimes look like an ulceration, rather than a mass, of the eyelid.
- Canine Meibomian adenoma
  - The typical mass is hairless, has an uneven surface, arises from the eyelid margin, and is variably pigmented.
  - Surrounding eyelid may be inflamed to variable degrees.
- Feline squamous cell carcinoma
  - The typical appearance is eyelid ulceration, thickening, and inflammation.

Clinical significance

- Dogs:
  - Eyelid masses are most often benign (Krehbiel & Langham, 1975; Roberts *et al.*, 1986).
  - The most common eyelid neoplasm is Meibomian adenoma (Krehbiel & Langham, 1975).
  - Many neoplasms have been documented in the canine eyelid, some of which include melanocytoma, papilloma, histiocytoma, and mast cell tumor (Bonney *et al.*, 1980; Krehbiel & Langham, 1975; Roberts *et al.*, 1986).
  - As they enlarge, eyelid masses become irritating because they come into contact with the ocular surface.
- Cats:
  - Eyelid masses are usually malignant and locally invasive.
  - Squamous cell carcinoma is the most common feline eyelid neoplasm (Newkirk & Rohrbach, 2009).
  - Many other neoplasms have been documented in the feline eyelid, some of which include mast cell tumor (Newkirk & Rohrbach, 2009), apocrine hidrocystoma (Chaitman *et al.*, 1999), and adenocarcinoma (Newkirk & Rohrbach, 2009).

Diagnosis

- The diagnosis of an eyelid neoplasm is initially made by visualizing an eyelid mass, thickening, or distortion.
- Histopathology is required to confirm neoplasia and to identify the tumor type.
  - For small masses, the sample is usually collected at the time of therapeutic mass removal.
  - For larger masses, an incisional biopsy is recommended prior to attempting complete removal.
    - A biopsy determines the tumor type and surgical margins required.
    - The potential for definitive diagnosis is superior to that of fine-needle aspirate.
- Masses that appear extensive or infiltrative should be evaluated with MRI or CT scan to determine their extent prior to treatment.
  - Also consider ruling out metastatic neoplasia (e.g., thoracic radiographs or CT, abdominal ultrasound or CT, and lymph node aspirates).

Treatment

- The goal of treatment is to remove the mass and therefore also eliminate ocular irritation.
- Treatment is most easily performed early in the course of disease, when the eyelid tumors are small.
- Wedge resection, debulking with cryotherapy, and CO_2 laser are three very common and effective treatments. Specifics for performing these techniques are published elsewhere, while an overview is included here.
- CO_2 laser
  - The laser is used to ablate the mass and adjacent tissue while preserving as much normal eyelid tissue as possible.
  - The surgical site heals by second intention.
  - Appropriate for small, benign neoplasms.
  - Referral to a veterinary ophthalmologist is advised.

- Debulking of the mass with cryotherapy
  - The mass is removed without attempting to achieve clean margins and cryotherapy is applied to the site of mass removal to destroy remaining neoplastic cells.
  - The surgical site heals by second intention.
  - Appropriate for small, benign neoplasms.
- Wedge resection
  - Appropriate for removal of small masses, where less than one-third of the eyelid length is lost to the excision.
  - Appropriate for incisional biopsy of larger masses.
- When tumor removal necessitates removal of a significant amount of eyelid tissue, referral to a veterinary ophthalmologist for more extensive blepharoplasty may be required.
  - For example, H-plasty, semicircular flap, axial pattern flaps, and lip-to-lid flap.
  - Advanced imaging (e.g., MRI or CT scan) is often recommended to determine the extent of the mass prior to any attempts at removal.
  - For very extensive tumors, imaging may indicate that exenteration is needed to achieve clean margins or that complete removal is not possible and adjunctive therapies (e.g., radiation therapy) are required.

Prognosis

- The prognosis is very good following removal of benign neoplasms such as canine Meibomian adenoma and melanocytoma and feline mast cell tumors.
- The prognosis can be fair for invasive tumors (e.g., squamous cell carcinoma) if excision is complete.
  - Patients should be monitored for recurrence.
- In general, the prognosis is guarded for invasive neoplasms or those with extensive eyelid involvement, especially if excision was incomplete.
  - Regrowth is common.
  - Regrowth can extend into adjacent areas such as the orbit.
    - Recurrence can be difficult to detect and pets sometimes do not present until this is advanced.
    - Additional treatment is more challenging.

Chalazion

What it is

- Retention of inspissated Meibomian gland secretions within the eyelid, usually accompanied by eyelid inflammation.
- As meibum accumulates, it leaks out of the glands, inciting inflammation and lipogranuloma formation.

Predisposed individuals

- Chalazia mainly affect dogs.
- Brachycephalic dogs appear to develop chalazia more often than other breeds.

Defining characteristics

- Round, white structures visible through the palpebral conjunctiva approximately 3 mm from the eyelid margin (Figures 2.10, 2.31, 2.32, 2.33).
- Flat or slightly elevated from the conjunctival surface.
- The surrounding conjunctiva and eyelid are inflamed to varying degrees.

Clinical significance

- In many cases, small chalazia are incidental findings on ophthalmic examination, without obvious signs of ocular irritation.
- Larger chalazia cause irritation by rubbing on the ocular surface.
- Leakage of meibum from chalazia incites lipogranulomatous conjunctivitis, which is uncomfortable.
- Chalazia often occur in association with Meibomian adenomas.

Diagnosis

- The diagnosis is based on clinical appearance.

Treatment

- The goal of treatment is to eliminate ocular irritation.
- Small chalazia may be treated by warm compress applied to the eyelids.
  - Application of heat encourages meibum to become fluid and can facilitate its exit from the glands.
- If this is unsuccessful, chalazia should be opened and drained under sedation or general anesthesia. Technique:
  - The chalazion is isolated with a chalazion clamp.
    - This clamp provides a solid surface to work against and also provides hemostasis during a procedure.
  - Using a 6400 blade or similar small blade, a superficial stab incision is made through the palpebral conjunctiva to expose the meibum.
  - The incision penetrates only through the palpebral conjunctiva overlying the chalazion. The incision does not penetrate through the entire thickness of the eyelid.
  - A curette is used to remove the meibum.
  - The wound is left to heal by second intention.
- An ophthalmic antibiotic-corticosteroid combination can be used postoperatively.
  - For example, neomycin, polymyxin B, and dexamethasone ophthalmic ointment (or ophthalmic suspension), 1/4″ strip (or one drop) applied three to four times daily for 3–5 days postoperatively.
  - Do not use in the presence of corneal ulceration.
- If there is a concurrent eyelid mass, this should be treated as per previous discussion.

Prognosis

- Although development of new chalazia is possible, the prognosis for resolution of an individual chalazion is very good.

Blepharitis

What it is

- Blepharitis is inflammation of the eyelids.

Predisposed individuals

- Dogs and cats of any breed, age, or sex can be affected.

Defining characteristics

- *Erythema* of the eyelid skin (Figures 2.34, 2.35, 2.36, 2.37, 2.38, 2.39, 2.40)
- *Swelling* of the eyelid skin (Figures 2.34, 2.35, 2.38, 2.40)
- *Alopecia* (Figures 2.34, 2.36, 2.37, 2.38, 2.39, 2.40)
- Crusting of the skin along the eyelid margins (Figures 2.39, 2.40)
- Ulceration of the eyelid skin (Figure 2.39)
- Erosion of the eyelid margin (Figure 2.39)
- Distortion of normal eyelid structure
- *Ocular discharge*
- Chemosis
- Conjunctival hyperemia

Clinical significance

- Blepharitis can arise from many different causes.
  - Allergic dermatitis is one of the more common underlying causes of blepharitis in dogs (Weingart *et al.*, 2019).
- Depending on the underlying cause, the significance of blepharitis may be limited to only the eyelids, may involve other ocular structures and threaten vision, or could involve other organ systems and threaten overall health.
- Some causes of blepharitis include the following:
  - Idiopathic inflammation (Collins *et al.*, 1992; Panich *et al.*, 1991)
  - Immune-mediated disease (Pena *et al.*, 2008)
    - For example, atopic dermatitis, food-induced atopic dermatitis, pemphigus foliaceus, cutaneous lupus erythematosus, uveodermatologic syndrome, and juvenile cellulitis (Pena *et al.*, 2008).
  - Infectious causes
    - For example, bacterial dermatitis, demodicosis, dermatophytosis, leishmaniasis (Pena *et al.*, 2000), FHV-1, and canine herpesvirus (Ledbetter, 2013).
  - Neoplasia
    - For example, Meibomian adenoma, squamous cell carcinoma, mast cell tumor, and lymphoma (Donaldson & May, 2000; Krehbiel & Langham, 1975).
  - Trauma
  - Miscellaneous
    - For example, reaction to ophthalmically-applied medications and insect bite/sting (Stades & van der Woerdt, 2021).

Diagnosis

- Blepharitis is diagnosed when the aforementioned clinical signs are observed.
- Once blepharitis is diagnosed, the clinician should attempt to identify the underlying cause. The following diagnostic tests are recommended:
  - Cytology

- Useful for the identification of bacteria, fungi/yeast, and cellular changes indicative of neoplasia or immune-mediated disease.
  - Culture and sensitivity
    - Should be performed when bacteria or fungi are identified on cytology.
  - Skin scraping
    - Used to identify skin parasites.
  - Histopathology
    - Wedge resection to obtain tissue for analysis.
    - Provides a diagnosis for most cases in which it is used.
    - Indicated when cytology, skin scrapings, and culture and sensitivity do not suggest a diagnosis; when cytology is suggestive of immune-mediated or neoplastic causes; or when blepharitis is nonresponsive to therapy.

Treatment

- The goal is to eliminate eyelid inflammation, thereby stopping its secondary effects on ocular health and improving patient comfort.
- Treatment involves (1) treatment of the underlying cause, if identified, and (2) treatment of the eyelid inflammation.
1. Treatment of the underlying cause
   - This will vary with the specific cause.
2. Treatment of eyelid inflammation
   - This involves nonspecific anti-inflammatory therapy, either applied directly to the affected skin or administered orally.
     - Corticosteroid ophthalmic ointment (e.g., dexamethasone in combination with neomycin and polymyxin B) applied to the affected skin is sufficient as sole therapy for mild to moderate cases of blepharitis.
       - Use a small amount of ointment applied two to three times daily; taper as clinical signs improve.
     - Oral administration of corticosteroids is required for many cases of blepharitis.
       - Prednisone or prednisolone administered at a dose of 0.5 mg/kg one to two times daily.
       - Can be used concurrently with topically applied medications.
       - Taper dose as clinical signs improve.
     - Oral therapy with veterinary-labeled NSAIDs at labeled doses is an alternative to oral corticosteroids when infectious disease or other contraindications to corticosteroids are present.
   - Tetracycline antibiotics can also be used to treat the inflammation of blepharitis.
     - These effects are separate from their antimicrobial properties.
     - Oral doxycycline is administered at a dose of 5–10 mg/kg PO q12h for 3–4 weeks.
     - In cats, administer doxycycline as a suspension, rather than a tablet, to reduce the potential for esophageal stricture.

The first recheck should be 1–2 weeks after starting therapy. The intervals between recheck examinations and the total number of rechecks are dependent on clinical progress.

Prognosis

- Idiopathic blepharitis has a very good prognosis for resolution of clinical signs, although recurrence is possible.
- Otherwise, prognosis depends on the underlying cause of blepharitis.
- With prolonged and/or severe blepharitis, eyelid distortion and cicatricial entropion can develop.

Additional information

- Blepharitis can be associated with Meibomian gland dysfunction, qualitative tear film abnormalities (see Chapter 12), and decreased tear production (see Chapter 14).
  - If the STT is low, then at minimum continued monitoring is indicated.
    - Lacrimostimulant therapy should be considered if the STT does not return to normal, or if decreased tear production is accompanied by clinical signs consistent with keratitis (see Chapter 14).
  - Ointment-based tear film replacements mimic the lipid portion of the tear film and can address any qualitative tear film deficiency that may be present.
    - Apply 1/4″ strip to the affected eye two to four times daily.
- Application of warm compresses to the eyelids for 5–10 minutes, two to three times daily, can improve patient comfort.
- Blepharitis is often accompanied by skin lesions elsewhere on the body (Weingart *et al.*, 2019).
  - When blepharitis is diagnosed, a full dermatologic examination is warranted and may assist with identifying the underlying cause.

Eyelid laceration

What it is

- A tear of the eyelids, usually the result of trauma (Figures 2.41, 2.42).

Predisposed individuals

- Dogs and cats of any age, breed, or sex can sustain eyelid lacerations.

Defining characteristics

- Discontinuity of the eyelid margin(s) accompanied by exposure of the subcutaneous tissue or conjunctiva.
- Depending on the extent of the laceration, the eyelid may be largely intact with minimal subcutaneous tissue visible or the eyelid could be hanging by a thin thread of tissue, with excessive corneal exposure.

Clinical significance

- Even small eyelid lacerations predispose to keratoconjunctivitis and corneal ulceration.
  - An irregular eyelid margin is a physical irritant to the ocular surface.
- Muscle damage, tissue loss, or eyelid distortion can lead to lagophthalmos and corneal exposure.
- Given the close proximity between the eyelids and the eyes themselves, eyelid lacerations may be accompanied by ocular injury.

Diagnosis

- The diagnosis of an eyelid laceration is based on appearance.
- The ophthalmic examination should be performed carefully to rule out concurrent ocular injury.
- Since trauma is usually involved, the patient should be checked for nonocular injuries.

Treatment

- Any serious nonocular injuries should be addressed before the eyelid laceration.
- The main goal of treatment is to correctly restore eyelid anatomy, especially the continuity of the eyelid margin.
  - Eyelid lacerations should therefore be closed primarily, not left to heal by second intention.
- Other treatment goals are to prevent/treat eyelid infection, provide analgesia, and address concurrent injuries to the eye itself.
- Parenteral, broad-spectrum antibiotic prophylaxis (such as intravenous cefazolin) should be administered prior to surgical repair (performed under general anesthesia).
- The eyelids, periocular skin, conjunctival sac, and ocular surface should be copiously lavaged with dilute (5%) povidone–iodine solution, sterile eyewash, sterile saline, or lactated Ringer's solution to cleanse the ocular surface and to remove any debris. This should be followed by surgical preparation of the eyelids using dilute povidone–iodine solution.
- Specific descriptions of the technique are published elsewhere; important considerations are as follows:
  - Eyelids require minimal debridement. If wound edges need to be "freshened," scraping with a scalpel blade is usually sufficient.
  - Avoid removing eyelid tissue, especially margin.
    - Preservation of eyelid tissue is superior to attempts at surgically recreating eyelids.
    - Robust vascular supply maximizes healing potential.
    - Even if the eyelid appears to be hanging by a minimal amount of tissue, include it in the repair rather than removing it.
  - Two layers should be closed: the tarsoconjunctival layer and the skin layer.
    - This avoids wound gaping, which occurs more often with closure of just one layer.

- When closing the tarsoconjunctival layer, take care not to penetrate through the conjunctiva because this allows suture to contact the eye.
  - Accurate apposition of the eyelid margins is crucial for maintenance of eyelid function.
    - To ensure alignment, place the first suture at the eyelid margin, then complete suturing of the remainder of the laceration.
    - Use figure-of-eight suture at the margin to decrease chances of suture knots rubbing on cornea.
- Postoperatively, an Elizabethan collar should be placed.
- Postoperative medications should include the following:
  1 Oral veterinary-labeled NSAID administered at the labeled dose for approximately 7 days.
    - Treatment duration depends on the severity of laceration and presence or absence of concurrent ocular injury.
  2 Analgesia
    - Addressed with NSAID therapy.
    - As needed, augment with medications such as gabapentin or opioids, used according to labeled doses.
    - Duration depends on the severity of laceration and presence or absence of concurrent ocular injury.
  3 Oral antibiotic therapy
    - Broad-spectrum antibiotics such as amoxicillin/clavulanic acid (Clavamox®) or cephalosporins at the labeled doses for approximately 7–10 days.

Recheck in 10–14 days, at the time of suture removal. A second recheck is advised 1–2 months later to monitor for postoperative changes to the eyelid.

Prognosis

- For most eyelid lacerations, the prognosis for return to eyelid function is very good if the laceration is repaired promptly.
- For lacerations involving the medial aspect of the eyelids, damage to the nasolacrimal puncta is possible and may result in chronic epiphora.
- For extensive eyelid lacerations, or lacerations associated with a large amount of tissue loss, altered eyelid function and decreased protection of the eye may result in chronic surface ocular disease.
  - Referral to a veterinary ophthalmologist for treatment of these injuries may be necessary.

Further reading

Eyelid neoplasia
Aquino, SM. 2007. Management of eyelid neoplasms in the dog and cat. *Clinical Techniques in Small Animal Practice.* 22(2):46–54.

References

Bonney, CH, et al. 1980. Papillomatosis of conjunctiva and adnexa in dogs. *Journal of the American Veterinary Medical Association.* 176(1):48–51.

Chaitman, J, et al. 1999. Multiple eyelid cysts resembling hidrocystomas in three Persian cats and one Himalayan cat. *Veterinary Pathology.* 36(5):474–476.

Collins, BK, et al. 1992. Idiopathic granulomatous disease with ocular adnexal and cutaneous involvement in a dog. *Journal of the American Veterinary Medical Association.* 201(2):313–316.

Donaldson, D & May, MJ. 2000. Epitheliotropic lymphoma (mycosis fungoides) presenting as blepharoconjunctivitis in an Irish setter. *Journal of Small Animal Practice.* 41(7):317–320.

Krehbiel, JD & Langham, RF. 1975. Eyelid neoplasms of dogs. *American Journal of Veterinary Research.* 36(1):115–119.

Ledbetter, EC. 2013. Canine herpesvirus-1 ocular diseases of mature dogs. *New Zealand Veterinary Journal.* 61(4):193–201.

McDonald, JE & Knollinger, AM. 2019. The use of hyaluronic acid subdermal filler for entropion in canines and felines: 40 cases. *Veterinary Ophthalmology.* 22(2):105–115.

Newkirk, KM & Rohrbach, BW. 2009. A retrospective study of eyelid tumors from 43 cats. *Veterinary Pathology.* 46(5):916–927.

Panich, R, et al. 1991. Canine cutaneous sterile pyogranuloma/granuloma syndrome: a retrospective analysis of 29 cases (1976 to 1988). *Journal of the American Animal Hospital Association.* 33(6):540–543.

Pena, MT, et al. 2000. Ocular and periocular manifestations of leishmaniasis in dogs: 105 cases (1993–1998). *Veterinary Ophthalmology.* 3(1):35–41.

Pena, MT, et al. 2008. Canine conjunctivitis and blepharitis. *Veterinary Clinics of North America Small Animal Practice.* 18(2):233–249.

Roberts, SM, et al. 1986. Prevalence and treatment of palpebral neoplasms in the dog: 200 cases (1975–1983). *Journal of the American Veterinary Medical Association.* 189(10):1355–1359.

Stades, FC & van der Woerdt, A. 2021. Diseases and surgery of the canine eyelid. In: Veterinary Ophthalmology (eds G Ben-Schlomo, BC Gilger, DV Hendrix, TJ Kern, & CE Plummer) 6th edn, p. 971. Wiley-Blackwell, Hoboken, NJ.

Weingart, C, et al. 2019. Blepharitis in dogs: a clinical evaluation in 102 dogs. *Veterinary Dermatology.* 30(3):222–e69.

Zimmerman, KL & Reinstein, SL. 2019. Evaluation of transconjunctival thermal electrocautery for treatment of canine distichiasis: 88 eyelids (2013–2016). *Veterinary Ophthalmology.* 22(1):50–60.

12 The third eyelid, nasolacrimal system, and precorneal tear film

Please see Chapter 3 for images of the third eyelid, nasolacrimal system, and precorneal tear film.

1 Third eyelid (Figure 3.1)
  ○ Also referred to as the nictitating membrane or nictitans.
  ○ A thin band of tissue located in the ventromedial orbit in cats and dogs.
  ○ The third eyelid "blinks" across the ocular surface.
    ▪ The direction of movement is diagonal, from ventromedially within the orbit in a dorsolateral direction.
    ▪ In dogs, movement of the third eyelid across the eye is passive, occurring when the eye is retracted into the orbit.
    ▪ In the cat, smooth muscle may contribute to movement.
  ○ Components
    ▪ Cartilage.
      □ T-shaped, with the horizontal portion of the cartilage along the leading edge of the third eyelid and the vertical cartilage perpendicular to this.
    ▪ Lymphoid tissue, particularly on the bulbar surface of the third eyelid.
    ▪ Glandular tissue (gland of the third eyelid), located at the base of the third eyelid.
    ▪ Conjunctiva overlying the anterior and bulbar surfaces.
  ○ Functions of the third eyelid
    ▪ Physical protection of the ocular surface.
    ▪ Formation of the precorneal tear film.
      □ Up to 50% of the aqueous component of the tears is produced by the gland of the third eyelid.
    ▪ Distribution of the precorneal tear film across the ocular surface (occurs each time the third eyelid sweeps across the ocular surface).
    ▪ Removal of debris from the ocular surface (by sweeping across the ocular surface).
    ▪ Immunologic protection to the ocular surface (lymphoid tissue).
  ○ Diseases of the third eyelid may appear as changes to the third eyelid itself or as surface ocular inflammation secondary to compromised function.
    ▪ Changes to the third eyelid itself include the following:
      □ Elevation of the third eyelid

      □ Swelling or thickening of the third eyelid (Figure 3.17)
      □ Folding or eversion of the third eyelid (scrolled cartilage) (Figures 3.4, 3.5, 3.6)
      □ Prolapse of the third eyelid gland (Figures 3.7, 3.8, 3.9, 3.10, 3.11, 3.12)
      □ Hyperemia of the conjunctiva overlying the third eyelid
      □ Depigmentation of the third eyelid (Figures 3.17, 3.18, 3.19)
    ▪ Clinical signs resulting from altered third eyelid function include the following:
      □ Conjunctival hyperemia
      □ Superficial corneal vascularization
      □ Corneal edema
      □ Corneal fibrosis
      □ Corneal melanosis
      □ A dry or roughened appearance to the cornea
2 The nasolacrimal secretory and drainage apparatus
  ○ For each eye, components are as follows:
    ▪ An orbital lacrimal gland and the gland of the third eyelid
      □ These glands produce the aqueous component of the precorneal tear film.
    ▪ Lacrimal puncta (Figures 2.1, 2.2)
      □ One punctum is located in the dorsal eyelid and one is in the ventral eyelid; each is approximately 2 mm from the medial canthus.
      □ These are the entry points to the nasolacrimal canaliculi.
    ▪ Nasolacrimal canaliculi
      □ Extending from each of the puncta, the canaliculi merge to form the nasolacrimal sac, which is a dilated entrance to the nasolacrimal duct.
    ▪ Nasolacrimal duct
      □ Extends from the lacrimal bone, through the maxillary bone, into the nasal mucosa, to exit within the nasal cavity.
      □ Terminates at the nasal punctum within the nasal cavity.

Small Animal Ophthalmic Atlas and Guide, Second Edition. Christine C. Lim.
© 2023 John Wiley & Sons, Inc. Published 2023 by John Wiley & Sons, Inc.
Companion website: www.wiley.com/go/lim/atlas

- Nasal punctum
  - A small opening in the nasal mucosa that is the exit point of the nasolacrimal drainage apparatus.
  - Located approximately 10 mm proximal to the opening of the corresponding nare, on the floor of the nasal cavity.
- Some individuals have an accessory opening located more posteriorly within the nasal cavity. This may be in addition to the nasal punctum, or it may be the only exit point of the nasolacrimal drainage apparatus (Sahr *et al.*, 2021).
  - Functions of the nasolacrimal system:
    - Production of the aqueous precorneal tear film (by the orbital and third eyelid glands).
    - Nutrition and oxygenation of the ocular surface (by the precorneal tear film).
    - Immune protection of the ocular surface (antimicrobial substances are dissolved within the precorneal tear film.)
    - Lubrication of the ocular surface (by tears).
    - Disposal of wastes (during each blink, older tears are pushed into the lacrimal puncta.)
      - Clinical signs of obstruction of the nasolacrimal apparatus include epiphora or other ocular discharge (mucoid and mucopurulent).

3 The precorneal tear film
  - Made up of three main components, which are as follows:
    - Mucin
      - Produced by conjunctival goblet cells (see Chapter 13).
      - Functions:
        - Adheres tears to the cornea.
        - Smooths irregularities of the corneal surface.
        - Binds particulate matter for disposal.
        - Stabilizes the tear film to prevent early evaporation.
    - Aqueous
      - Produced by the third eyelid gland and the orbital lacrimal gland.
      - Functions:
        - Hydrates the ocular surface.
        - Lubricates movement of eyelids across the ocular surface.
        - Immunologic (dissolved antimicrobial substances within the aqueous tears).
        - Nutrition to the cornea.
        - Removal of waste from the ocular surface.
    - Lipid
      - Produced by Meibomian glands.
      - Function: to prevent early evaporation of the precorneal tear film.
- When the tear film is compromised, nutrition to the ocular surface is impaired, as are immunologic functions and the removal of waste material. Tear film deficiency or dysfunction also increases friction between the eyelids and the cornea and promotes drying of the cornea. Therefore, clinical signs

of tear film deficiency and dysfunction are compatible with clinical signs of ocular surface inflammation, including the following:
  - Blepharospasm
  - *Conjunctival hyperemia*
  - *Superficial corneal vascularization*
  - Corneal edema
  - Corneal fibrosis
  - Corneal melanosis
  - *A dry, roughened corneal surface*
  - *Mucoid or mucopurulent ocular discharge*

Disorders of the third eyelid, nasolacrimal system, and precorneal tear film can alter the production, distribution, and removal of tears. This affects protection, nourishment, and hydration of the eye, which is why disorders of these structures can have a significant impact on corneal and conjunctival health. Effects range from mild to marked surface ocular irritation and inflammation (superficial keratitis, conjunctivitis, and keratoconjunctivitis) (see Chapters 13 and 14) and can even include corneal ulceration (Chapter 14).

Diseases of the third eyelid, nasolacrimal system, and precorneal tear film

Third eyelid gland prolapse ("cherry eye")

What it is
- Displacement of the gland of the third eyelid from its normal position in the ventromedial orbit.

Predisposed individuals
- Third eyelid gland prolapse occurs in young animals, usually manifesting by 1–2 years of age.
  - Third eyelid neoplasia and orbital disease should be ruled out when older animals present with apparent third eyelid gland prolapse.
- This occurs most often in dogs.
  - Third eyelid gland prolapse is seen often in brachycephalic dogs and dogs with excessive facial skin (e.g., mastiff, Newfoundland, and St. Bernard).
- Prolapse of the third eyelid gland is uncommon in cats.
  - Burmese are affected most often.
- Individuals with eversion of the third eyelid cartilage (Figures 3.4, 3.5, 3.6), also referred to as scrolled cartilage, are at higher risk of third eyelid gland prolapse.
  - The vertical or horizontal portion of the third eyelid cartilage bends and causes the third eyelid to fold on itself.
  - This increases the risk of third eyelid gland prolapse by placing abnormal forces on the gland and tissues surrounding it.
  - Predisposed breeds include the great Dane, Newfoundland, and German shorthaired pointer.

Defining characteristics

- A swollen, pink round mass (the gland of the third eyelid) is seen at the medial canthus, anterior to the eye (Figures 3.7, 3.8, 3.9, 3.10, 3.11, 3.12).
  - The surface of the gland overall is relatively smooth.
- The leading edge of the third eyelid is ventral to the prolapsed gland and may or may not be visible initially.
- The leading edge will become visible when the lower eyelid is lowered.
- Conjunctivitis is usually present, ranging from mild to marked.
  - Conjunctival hyperemia
  - Chemosis
  - Mucoid ocular discharge
- Cartilage eversion, if present, may or may not be visible on initial examination.
  - A very swollen third eyelid gland can make it difficult to fully visualize the cartilage.

Clinical significance

- A prolapsed gland is inflamed and uncomfortable.
- Chronic inflammation leads to fibrosis of the glandular tissue.
  - Chronic fibrosis decreases the amount of functional glandular tissue, predisposing to KCS.
- In older animals, a prolapsed third eyelid gland may be a symptom of third eyelid or orbital neoplasia.

Diagnosis

- The diagnosis is based on clinical appearance.

Treatment

- This refers to treatment of third eyelid gland prolapse in the absence of concurrent neoplastic or orbital disease.
- For treatment of third eyelid neoplasia, see the next section ("Third eyelid neoplasia").
- For treatment of orbital disease, see Chapter 10.
- The goals are to reduce inflammation of the third eyelid gland, to replace the gland in the orbit, to maintain the gland in this position, and to minimize the effects of gland prolapse on surface ocular hydration.
- Anti-inflammatory therapy should be employed preoperatively and postoperatively.
  - Improves patient comfort.
  - Reduces gland swelling, facilitating its repositioning.
  - Decreases postsurgical inflammation.
  - Use both ophthalmically applied and systemically administered drugs.
    - For example, prednisolone acetate 1% ophthalmic suspension or dexamethasone (available as a 0.1% ophthalmic solution or in combination with neomycin and polymyxin B in both ointment and suspension forms) applied to the affected eye two to four times daily prior to surgery and for 7–14 days postoperatively.
      - Do not use if corneal ulceration is present.
    - For example, oral veterinary-labeled NSAIDs at the labeled dose prior to surgery and for 7–10 days postoperatively.
- Tear film replacement.
  - Corneal exposure, keratitis, or corneal ulceration can occur when the prolapsed gland prevents full eyelid closure.
  - Chronic conjunctivitis leads to instability and premature evaporation of the precorneal tear film, causing corneal drying, development of keratitis, and a predisposition to corneal ulceration.
- *A prolapsed third eyelid gland, in the absence of concurrent neoplastic disease, should not be excised.*
  - Excision is an unacceptable treatment that greatly increases the potential for development of KCS.
- The gland should be replaced to its original position within the ventromedial orbit.
  - Specific surgical techniques are numerous and published elsewhere. Most involve either tacking the gland down (e.g., to the orbital periosteum) with nonabsorbable suture or tucking the gland into a pocket created in the conjunctiva.
- Third eyelid cartilage eversion should be corrected at the time of third eyelid gland replacement.
  - Various techniques are published elsewhere and involve resection of the bent portion of the cartilage or use of cautery to alter the shape of the cartilage.

Prognosis

- For prolapse of short duration, the prognosis for replacement of the gland is good.
- Recurrent prolapse is the most common postoperative complication.
  - The likelihood of recurrent prolapse increases in glands that have been chronically prolapsed and glands that have undergone previous surgical repair.
- Surgery should be repeated if the prolapse recurs.
- In some cases, surgery may have to be repeated several times.
  - Individuals experiencing multiple prolapses should be referred to a veterinary ophthalmologist for treatment.
- Dogs with third eyelid gland prolapse are at risk of KCS even with successful replacement of the gland.
  - The risk of KCS is higher when gland prolapse is more chronic or when multiple surgeries have been performed, in part due to the large amount of scar tissue that develops.
  - The STT values should be monitored for several months following gland replacement.
  - Therapy for KCS should be initiated if the STT values fall below 15 mm/min (see Chapter 14).

Third eyelid neoplasia

What it is

- Neoplasms arising from the third eyelid or overlying conjunctiva, or neoplasms metastasizing to the third eyelid.

Predisposed individuals

- Dogs and cats of any age, breed, or sex can develop third eyelid neoplasia, but it occurs more often in patients over 10 years of age (Dees *et al.*, 2016).

Defining characteristics

- Superficial neoplasms are usually small, raised masses arising from the conjunctiva of the anterior or bulbar surfaces of the third eyelid (Figures 3.13, 3.14).
- Neoplasms of the gland of the third eyelid may initially appear as a prolapse of the third eyelid gland.
- Because of their location, neoplasms of the gland may not present for evaluation until they are quite large.
- These are often fleshy orbital masses located anterior to the eye but posterior to the third eyelid (Figures 3.15, 3.16).
- Although these originate from the ventromedial orbit, this can be difficult to determine when the tumor is large.

Clinical significance

- Small, benign, superficial neoplasms are often clinically insignificant (see Chapter 13 for conjunctival neoplasia).
- Malignant neoplasms can be locally invasive.
- Third eyelid neoplasms can also be a part of a larger, systemic neoplastic process.
- Many different third eyelid neoplasms have been reported.
  - Some malignant and/or invasive neoplasms include adenocarcinoma (Wilcock & Peiffer, 1988), lymphoma (Hong *et al.*, 2011; Newkirk & Rohrbach, 2009), melanoma (Schobert *et al.*, 2010), and squamous cell carcinoma (Lavach & Snyder, 1984), with adenocarcinoma being most common among dogs and cats (Dees *et al.*, 2016).
  - Some benign neoplasms include papilloma, hemangioma/hemangiosarcoma (Pirie & Dubielzig, 2006; Pirie *et al.*, 2006), and extramedullary plasmacytoma (Perlmann *et al.*, 2009).

Diagnosis

- The diagnosis of third eyelid neoplasia is made by visualizing a mass on the anterior or bulbar surface of the third eyelid, a diffuse thickening of the third eyelid and/or third eyelid gland, or a mass arising from the third eyelid gland.
  - Masses arising from the gland of the third eyelid tend to be significantly larger and more inflamed than a gland that is simply prolapsed.
  - Masses arising from the gland of the third eyelid tend to appear much more irregular in texture or shape when compared with a gland that is simply prolapsed.
- Histopathology is required to diagnose the type of neoplasm affecting the third eyelid.
  - Small conjunctival masses can be removed completely and submitted as excisional biopsy samples. The technique for excision of small masses is as follows:
    - A cotton swab is saturated with proparacaine 0.5% ophthalmic solution or 2% lidocaine and applied to the biopsy site for 1 minute. This provides anesthesia to the conjunctival surface.
    - Small forceps, such as Bishop Harmon forceps, are used to grasp the conjunctiva adjacent to the mass. The forceps are pulled up to tent the conjunctiva, elevating the mass and some normal surrounding conjunctiva.
    - At the base of the tent, where the conjunctiva attaches to the surface of the third eyelid and below the level of the mass, the conjunctiva is snipped with tenotomy scissors.
    - The sample is placed onto a flat surface such as a tongue depressor, a piece of paper, or the inside of a tissue cassette to keep it flat and maintain orientation.
    - The sample with the tongue depressor/paper/tissue cassette is then placed into 10% neutral buffered formalin and submitted for histopathology.
  - For larger masses, incisional biopsies can be performed before attempting complete removal.
- Advanced imaging, such as an MRI or a CT, is recommended for larger masses, especially those involving the gland, prior to pursuing removal.
  - Imaging helps to determine the extent of the mass within the orbit and whether more aggressive surgery or adjunctive therapies are required.

Treatment

- The goal of treatment is to completely remove the neoplasm while minimizing damage to adjacent structures.
- For small conjunctival masses:
  - If histopathology indicates a benign lesion and complete removal, then the excisional biopsy is adequate therapy.
  - If histopathology indicates a benign lesion and incomplete removal, options include the following:
    - Monitoring for regrowth.
    - Adjunctive therapy at the site of mass removal.
    - Resection of a larger area of conjunctiva to remove any remaining neoplastic tissue.
  - If histopathology indicates a malignant lesion, monitoring for regrowth, adjunctive therapy, and further resection (including removal of the third eyelid) are all options.
    - Which option to choose is influenced by tumor type, whether the resection was complete or incomplete, and imaging that indicates tumor extent.
    - Rule out metastatic disease (e.g., thoracic radiographs or CT, abdominal ultrasound or CT, and lymph node aspirates).
- For larger masses where incisional biopsy was used to obtain a diagnosis, the treatment depends on the tumor type.
  - Further surgical resection to obtain clean margins can include third eyelid removal, exenteration, or more invasive surgery that may require referral to a veterinary ophthalmologist.
  - Adjunctive therapies such as radiation therapy, chemotherapy, or a combination of these may be required instead of or in addition to surgical excision.

Prognosis

- The prognosis is very good following removal of benign neoplasms.
- For malignant neoplasms, such as adenocarcinoma, the prognosis is good if the tumor is confined to the third eyelid and excision is complete.
- If removal of a malignant neoplasm was not complete, then recurrence is likely and prognosis for overall survival depends on the tumor type (this determines behavior and responsiveness to other therapies).

Additional information

- Prolapse of the third eyelid gland is a disease of young animals (usually within the first 1–2 years of life). If this condition is diagnosed in older animals, third eyelid neoplasia should be suspected and diagnostics pursued.
- KCS can occur following third eyelid removal. Periodic monitoring of the STT values is recommended so that if KCS develops, it is diagnosed and treated early.

Nasolacrimal duct obstruction

What it is

- Blockage at any point along the nasolacrimal drainage system that prevents flow of tears from the conjunctival sac into the nasal cavity.
- The blockage may be due to a physical impairment of drainage (e.g., foreign material trapped within the nasolacrimal duct).
- The blockage can also be a result of conformation (e.g., ventromedial entropion causing misalignment of the punctum with the ocular surface such that tears are unable to enter the nasolacrimal duct).

Predisposed individuals

- Brachycephalic individuals are predisposed to nasolacrimal duct blockage as a result of their conformation (see Chapter 10 for discussion of brachycephalic ocular syndrome).
- Hunting dogs and other highly active, outdoor dogs have a higher likelihood of developing nasolacrimal duct obstruction following entrapment of foreign material within the duct.

Defining characteristics

- Epiphora and tear staining near the medial canthus of the affected eye.
  - If dacryocystitis is present, there may also be mucoid or mucopurulent discharge arising from the nasolacrimal puncta.
- If the obstruction is due to eyelid conformation, entropion of the medial aspect of the ventral eyelid is visible.

Clinical significance

- Clinical significance depends on both the amount of facial moisture resulting from the nasolacrimal duct blockage and the underlying cause of the obstruction.

- Mild periocular wetness may not cause clinical problems, but as periocular moisture increases, the risk of dermatitis rises.
- Potential causes of obstruction:
  - Punctal atresia
    - Congenital absence of the puncta.
  - Imperforate punctum
    - A congenital defect where a thin layer of conjunctiva occludes the punctal opening.
  - Obstruction of the nasolacrimal punctum secondary to conformational entropion.
    - Common in brachycephalic individuals.
  - Nasolacrimal duct atresia
    - Congenital absence of all or a portion of the nasolacrimal duct.
  - Foreign body obstruction
  - Dacryocystitis
    - Swelling of the nasolacrimal drainage apparatus can occlude the nasolacrimal duct.
  - Scar tissue
    - Scarring following conjunctivitis can result in stenosis or occlusion of the puncta.
    - Scarring following dacryocystitis can result in stenosis or occlusion of the nasolacrimal duct.
  - Neoplasia
    - Neoplasia of the surrounding soft tissue or bony structures can cause obstruction.
  - Trauma
    - For example, the nasolacrimal drainage system components can be damaged with eyelid laceration or skull fractures.
- Diseases of structures through which the nasolacrimal duct passes have potential to cause obstruction.
  - For example, proximity of the nasolacrimal duct to the roots of the maxillary teeth, particularly the canine teeth, means that primary dental disease can result in nasolacrimal duct obstruction.
  - For example, extension of nasal disease may compress the nasolacrimal duct, resulting in obstruction.
- In many cases, the cause of the nasolacrimal duct obstruction cannot be identified.
  - Clinical significance then depends on the degree of epiphora and periocular moisture (mentioned earlier) and whether this is causing discomfort to the patient.
- Regardless of underlying cause, many pet owners, particularly those with white dogs, find epiphora esthetically objectionable.

Diagnosis

- Diagnostics are aimed at (1) confirming obstruction and (2) determining the underlying cause of obstruction.
- **1** Confirming obstruction
- Jones test.

- A positive Jones test occurs when fluorescein placed into the conjunctival sac is visualized at the ipsilateral nostril or in the mouth (Figures 3.2, 3.3).
  - This usually occurs within 2 minutes of fluorescein placement into the conjunctival sac, but nasolacrimal transit times of as long as 30 minutes are possible (Binder & Herring, 2010).
  - A positive Jones test rules out nasolacrimal duct obstruction.
  - The Jones test is negative if fluorescein fails to appear at the nostril or in the mouth (Figure 3.3).
  - A negative Jones test supports conformational or physical obstruction of the duct.
- Nasolacrimal duct flush.
  - Should be performed when the Jones test is negative.
- For obstructions secondary to physical obstruction, attempts at flushing the nasolacrimal ducts are either difficult (resistance encountered during attempts at flushing) or unsuccessful.
- For conformational obstructions, the Jones test is negative but the nasolacrimal duct is easily flushed.
2 Determining the cause of obstruction
- Visualization of eyelid puncta can rule out obstructions at this level.
- Imaging.
  - Indicated when nasolacrimal duct flushing is unsuccessful.
  - Dental radiographs may identify any maxillary bone or tooth root lesions contributing to obstruction.
  - Skull radiographs with contrast injected into nasolacrimal duct.
    - Can identify bony lesions contributing to obstruction.
    - Can identify the site of obstruction, dilations within the nasolacrimal duct, or perforation of the nasolacrimal duct.
  - Computed tomography with contrast injected into nasolacrimal duct.
    - Can identify bony lesions contributing to obstruction.
    - Can identify the site of obstruction, dilations within the nasolacrimal duct, nature of obstruction, perforation of the nasolacrimal duct, or other physical alterations of the nasolacrimal duct.
    - Image quality and level of detail visible is superior to those of radiographs.
    - Indicated when previous tests have not identified the nature of the obstruction.
- Cytology and culture and sensitivity of any discharge are also recommended to identify infectious components.

Treatment

- The main goal of treatment is to reestablish patency of the nasolacrimal duct.
- Treatment must therefore address the underlying cause of obstruction.
  - Punctal and nasolacrimal duct atresia are addressed surgically, and referral is advised.

- Treatment usually involves creating alternative drainage pathways.
  - Imperforate punctum
    - Flushing of the nasolacrimal duct through the other, patent punctum for the same eye can result in a visible conjunctival bulge where the imperforate punctum is present.
    - If this bulge is visible, the conjunctiva can be carefully snipped with small scissors to open up the punctum.
    - Ophthalmically applied corticosteroid suspensions (e.g., prednisolone acetate or dexamethasone) are applied to the conjunctival sac two to four times daily for 7–10 days to inhibit scarring and reocclusion of the punctum.
  - Conformation can be improved surgically by repairing ventromedial entropion.
  - Foreign body obstruction requires referral for surgical removal.
  - Dacryocystitis should be treated with systemic veterinary-labeled NSAIDs and ophthalmically applied antibiotics (chosen according to cytology and culture and sensitivity).
  - Treatment for neoplasia is based on the type of neoplasia present and the extent of the neoplasm.
  - Following repair of skull fractures or eyelid lacerations, and for cases of obstruction secondary to scarring, the patient may require referral for surgical reconstruction of the nasolacrimal duct.

Prognosis

- Prognosis depends on the underlying cause.
- The prognosis is good for alleviating the obstruction when it is secondary to conformation, imperforate punctum, or dacryocystitis.
- It is more difficult to establish and maintain patency when surgery is required to reconstruct a new drainage pathway, as postoperative scarring can lead to recurrence of obstruction.

Additional information

- In many cases, especially when epiphora is due to conformation, tearing can only be reduced, but not completely eliminated, by treatment.
  - Managing client expectations is important.
- Perform the Jones test on one eye at a time, with several minutes between each eye.
  - This way, if fluorescein appears in the mouth instead of at the nares, one can determine from which side the fluorescein emerged (and therefore which side is patent).
- The anatomy of the nasolacrimal drainage apparatus is altered in brachycephalic dogs and cats when compared to non-brachycephalics, and may therefore increase the potential for impaired drainage (Sahr et al., 2021; Schleuter, 2021).

Tear film disorders—KCS

- Because many of the clinical signs of KCS are corneal changes, this condition is discussed in Chapter 14.

Qualitative tear film abnormality

What it is

- An abnormality of the lipid or mucin portion of the precorneal tear film resulting in instability of the precorneal tear film, premature evaporation of the precorneal tear film, and ocular surface irritation.

Predisposed individuals

- Cats and dogs with active or recent conjunctivitis are likely to have a mucin deficiency of the precorneal tear film.
  - Inflammation of the conjunctiva leads to atrophy of the conjunctival goblet cells (Johnson *et al.*, 1990; Lim *et al.*, 2009; Moore & Collier 1990).
- Cats and dogs with blepharitis are likely to have abnormalities of the lipid portion of the tear film.
  - Inflamed Meibomian glands produce abnormal lipid products (Nelson *et al.*, 2011).

Defining characteristics

- Clinical signs are consistent with those of surface ocular irritation, which are as follows:
  - Blepharospasm
  - Mucoid ocular discharge
  - *Conjunctival hyperemia*
  - *Superficial corneal vascularization*
- The tear production, as measured by the STT, is usually within normal limits.

Clinical significance

- Although the aqueous component of the precorneal tear film is adequate, premature evaporation of the tear film leads to drying of the corneal surface.
- The chronic irritation resulting from a dry corneal surface is uncomfortable.
- The chronic irritation resulting from a dry corneal surface predisposes to keratoconjunctivitis and even corneal ulceration.
- Underlying causes of blepharitis and conjunctivitis may be present and, if so, should be treated (see Chapters 11 and 13).
- Mucin deficiency can result from conjunctivitis, but can also perpetuate conjunctivitis after the original cause of inflammation has resolved.
  - Treatment of the mucin deficiency is then needed to decrease conjunctival inflammation.
- Mucin deficiency can persist for weeks after clinically visible signs of conjunctivitis have resolved (Lim *et al.*, 2009).

Diagnosis

- When active blepharitis is present, an abnormality of the lipid portion of the tear film should be assumed.
- When active conjunctivitis is present, mucin deficiency should be assumed.

- Although meibometry exists and can be used to assess tear film lipids, it is not routinely available for the practice setting.
- Goblet cell atrophy can be diagnosed by conjunctival biopsy.
  - See Chapter 13 for technique.
- The TFBUT is an assessment of tear film stability and is considered an indirect measure of the mucin content of the precorneal tear film. It is less invasive to perform than conjunctival biopsy.
  - This is a measurement of how long the tears remain as a stable film over the cornea.
  - Therefore, a shorter TFBUT means the tear film is less stable (evaporates early), while a longer TFBUT indicates a very stable tear film (it remains as an intact film over the cornea.)
  - Normal TFBUT for cats ranges from approximately 12 to 21 seconds (Cullen *et al.*, 2005).
  - Normal TFBUT for dogs ranges from approximately 15 to 20 seconds (Moore *et al.*, 1987).
  - Qualitative tear film deficiency is diagnosed when the TFBUT is shorter than the reference range and clinical signs of surface ocular disease are present.
  - Technique for TFBUT:
    - This test should be performed in a darkened room, as for the ophthalmic examination. It requires the use of magnification (e.g., loupes), cobalt blue light, a stopwatch or other method of timing, fluorescein stain, and at least one assistant to restrain the pet and control the timer. Timing begins when the tears are first spread over the cornea and ends when the first sign of evaporation (visible as a break in the tear film) is seen.
    - Place a drop of concentrated fluorescein solution into the conjunctival sac, then close the eye.
    - Looking through the loupes or other source of magnification, direct the cobalt blue light source toward the eye and ready the timer for use. Timing will begin when the eyelids are opened.
    - Open the eyelids and observe the dorsolateral corneal surface (this is where timing begins.) Continue to observe the cornea until the first sign of evaporation is seen.
    - The corneal surface will initially appear green due to the fluorescein in the tear film that covers the corneal surface. Eventually, a black spot will appear within the tear film. This represents the first spot of evaporation within the precorneal tear film. This is when timing ends.

Treatment

- If active conjunctivitis is present, it should be treated as per the discussion in Chapter 13.
  - Ophthalmically applied CsA (Optimmune®) is a good choice for treating the qualitative tear film deficiency associated with conjunctivitis because it increases mucin stores within the conjunctiva (Moore *et al.*, 2001).
  - Application of mucinomimetic tear film replacements will also reduce corneal drying and irritation.

∘ Hyaluronan 0.25% or higher (e.g., I-Drop®Vet, an-HyPro) is a mucinomimetic tear film replacement.
  ▪ Hyaluronan has superior corneal retention time when compared with other lacrimomimetics (Snibson *et al.*, 1992).
  ▪ If frequent application is needed, preservative-free formulations are preferred over multi-dose vials because ophthalmic preservatives can be toxic to the epithelial surface.
  ▪ Administer two to four times daily (or more, if preservative-free formulation is used) and continue for 3–4 weeks beyond resolution of clinical signs.
• If active blepharitis is present, it should be treated as per the discussion in Chapter 11.
  ∘ Application of tear film substitutes that mimic the lipid portion of the tears will reduce corneal irritation and discomfort.
    ▪ These are generally available as ophthalmic ointments.
    ▪ The ingredients that mimic lipid include petrolatum, lanolin, and mineral oil.
    ▪ Administer two to four times daily during active blepharitis.

Prognosis

• Following resolution of the original inflammatory insult (blepharitis and conjunctivitis), the prognosis for resolution of the qualitative tear film abnormality is very good.
  ∘ Because recovery of the goblet cells is delayed, resolution of mucin deficiency lags behind resolution of clinical conjunctivitis.

Other third eyelid disorders—Pannus

Please see Chapter 14.

References

Binder, DR & Herring, IP. 2010. Evaluation of nasolacrimal fluorescein transit time in ophthalmically normal dogs and nonbrachycephalic cats. *American Journal of Veterinary Research.* 71(5):570–574.

Cullen, CL, *et al.* 2005. Tear film breakup times in young healthy cats before and after anesthesia. *Veterinary Ophthalmology.* 8(3):159–165.

Dees, DD, *et al.* 2016. Third eyelid gland neoplasms of dogs and cats: a retrospective histopathologic study of 145 cases. *Veterinary Ophthalmology.* 19(2):138–143.

Hong, IH, *et al.* 2011. Mucosa-associated lymphoid tissue lymphoma of the third eyelid conjunctiva in a dog. *Veterinary Ophthalmology.* 14(1):61–65.

Johnson, BW, *et al.* 1990. Effects of inflammation and aqueous tear film deficiency on conjunctival morphology and ocular mucus composition in cats. *American Journal of Veterinary Research.* 51:820–824.

Lavach, JD & Snyder, SP. 1984. Squamous cell carcinoma of the third eyelid in a dog. *Journal of the American Veterinary Medical Association.* 184(8):975–976.

Lim, CC, *et al.* 2009. Effects of feline herpesvirus type 1 on tear film break-up time, Schirmer tear test results, and conjunctival goblet cell density in experimentally infected cats. *American Journal of Veterinary Research.* 70(3):394–403.

Moore, CP & Collier, LL. 1990. Ocular surface disease associated with loss of conjunctival goblet cells in dogs. *Journal of the American Animal Hospital Association.* 26(5):458–466.

Moore, CP, *et al.* 1987. Density and distribution of canine conjunctival goblet cells. *Investigative Ophthalmology and Visual Science.* 28(12):1925–1932.

Moore, CP, *et al.* 2001. Effect of cyclosporine on conjunctival mucin in a canine keratoconjunctivitis sicca model. *Investigative Ophthalmology and Visual Science.* 42(3):653–659.

Nelson, JD, *et al.* 2011. The international workshop on meibomian gland dysfunction: report of the definition and classification subcommittee. *Investigative Ophthalmology and Visual Science.* 52(4):1930–1937.

Newkirk, KM & Rohrbach, BW. 2009. A retrospective study of eyelid tumors from 43 cats. *Veterinary Pathology.* 46(5):916–927.

Perlmann, E, *et al.* 2009. Extramedullary plasmacytoma of the third eyelid gland in a dog. *Veterinary Ophthalmology.* 12(2):102–105.

Pirie, CG & Dubielzig, RR. 2006. Feline conjunctival hemangioma and hemangiosarcoma: a retrospective evaluation of eight cases (1993–2004). *Veterinary Ophthalmology.* 9(4):227–231.

Pirie, CG, *et al.* 2006. Canine conjunctival hemangioma and hemangiosarcoma: a retrospective evaluation of 108 cases (1989–2004). *Veterinary Ophthalmology.* 9(4):215–226.

Sahr, S, *et al.* 2021. Evaluating malformations of the lacrimal drainage system in brachycephalic dog breeds: a comparative computed tomography analysis. *PLOS One.* doi:10.1371/journal.pone.0257020

Schleuter, C, *et al.* 2009. Brachycephalic feline noses: CT and anatomical study of the relationship between head conformation and the nasolacrimal drainage system. *Journal of Feline Medicine and Surgery.* 11(11):891–900.

Schobert, CS, *et al.* 2010. Feline conjunctival melanoma: histopathological characteristics and clinical outcomes. *Veterinary Ophthalmology.* 13(1):43–46.

Snibson, GR, *et al.* 1992. Ocular surface residence times of artificial tear solutions. *Cornea.* 11(4):288–293.

Wilcock, B & Peiffer, R. 1988. Adenocarcinoma of the gland of the third eyelid in seven dogs. *Journal of the American Veterinary Medical Association.* 193(12):1549–1550.

13 Conjunctiva

Please see Chapter 4 for images of the conjunctiva.

- The conjunctiva covers the external ocular surface except for the cornea (Figure 4.1).
  - The conjunctiva overlying the sclera is referred to as the bulbar conjunctiva.
  - The conjunctiva that lines the inner surfaces of the eyelids is referred to as the palpebral conjunctiva.
  - The dorsal conjunctival fornix is the area at which the dorsal palpebral and the dorsal bulbar conjunctiva merge, and the ventral conjunctival fornix is the area at which the ventral palpebral and the ventral bulbar conjunctiva merge.
  - The conjunctiva also covers the anterior and posterior surfaces of the third eyelid.
- Components of the conjunctiva include the following:
  - Blood vessels
  - Nerves
  - Lymphoid tissue
  - Lymphatic vessels
  - Goblet cells
  - Fibrous tissue
  - Melanocytes
- Various microbes inhabit the conjunctival surface in health.
  - The population consists of a mixture of Gram-positive and Gram-negative bacteria, with greater numbers of Gram-positive aerobes (Gerding & Kakoma, 1990).
  - *Staphylococcus* spp. predominate (Gerding & Kakoma, 1990).
  - Other bacteria that have been found in the healthy conjunctival sac include *Streptococcus* spp., *Corynebacterium* spp., *Bacillus* spp., *Neisseria* spp., and *Pseudomonas* spp. (Gerding & Kakoma, 1990).
  - *Chlamyophila felis* has been recovered from the conjunctival sacs of normal cats (Low *et al.*, 2007).
  - *Mycoplasma* spp. have been recovered from the conjunctival sacs of normal cats and dogs (Campbell *et al.*, 1973; Rosendal, 1973).
  - Fungal organisms are occasionally isolated from the conjunctival sacs of healthy dogs and cats (Samuelson *et al.*, 1984).

- Functions of the conjunctiva:
  - Conjunctival goblet cells produce the mucous component of the precorneal tear film.
    - Mucin stabilizes the precorneal tear film and prevents early evaporation.
    - Goblet cells are most highly concentrated in the ventromedial conjunctival fornix.
  - Provides immunologic protection to the ocular surface.
    - By the conjunctiva-associated lymphoid tissue.
  - Allows movement of the eye while minimizing friction between it and the eyelids.
- Signs of conjunctival disease include the following:
  - *Ocular discharge*: mucoid, serous, sanguineous, or purulent.
  - *Conjunctival hyperemia* (Figures 4.2, 4.3, 4.4, 4.5)
  - Chemosis (Figures 4.4, 4.5, 4.6, 4.7)
  - Conjunctival lymphoid follicle formation (Figures 4.5, 4.10, 4.11, 4.12, 4.13)
  - Thickening of the conjunctiva (Figures 4.4, 4.14)
  - Mass formation on the conjunctiva (Figures 4.15, 4.16, 4.17, 4.18, 4.19, 4.20)
  - Subconjunctival hemorrhage (Figures 4.8, 4.9)

Diseases of conjunctiva

Canine conjunctivitis

What it is
- Conjunctivitis refers to inflammation of the conjunctiva.

Predisposed individuals
- Dogs of any age, breed, or sex can develop conjunctivitis.
- Immune-mediated conjunctivitis is seen more often in younger individuals.
- Infectious conjunctivitis is seen more often in dogs who are exposed to other dogs (for example, at dog parks or day care centers) or who are immunocompromised (Gervais *et al.*, 2012; Ledbetter *et al.*, 2009).
- Neoplastic conditions are seen more often in older individuals.

Small Animal Ophthalmic Atlas and Guide, Second Edition. Christine C. Lim.
© 2023 John Wiley & Sons, Inc. Published 2023 by John Wiley & Sons, Inc.
Companion website: www.wiley.com/go/lim/atlas

Defining characteristics

- Clinical signs of conjunctivitis that are consistently present include the following:
  - *Ocular discharge,* usually mucoid
  - *Conjunctival hyperemia* (Figure 4.2)
- Signs of conjunctivitis that are variably present include the following:
  - Chemosis (Figures 4.6, 4.7)
  - Conjunctival lymphoid follicle formation (Figures 4.10, 4.11)
  - Hemorrhage (Figures 4.8, 4.9)
  - Conjunctival thickening (Figure 4.14)
- Neoplastic conjunctivitis tends to have one of two appearances:
  - Diffuse thickening of the conjunctiva (Figure 4.14).
  - Mass lesions elevated from the conjunctival surface (Figures 4.15, 4.16, 4.17, 4.18, 4.19, 4.20).

Clinical significance

- Conjunctivitis is irritating and causes patient discomfort.
- Chronic conjunctivitis leads to goblet cell atrophy, mucin deficiency in the precorneal tear film (qualitative tear film abnormality or deficiency, see Chapter 12), and instability of the precorneal tear film.
  - Instability of the precorneal tear film is associated with early evaporation of tears. This in turn dries the ocular surface in spite of adequate or even excessive tear production.
  - Tear film instability perpetuates further ocular surface irritation and inflammation, even if the inciting cause of conjunctivitis is no longer present.
- *Canine conjunctivitis tends to be noninfectious in etiology.*
- Conjunctivitis has many potential causes. Some include the following:
  - Idiopathic
  - Immune-mediated
    - Atopy (Pena *et al.,* 2008)
    - Follicular conjunctivitis in young dogs (Pena *et al.,* 2008)
      - This is thought to be due to an immature immune system
    - KCS (see Chapter 14) (Kaswan & Salisbury, 1990)
    - Pannus or chronic superficial keratitis (see Chapter 14) (Bedford & Longstaffe, 1979)
  - Infectious
    - Canine herpesvirus (Ledbetter *et al.,* 2009)
      - Ocular disease resulting from herpetic infection occurs more often to dogs who are exposed to other dogs or who are immunocompromised (Gervais *et al.,* 2012; Ledbetter *et al.,* 2009).
      - Parasitic (Beckwith-Cohen, *et al.,* 2016; Sanchez *et al.,* 2012)
  - Neoplastic (see Conjunctival Neoplasia later in this chapter)
  - Trauma
    - Including entropion, aberrant hairs (distichiae, ectopic cilia, and trichiasis), and eyelid masses (see Chapter 11)

Diagnosis

- Diagnosis is two-part and involves the (1) diagnosis of conjunctivitis and (2) diagnosis of the underlying cause.
1 Conjunctivitis is diagnosed by observation of clinical signs as mentioned earlier.
2 Determining the underlying cause of conjunctivitis requires careful ophthalmic examination and, often, additional diagnostic testing.
- Ophthalmic examination will rule out foreign material within the conjunctival fornices, as well as eyelid abnormalities such as entropion, aberrant hairs (distichiae, ectopic cilia, trichiasis), and eyelid masses.
- The STT will determine if low aqueous tear production (see Chapter 14 for KCS) is contributing to conjunctivitis.
- The TFBUT can identify if a qualitative tear film abnormality is present (see Chapter 12).
- In the absence of eyelid and precorneal tear film abnormalities, the underlying cause of conjunctivitis is often not definitively identified.
- Conjunctival culture is often of limited utility.
  - Bacteria can be cultured from the conjunctiva of dogs and cats without ocular disease.
  - Primary bacterial conjunctivitis is rare in dogs.
    - Bacterial overgrowth can occur secondary to other etiologies such as KCS.
- Cytology of conjunctival scrapings can be nondiagnostic, but also can be more informative than culture.
  - A diagnosis of atopic conjunctivitis in dogs can be supported by changes in cells visualized on cytology.
  - Neoplastic cells can be identified by cytology.
- Histopathologic evaluation of a conjunctival sample is often the most useful diagnostic test.
  - Indicated for severe conjunctivitis, when neoplasia is suspected, or when conjunctivitis is unresponsive to therapy.
  - See Diagnosis under Conjunctival Neoplasia later in this chapter for technique of conjunctival biopsy.
  - In dogs, lymphoplasmacytic conjunctivitis without an obvious etiology is a very common diagnosis.
  - Histopathology is very useful for ruling out the uncommon and potentially more serious causes of conjunctivitis.

Treatment

- The goal of treatment is to eliminate conjunctival inflammation.
- Treatment can be divided into (1) nonspecific anti-inflammatory therapy, (2) therapy directed at the underlying cause of conjunctivitis (if identified), and (3) supplementation of the precorneal tear film.
1 Anti-inflammatory therapy
  - This is indicated whether or not the underlying cause is identified.
  - Anti-inflammatory therapy involves ophthalmically applied corticosteroids, CsA, or a combination of these drugs.

- Corticosteroids
  - Prednisolone acetate ophthalmic suspension 1% or dexamethasone (0.1% ophthalmic solution or, if antibiotics needed, in combination with neomycin and polymyxin B in both ointment and suspension forms).
  - Do not use when infectious etiologies are suspected.
  - Do not use in the presence of corneal ulceration.
  - Dose: one drop of suspension/solution or 1/4″ strip of ointment applied to the affected eye two to four times daily, as determined by the severity of inflammation. As clinical signs improve, the dose should be gradually tapered.
  - Improvement is usually noted within 1–2 weeks of starting treatment.
  - If long-term management is required, use no more than one to two times daily.
- CsA
  - CsA 0.2% ophthalmic ointment (Optimmune®)
  - Dose: 1/4″ strip applied to the affected eye q12h.
  - If clinical signs of conjunctivitis are controlled with this dose of CsA and it is used for long-term control of idiopathic conjunctivitis, it may be possible to decrease the frequency of dosing to once daily.
  - CsA can be used in the presence of corneal ulceration.
  - Clinical improvement may not be noted before 3–4 weeks of therapy.
  - In addition to anti-inflammatory effects, CsA improves mucin production by the conjunctival goblet cells.
  - For long-term use, CsA is preferred over corticosteroids due to lower risk of complications.

2 Therapy for the underlying cause.
  - Varies according to the underlying cause.
    - Atopy—address overall atopic syndrome.
    - KCS—see Chapter 14.
    - Pannus/chronic superficial keratitis—see Chapter 14.
    - Conjunctival neoplasia—later in this chapter.
    - Infectious—address specific underlying etiology.

3 Tear film supplementation
  - Tear film instability (see Chapter 12) associated with goblet cell atrophy can persist for weeks after resolution of visible clinical signs.
  - Tear film supplements should therefore be mucinomimetic and maintained for several weeks beyond resolution of clinical signs.
  - Hyaluronan 0.2% or higher (ex. I-Drop®Vet, an-HyPro) is a mucinomimetic tear film replacement.
  - Hyaluronan has superior corneal retention time when compared with other lacrimomimetics (Snibson *et al.*, 1992).
  - If frequent application is needed, preservative-free formulations are preferred over multidose vials because ophthalmic preservatives can be toxic to the epithelial surface.
    - Administer two to four times daily (or more if preservative-free formulation is used) and continue for 3–4 weeks beyond resolution of clinical signs.

A recheck examination is recommended for approximately 2 weeks after initiating treatment. The time interval between future rechecks, and the total number of rechecks required, is determined by patient progress (i.e., degree and time course to improvement of clinical signs).

Prognosis

- Prognosis depends on the underlying cause of conjunctivitis.
- Idiopathic and immune-mediated conjunctivitides usually respond well to treatment with ophthalmic corticosteroids and/or CsA.
  - After control of clinical signs, treatment can often be discontinued completely after tapering.
  - However, it is possible for some patients to require low-dose (e.g., once to twice daily) long term therapy to prevent recurrence/progression.

Additional information

- If copious ocular discharge is present, rinsing of the conjunctival sac with sterile eyewash and cleansing of the eyelids/periocular hairs is advised.
  - This reduces antigens within the conjunctival sac.
  - Removal of discharge from the conjunctival sac prior to application of medications improves ocular penetration of ophthalmically applied medications.
  - This improves patient comfort.

Feline conjunctivitis

What it is

- Conjunctivitis refers to inflammation of the conjunctiva.

Predisposed individuals

- Kittens are usually exposed to infectious disease such as FHV-1 early in life and develop upper respiratory illness and eye disease secondary to this.
- Cats living in group situations (catteries, animal shelters, and multi-cat households) are at higher risk for developing conjunctivitis.
  - This is because the most common causes of conjunctivitis in cats are infectious agents.
  - This type of living situation also increases stress, which can predispose to FHV-1 recurrence.

Defining characteristics

- Clinical signs of conjunctivitis that are consistently present include the following:
  - *Ocular discharge,* usually mucoid or mucopurulent
  - *Conjunctival hyperemia* (Figures 4.3, 4.4, 4.5)

- Signs of conjunctivitis that are variably present include the following:
  - Chemosis (Figures 4.3, 4.4, 4.5)
  - Conjunctival lymphoid follicle formation (Figures 4.5, 4.12, 4.13)
  - Hemorrhage
  - Conjunctival thickening (Figure 4.4)
- Some general rules have been used to raise the index of suspicion for specific etiologic agents of feline conjunctivitis:
  - Noticeable lymphoid follicle development is often attributed to C. *felis* conjunctivitis.
  - Conjunctivitis secondary to *C. felis* tends to have more chemosis than hyperemia.
  - Conjunctivitis secondary to FHV-1 tends to have more hyperemia than chemosis.
  - Unilateral conjunctivitis is more likely to be related to FHV-1 than C. *felis*.
  - Conjunctivitis with concurrent upper respiratory infection is more likely due to FHV-1.
  - When keratitis and/or corneal ulceration is present, conjunctivitis is presumed to be due to FHV-1.
- As with dogs, cats can also develop neoplastic conjunctivitis, and this tends to have one of the two appearances:
  - Diffuse thickening of the conjunctiva.
  - Mass lesions elevated from the conjunctival surface.

Clinical significance

- Conjunctivitis is irritating and causes patient discomfort.
- Chronic conjunctivitis leads to goblet cell atrophy, mucin deficiency in the precorneal tear film (qualitative tear film abnormality or deficiency), and instability of the precorneal tear film.
  - Instability of the precorneal tear film is associated with early evaporation of tears. This in turn dries the ocular surface in spite of adequate or even excessive tear production.
  - Tear film instability perpetuates further ocular surface irritation and inflammation, even if the inciting cause of conjunctivitis is no longer present.
- *Feline conjunctivitis is usually caused by an infectious agent.*
  - FHV-1, C. *felis*, and *Mycoplasma* spp. are implicated most often.
  - Other infectious causes, such as parasitic or fungal diseases, are uncommon.
- Noninfectious causes of feline conjunctivitis are less common.
  - One noninfectious syndrome, EK, is discussed in Chapter 14.

Diagnosis

- Diagnosis is two-part and involves (1) diagnosis of conjunctivitis and (2) diagnosis of the underlying cause.
1 Conjunctivitis is diagnosed by observation of clinical signs as mentioned earlier.
2 Determining the underlying cause of conjunctivitis requires careful ophthalmic examination and, often, additional diagnostic testing.

- Although these are uncommon in the cat, a careful ophthalmic examination should still be conducted to rule out eyelid abnormalities such as entropion, ectopic cilia, distichiasis, trichiasis, and eyelid masses.
- The TFBUT can identify if a qualitative tear film abnormality is present (see Chapter 12.)
- Obtaining a definitive diagnosis for feline conjunctivitis is challenging because laboratory tests are difficult to interpret.
  - FHV-1, C. *felis*, and *Mycoplasma* spp. are difficult to culture successfully.
  - There are inclusion bodies associated with FHV-1, C. *felis*, and *Mycoplasma* spp.; however, they are easily missed (because they appear on specific days of infection) or are not visible on routine cytological stains.
  - Techniques such as virus isolation and immunofluorescent antibody assays lack sensitivity, resulting in many false negatives.
  - Detection of viral DNA by polymerase chain reaction is highly sensitive.
    - The DNA of infectious organisms like FHV-1 can be found in normal, healthy cats; therefore, the significance of a positive test result is sometimes unclear.
- Therefore, in cats, conjunctivitis is often presumed to be due to either FHV-1, C. *felis*, or *Mycoplasma* spp. and response to treatment is used in the same manner as a diagnostic tool.
  - For example, response to the specific therapy is used to support the presumptive diagnosis.
  - Clinical signs as listed under "Defining characteristics" are used to weigh the likelihood of the etiologic agent being viral or bacterial.

Treatment

- The goals of treatment are to eliminate conjunctival inflammation and to treat the underlying infectious agent.
- Treatment is divided into (1) antiviral or antibacterial therapy, (2) supplementation of the precorneal tear film, and, if needed, (3) nonspecific anti-inflammatory therapy. For FHV-1, elimination of known stressors is also a component of therapy.
1 Antiviral or antibacterial therapy
  If FHV-1 is determined or suspected to be the cause of feline conjunctivitis, ophthalmic and/or systemic antiviral therapy is required.
  (a) L-lysine
    - Amino acid supplement that inhibits viral replication.
    - 500 mg PO q12h can reduce the severity of clinical signs (Stiles *et al.*, 2002).
    - Twice-daily dosing is preferred over free-feeding of powder sprinkled on food, due to association of latter method with worsened clinical disease and viral shedding (Drazenovich *et al.*, 2009).
    - More effective if administration begins prior to clinical disease onset (Stiles *et al.*, 2002).
      - Daily administration is the only way to ensure this. Therefore, indefinite, daily supplementation is

recommended for cats who experience recurrent herpetic disease (rather than for cats presenting for the first outbreak and rather than administration only during clinical disease).

(b) Ophthalmically applied antiviral medications

- Cidofovir 0.5% ophthalmic solution, idoxuridine 0.1% ophthalmic solution or 0.5% ophthalmic ointment, ganciclovir 0.15% ophthalmic gel, trifluridine 1% ophthalmic solution, and many others.
- Most antiviral eye medications must be compounded.
- Cats appear to frequently react adversely to application of trifluridine; thus, this is usually not the first choice.
- Cidofovir is most convenient because it is applied at one drop to the affected eye q12h.
- Ganciclovir appears clinically efficacious when applied 3 times daily (Ledbetter *et al.,* 2021).
- Idoxuridine must be applied at least four times daily but has more *in vitro* efficacy against FHV-1 than cidofovir (Maggs & Clarke, 2004).
- Apply until one week past resolution of clinical signs, without tapering the dose.
  - □ Due to potential for corneal toxicity with antiviral medications, total duration of treatment should be no longer than approximately four weeks, even if clinical signs persist.

(c) Systemic antiviral medication

- Famciclovir is an alternative to ophthalmically applied antiviral medications.
- Evidence supports doses of 40–90 mg/kg PO q12h to q8h (Sebbag *et al.,* 2016; Thomasy *et al.,* 2016).
- Do not use acyclovir or valacyclovir due to poor bioavailability and potential for fatal toxicity.
- Visible improvement is usually noticed within 3–4 days of starting famciclovir treatment.
- Treat for one week beyond resolution of clinical signs.
- Side effects appear to be infrequent and are mainly gastrointestinal (vomiting, anorexia, and diarrhea).

If *C. felis* or *Mycoplasma* spp. are determined or suspected to be the underlying cause, systemic antibiotic therapy is needed.

- Because this organism can be sequestered at nonocular sites, ophthalmic therapy alone will not clear *C. felis* (Sparkes *et al.,* 1999).
- Doxycycline 5 mg/kg PO q12h for 3–4 weeks.
  - Oral suspension, rather than tablets or capsules, should be used due to risk of esophageal strictures.

2 Tear film supplementation

- Tear film instability (see Chapter 12) associated with goblet cell atrophy can persist for weeks after resolution of visible clinical signs.
- Tear film supplements should therefore be mucinomimetic and maintained for several weeks beyond resolution of clinical signs.

- Hyaluronan 0.2% or higher (ex. I-Drop®Vet, an-HyPro) is the preferred mucinomimetic tear film replacement because of its superior corneal retention time when compared with other lacrimomimetics (Snibson *et al.,* 1992).
  - If frequent application is needed, preservative-free formulations are preferred over multidose vials because ophthalmic preservatives can be toxic to the epithelial surface.
- Administer two to four times daily (or more if preservative-free formulation is used) and continue for 3–4 weeks beyond resolution of clinical signs.

3 Anti-inflammatory therapy

- In cats, anti-inflammatory agents are not necessarily employed as first-line therapy for conjunctivitis.
  - Anti-inflammatory therapy is used as an adjunct to antiviral/antibacterial therapy and tear film supplementation when conjunctivitis is severe or when response to these therapies is less than expected.
- In contrast to the recommended treatment for dogs, ophthalmically applied corticosteroids are not recommended for cats due to the likelihood of infectious etiology.
- CsA (Optimmune®) is preferred over corticosteroids for anti-inflammatory treatment in cats.
  - Dose: 1/4″ strip applied to the affected eye q12h during active episodes of conjunctivitis.
  - CsA can be used in the presence of corneal ulceration.

4 Elimination of stress

- After initial infection, FHV-1 becomes latent within the trigeminal ganglion.
- Stress can induce reactivation of the latent virus.
  - For example, stressors can include corticosteroid treatment, inter-cat aggression, and changes in pet owner schedule.
- If a stressor can be identified and eliminated, then this is a recommended "treatment" (also recommended to prevent future episodes of herpetic disease).

A recheck examination is recommended approximately one to two weeks after initiating treatment. The time interval between future rechecks, and the total number of rechecks required, is determined by patient progress (i.e., degree and time course to improvement of clinical signs).

Prognosis

- The prognosis for resolution of a single episode of herpetic conjunctivitis is good.
  - However, because FHV-1 remains latent within the trigeminal ganglion, the risk of recurrence exists.
  - Recurrence is more likely to occur during times of stress.
  - Some cats develop recurrent diseases without apparent triggers.
- The prognosis for resolution of conjunctivitis due to *C. felis* or *Mycoplasma* spp. is good.
  - However, in a group-housing situation, reexposure can occur if the disease is not eliminated from the population.

Conjunctival neoplasia

What it is
- Neoplastic proliferation of cells on or within the conjunctiva.

Predisposed individuals
- Middle-aged to older dogs and cats develop conjunctival neoplasia more often than younger individuals.
- Dogs that spend more time outdoors, exposed to ultraviolet light, are at higher risk of developing hemangioma and hemangiosarcoma.
- Dogs with little periocular pigment are at higher risk of developing hemangioma/hemangiosarcoma.
- Cats with little periocular pigment are at higher risk of developing squamous cell carcinoma.

Defining characteristics
- Many neoplasms are raised masses on the conjunctival surface (Figures 4.15, 4.16, 4.17, 4.18, 4.19).
- Some neoplasms, especially lymphoma, appear as a diffuse thickening of the conjunctiva (Figure 4.14).
  - The thickening often has a "meaty" appearance.
- Clinical signs of conjunctivitis are present (see beginning of this chapter).
  - With mass-like lesions, conjunctivitis may be confined to the area immediately around the mass or may be diffuse.
  - With diffuse neoplasms, conjunctivitis tends to be more widespread.
- Ulceration of the conjunctiva or hemorrhage within the conjunctiva can also be present.

Clinical significance
- Although many tumor types have been documented in the conjunctiva, overall, conjunctival neoplasia in the dog and cat is much less common than conjunctivitis of other causes.
- Conjunctival neoplasia may exhibit benign or malignant behavior. Specific tumor types that occur more commonly are listed below.
  - Tumors with benign behavior:
    - Papilloma (dogs) (Figures 4.17, 4.19) (Sansom *et al.*, 1996)
    - Hemangioma/hemangiosarcoma (Pirie & Dubielzig, 2006; Pirie *et al.*, 2006)
    - Mast cell tumor (mainly dogs) (Figure 4.20) (Fife *et al.*, 2011)
  - Tumors with invasive or malignant behavior:
    - Squamous cell carcinoma (mainly cats) (Stiles & Townsend, 2007)
    - Melanoma (Reilly *et al.*, 2005; Schobert *et al.*, 2010)
    - Lymphoma (Figure 4.14)
      - Primary conjunctival lymphoma without ocular or systemic involvement may not behave aggressively (Holt *et al.*, 2006; Hong *et al.*, 2011).
- Conjunctival neoplasia may be limited to the conjunctiva or may represent only a portion of disseminated neoplastic disease.

Diagnosis
- Clinical suspicion of neoplasia is based on ophthalmic examination findings.
- Cytologic evaluation of a conjunctival scraping may identify neoplastic cells.
  - Absence of neoplastic cells on cytology does not rule out neoplasia.
- Histopathologic evaluation of the conjunctiva is required for definitive diagnosis.
  - Technique for conjunctival biopsy:
    - A cotton swab is saturated with proparacaine 0.5% ophthalmic solution or 2% lidocaine and applied to the biopsy site for 1 minute. This provides anesthesia to the conjunctival surface.
    - Small forceps, such as Bishop Harmon forceps, are used to grasp the conjunctiva adjacent to the mass. The forceps are pulled up to tent the conjunctiva, elevating the mass and some normal surrounding conjunctiva.
    - Using tenotomy scissors, snip the conjunctiva at the base of the tent, ensuring that the sample includes substantia propria as well as epithelium.
    - The sample is placed onto a flat surface such as a tongue depressor, a piece of paper, or the inside of a tissue cassette to keep it flat and maintain orientation.
    - The sample with the tongue depressor/paper/tissue cassette is then placed into 10% neutral buffered formalin and submitted for histopathology.

Treatment
- For primary conjunctival tumors (as opposed to conjunctival tumors that are a result of metastatic disease), the main goal of treatment is to completely remove the tumor while minimizing damage to adjacent structures and minimizing potential for localized or metastatic tumor spread.
- Treatment depends on the tumor type and behavior. (See Chapter 12 for treatment of third eyelid neoplasia, as same principles apply)

Prognosis
- Prognosis depends on the type of neoplasia.
  - The prognosis is excellent for benign neoplasms such as papilloma, hemangioma/hemangiosarcoma, and mast cell tumors.
    - Excision is usually curative (Fife *et al.*, 2011; Pirie & Dubielzig, 2006; Pirie *et al.*, 2006; Sansom *et al.*, 1996).
  - Conjunctival melanoma
    - The prognosis for cats is poor due to metastasis (Schobert *et al.*, 2010).
    - The prognosis for dogs is guarded due to high potential for recurrence and metastasis (Reilly, *et al.* 2005).
- For squamous cell carcinoma, prognosis is guarded to fair due to recurrence and local invasion.
- Conjunctival lymphoma often represents disseminated disease and prognosis is therefore poor.

∘ However, if localized to the conjunctiva only, excision or adjunctive therapies may be curative (Holt *et al.,* 2006; Hong *et al.,* 2011).

Further reading

Thomasy, SM & Maggs, DJ. 2016. A review of antiviral drugs and other compounds with activity against feline herpesvirus type 1. *Veterinary Ophthalmology.* 19(S1):119-130.

References

Beckwith-Cohen, B, *et al.* 2016. Protozoal infections of the cornea and conjunctiva in dogs associated with chronic ocular surface disease and topical immunosuppression. *Veterinary Ophthalmology.* 19(3):206-213.

Bedford, PGC & Longstaffe, JA. 1979. Corneal pannus (chronic superficial keratitis) in the German shepherd dog. *Journal of Small Animal Practice.* 20(1):41.

Campbell, LH, *et al.* 1973. Ocular bacteria and mycoplasma of the clinically normal cat. *Feline Practice.* 3(1)10–12.

Drazenovich, TL, *et al.* 2009. Effects of dietary lysine supplementation on upper respiratory and ocular disease and detection of infectious organisms in cats within an animal shelter. *American Journal of Veterinary Research.* 70(11):1391–1400.

Fife, M, *et al.* 2011. Canine conjunctival mast cell tumors: a retrospective study. *Veterinary Ophthalmology.* 14(3):153–160.

Gerding, PA & Kakoma, I. 1990. Microbiology of the canine and feline eye. *Veterinary Clinics of North America: Small Animal Practice.* 20(3):615 625.

Gervais, KJ, *et al.* 2012. Acute primary canine herpevirus-1 dendritic ulcerative keratitis in an adult dog. *Veterinary Ophthalmology.* 15(2):133-138.

Holt, E, *et al.* 2006. Extranodal conjunctival Hodgkin's-like lymphoma in a cat. *Veterinary Ophthalmology.* 9(3):141–144.

Hong, IH, *et al.* 2011. Mucosa-associated lymphoid tissue lymphoma of the third eyelid conjunctiva in a dog. *Veterinary Ophthalmology.* 14(1):61–65.

Kaswan, RL & Salisbury, MA. 1990. A new perspective on canine keratoconjunctivitis sicca. *Veterinary Clinics of North America: Small Animal Practice.* 20(3):583–613.

Ledbetter, EC, *et al.* 2009. Virologic survey of dogs with naturally acquired idiopathic conjunctivitis. *Journal of the American Veterinary Medical Association.* 235(8):954-959.

Ledbetter, EC, *et al.* 2021. Comparative efficacy of topical ophthalmic ganciclovir and oral famciclovir in cats with experimental ocular feline herpesvirus-1 infection. *Proceedings of the 52nd Annual ACVO Scientific Conference*, Indianapolis, USA, September 29-October 2, 2021.

Low, HC, *et al.* 2007. Prevalence of feline herpes virus 1, *Chlamydophila felis*, and *Mycoplasma* spp DNA in conjunctival cells collected from cats with and without conjunctivitis. *American Journal of Veterinary Research.* 68(6):643–648.

Maggs, DJ & Clarke, HE. 2004. In vitro efficacy of ganciclovir, cidofovir, penciclovir, foscarnet, idoxuridine, and acyclovir against feline herpesvirus type-1. *American Journal of Veterinary Research.* 65(4):399–403.

Pena, MT, *et al.* 2008. Canine conjunctivitis and blepharitis. *Veterinary Clinics of North America Small Animal Practice.* 18(2):233–249.

Pirie, CG & Dubielzig, RR. 2006. Feline conjunctival hemangioma and hemangiosarcoma: a retrospective evaluation of eight cases (1993–2004). *Veterinary Ophthalmology.* 9(4):227–231.

Pirie, CG, *et al.* 2006. Canine conjunctival hemangioma and hemangiosarcoma: a retrospective evaluation of 108 cases (1989–2004). *Veterinary Ophthalmology.* 9(4):215–226.

Reilly, CM, *et al.* 2005. Abstract no. 39. Features of canine conjunctival melanocytic tumors. *Veterinary Ophthalmology.* 8(6):443.

Rosendal, S. 1973. Canine mycoplasmas I: cultivation from conjunctivae, respiratory- and genital tracts. *Acta Pathologica Microbiologica Scandinavica.* 81B(4):441–445.

Samuelson, DA, *et al.* 1984. Conjunctival fungal flora in horses, cattle, dogs, and cats. *Journal of the American Veterinary Medical Association.* 184(10):1240–1242.

Sanchez, MD, *et al.* Pathology in Practice. *Journal of the American Veterinary Medical Association.* 240(4):385-387.

Sansom, J, *et al.* 1996. Canine conjunctival papilloma: a review of five cases. *Journal of Small Animal Practice.* 37(2):84–86.

Schobert, CS, *et al.* 2010. Feline conjunctival melanoma: histopathological characteristics and clinical outcomes. *Veterinary Ophthalmology.* 13(1):43–46.

Sebbag, L, *et al.* 2016. Pharmacokinetic modeling of penciclovir and BRL42359 in the plasma and tears of healthy cats to optimize dosage recommendations for oral administration of famciclovir. *American Journal of Veterinary Research.* 77(8):833-845.

Snibson, GR, *et al.* 1992. Ocular surface residence times of artificial tear solutions. *Cornea.* 11(4):288–293.

Sparkes, AH, *et al.* 1999. The clinical efficacy of topical and systemic therapy for the treatment of feline ocular chlamydiosis. *Journal of Feline Medicine and Surgery.* 1(1):31–35.

Stiles, J & Townsend, WM. 2007. Feline ophthalmology. In: Veterinary Ophthalmology (ed KN Gelatt), 4th edn, p. 1098–1099. Blackwell Publishing, Ames, LA.

Stiles, J, *et al.* 2002. Effect of oral administration of L-lysine on conjunctivitis cause by feline herpesvirus in cats. *American Journal of Veterinary Research.* 63(1):99–103.

Thomasy, SM, *et al.* 2016. Oral administration of famciclovir for treatment of spontaneous ocular, respiratory, or dermatologic disease attributed to feline herpesvirus type 1: 59 cases (2006–2013). *American Journal of Veterinary Research.* 249 (5):526-538.

CHAPTER 13

14 Cornea

Please see Chapter 5 for images of the cornea.

The cornea is the clear portion of the outer, fibrous tunic of the eye. From external to internal (i.e., from anterior to posterior or from superficial to deep), the four layers of the cornea are as follows:
- Epithelium
  - Five to seven cell layers thick
  - Hydrophobic
- Stroma
  - The majority of the corneal thickness
  - Hydrophilic
  - Nerves are found within the corneal stroma; the density of fibers is highest in the superficial one-third of the stroma.
- Descemet's membrane
  - Thin basement membrane secreted by the endothelium
  - Hydrophobic
- Endothelium
  - Single layer of cells lining the inner cornea

With the sclera, the cornea contributes to the physical shape of the globe. Another important function is to focus light entering the eye. A third function is light transmission, which is maximized by the clear, colorless nature of the cornea.

In health, the cornea is clear, smooth, and colorless. Factors contributing to this state include the following:
- Smooth corneal surface
  - The epithelium is nonkeratinized.
  - Surface irregularities are smoothed out by mucin in the precorneal tear film.
- Relative dehydration (also referred to as deturgescence)
  - The hypertonic precorneal tear film draws fluid out of the cornea.
  - The hydrophobic corneal epithelium is a barrier to entry of fluid into the cornea.
  - Pumps in the corneal endothelium actively remove fluid from the corneal stroma.
- Arrangement of the stromal collagen
  - Bundles of collagen are closely aligned in an orderly fashion.
  - This arrangement reduces scatter of light passing through the cornea.

- Lack of blood vessels
  - Lack of blood vessels increases corneal clarity; nutrition is obtained through the precorneal tear film and aqueous humor.
- Lack of pigment
- Low cellularity

In disease, the cornea loses its clear, colorless character. Signs of corneal disease include the following:
- A dry or roughened corneal surface (Figures 5.1, 5.2, 5.3)
  - When diffuse, this often indicates a deficiency of the precorneal tear film (see the section about KCS later in this chapter, and the section on qualitative tear film abnormalities in Chapter 12).
  - Focal corneal irregularities may indicate a localized irritant (e.g., eyelid mass) and/or corneal ulceration.
    - Location of the lesion usually correlates with location of the irritant.
- Corneal vascularization
  - Vessels enter the cornea from the limbus approximately 3 days following an insult, then lengthen by approximately 1 mm/day.
  - Superficial corneal vessels (Figures 5.1, 5.4, 5.5, 5.6, 5.7, 5.8)
    - This indicates superficial keratitis.
    - Disease primarily affects the ocular surface and superficial layers of the cornea.
    - Some causes of superficial corneal vascularization include extraocular diseases (eyelid diseases and diseases of the precorneal tear film) and superficial corneal ulceration.
    - Superficial corneal vessels appear red, long, thin, with regular branching ("tree-like").
  - Deep corneal vessels (Figures 5.9, 5.19, 5.21)
    - This indicates deep keratitis (stromal keratitis).
    - Disease involves deeper layers of the cornea and/or the intraocular structures.
    - Some causes of deep corneal vascularization include deep or perforating corneal ulcers, anterior uveitis, and glaucoma.

Small Animal Ophthalmic Atlas and Guide, Second Edition. Christine C. Lim.
© 2023 John Wiley & Sons, Inc. Published 2023 by John Wiley & Sons, Inc.
Companion website: www.wiley.com/go/lim/atlas

- When compared with superficial corneal vessels, deep vessels are thicker and have less branching ("hedge-like").
- Corneal edema (Figures 5.10, 5.11, 5.12)
  - Corneal edema appears bluish-white to white and hazy, with a "cobblestone" or "chicken-wire" pattern.
  - Fluid influx causes corneal swelling; distortion of the normal, orderly arrangement of the stromal lamellae; and increased spacing between lamellae.
  - Corneal edema indicates compromised corneal epithelium, endothelium, or both.
    - Edema associated with superficial epithelial defects tends to be concentrated around the epithelial defect (e.g., the edges of a corneal ulcer) (Figures 5.37, 5.39).
    - When associated with endothelial defects, edema tends to diffusely affect the cornea (Figures 5.10, 5.11, 5.12).
      - For example, edema caused by uveitis, glaucoma, and primary endothelial dysfunction (e.g., endothelial dystrophy and degeneration).
- Brown discoloration
  - Corneal melanosis (occurs more often in dogs than cats) (Figures 5.13, 5.14, 5.15, 5.16, 5.18, 5.30, 5.31, 5.32, 5.33)
    - A result of chronic corneal irritation.
    - Causes include eyelid diseases, KCS, brachycephalic conformation, and pannus.
    - Location of the melanin often correlates with source of irritation.
  - Corneal sequestrum (mostly affects cats; rare in dogs) (see section on corneal sequestrum later in this chapter) (Figures 5.69, 5.70, 5.71, 5.72, 5.73, 5.74)
    - A result of chronic corneal irritation.
    - Common causes are brachycephalic conformation and corneal ulceration.
  - Uveal prolapse (Figures 5.49, 5.50, 5.51, 5.52, 5.53, 5.54, 5.55)
    - Full-thickness corneal defect with protrusion of iris (see section on deep and perforating corneal ulceration later in this chapter).
- Corneal fibrosis (Figures 5.17, 5.18)
  - Fibrosis causes a white to gray discoloration of the cornea.
  - Can indicate chronic, active inflammation or a previous corneal inflammatory episode.
- Stromal white cell infiltrate (Figures 5.19, 5.20, 5.21, 5.55, 5.56, 5.57, 5.58, 5.59)
  - Densely white to yellow–white, sometimes referred to as having a "creamy" appearance.
    - Can appear similar to purulent discharge, but it is embedded within the cornea.
  - When present, corneal white cell infiltrate should raise suspicion for corneal infection.
- Refractile, white corneal deposits (Figures 5.22, 5.23, 5.24, 5.25, 5.26, 5.27, 5.28, 5.29)
  - Lipid or mineral deposits have a crystalline appearance often described as "sparkly" or like "ground glass."

- Potential causes include breed-related corneal dystrophy and lipid and/or mineral deposits secondary to concurrent ocular or systemic disorders.

Careful ophthalmic examination will help determine the underlying cause of the aforementioned corneal changes.

- Because of their roles in nutrition and protection to the ocular surface, diseases of the eyelids, the third eyelid, and the precorneal tear film often cause superficial corneal disease.
- Through alterations of aqueous humor dynamics, corneal nutrition, and corneal function, intraocular diseases can cause deep corneal disease.

Corneal diseases

Corneal dystrophy

What it is
- Breed-related corneal lipid deposits without accompanying inflammation.

Predisposed individuals
- Corneal dystrophy mainly affects dogs.
- Some predisposed breeds include rough collies, Siberian huskies, and Cavalier King Charles spaniels.

Defining characteristics
- Bilaterally symmetrical, round to oval corneal opacities (Figures 5.22, 5.23, 5.24, 5.25).
- Central or paracentral location.
- The opacities are refractile and white to gray in color.
- The lesions occupy less than 50% of the corneal surface area.
- Other ocular abnormalities are absent.

Clinical significance
- Corneal dystrophy may be heritable.
- The corneal opacities are usually clinically insignificant for the affected individual, as corneal dystrophy is rarely associated with detectable ocular discomfort or visual compromise.

Diagnosis
- The diagnosis of corneal dystrophy is based on characteristic appearance (see "Defining characteristics") of ocular lesions in a predisposed breed.
- Although development of corneal dystrophy is not associated with ocular or systemic disease, concurrent disease can alter the appearance of corneal dystrophy (Crispin, 2002).
  - Beyond the ophthalmic examination, further diagnostics as dictated by clinical suspicion include the following:
    - Assessment of serum triglycerides and cholesterol.
    - Testing for endocrinopathies such as hypothyroidism, hyperadrenocorticism, and diabetes mellitus.

Treatment
- Corneal dystrophy rarely requires treatment.

Prognosis

- The prognosis for maintenance of vision and ocular comfort is very good.
- Lesions are not associated with visual deficits or other ocular disease.

Additional information

- Refractile, white corneal deposits associated with corneal vascularization are not corneal dystrophy (Figures 5.26, 5.27, 5.28, 5.29).
  - Lesions of this type are referred to as corneal degeneration and may be due to lipid or mineral deposits.
  - Lesions may be unilateral or bilateral.
    - If bilateral, they are not symmetrical.
  - Concurrent ocular and/or systemic disorders are present.
    - Diagnostics as for corneal dystrophy are recommended.
    - Treatment for specific concurrent disease is required for improvement of corneal degeneration.
    - Treatment for keratitis is also indicated (see the section discussing keratitis).
  - If the deposits are substantial, they can become irritating to the cornea and incite further keratitis.

Corneal endothelial dysfunction

What it is

- Impaired function of and/or reduced numbers of corneal endothelial cells, resulting in corneal edema.
  - The altered endothelium is unable adequately remove fluid from the cornea.

Predisposed individuals

- Some breeds predisposed to corneal edema as a result of dystrophic endothelial cells include Boston terriers and German short-haired pointers.
- Dogs of advanced age are more likely to develop corneal edema secondary to age-related endothelial cell loss.
- Previous intraocular disease (e.g., uveitis, anterior lens luxation) increases the risk of corneal endothelial cell damage and resultant corneal edema.

Defining characteristics

- Corneal edema (Figures 5.10, 5.11, 5.12)
  - In early disease, edema may be localized and relatively faint.
  - Over time, edema becomes diffuse and more opaque.
  - Dystrophic endothelium and age-related endothelial loss usually cause bilateral corneal edema, which may or may not be symmetrical between eyes.

Clinical significance

- Progressive opacification of the cornea will progressively reduce vision.

- Corneal bullae (Figure 5.12), which can occur with fluid buildup, can rupture and lead to corneal ulceration.
  - The healing course of these ulcers may be protracted and ulcers may be recurrent; patients with endothelial dysfunction may therefore become chronically painful.

Diagnosis

- The diagnosis is made by visualizing corneal edema as mentioned earlier.
- Because serious ocular disease such as uveitis and glaucoma can also cause corneal edema, these must be ruled out at the time of diagnosis.

Treatment

- The goal of treatment is to reduce corneal edema, thereby improving vision and decreasing potential for complications such as bullae and ulcers.
- Hypertonic saline (5% NaCl) may be applied to the affected cornea q8h–q6h, or more often, with the goal of drawing fluid out of the cornea.
  - The effect is usually small and does not result in visible change to the edema.
  - This does not stop progression of disease; corneal edema will worsen over time.
  - This therapy becomes insufficient as disease progresses.
  - Hypertonic saline ointment may be more effective than solution at reducing corneal edema (Samuel *et al.*, 2019).
  - This treatment can be initiated while the patient awaits referral to a veterinary ophthalmologist.
- Because corneal edema will progress, surgical intervention on a referral basis should be considered.
  - Palliative therapy, such as thermokeratoplasty, can be performed with the goal of improving comfort but not vision (Miller *et al.*, 2003).
  - Other procedures, such as conjunctival grafting or endothelial transplantation, can be performed with the goal of also improving corneal clarity (Armor *et al.*, 2019; Giannikaki *et al.*, 2020).

Prognosis

- Endothelial cell dysfunction is progressive, although the rate varies between individuals.
- While patients may be comfortable and visual early in the disease process, the severity of the edema will worsen over time, leading to deterioration of visual function and increasing the risk of corneal ulceration.

Additional information

- Although patients may not be uncomfortable or visually compromised early on, referral to a veterinary ophthalmologist before disease becomes advanced can improve outcome should surgery be performed.

Canine keratitis

What it is
- Inflammation of the cornea.
- Superficial keratitis: inflammation of the corneal epithelium and/or superficial stroma.
- Deep or stromal keratitis: inflammation of the deeper stromal layers of the cornea.
- Nonulcerative keratitis refers to keratitis that is not associated with a break in the corneal epithelium.
- Ulcerative keratitis refers to keratitis that is associated with a disruption of the corneal epithelium, that is, a corneal ulcer.

Predisposed individuals
- Individual and breed predispositions vary with the cause of keratitis.
- Brachycephalic dogs are predisposed to superficial exposure keratitis resulting from their conformational defects and are also more prone to keratitis induced by external trauma.
- Some breeds that are predisposed to KCS include the following:
  - West Highland white terrier
  - English bulldog
  - Lhasa apso
  - Shih tzu
  - Cavalier King Charles spaniel
  - Pug
- Dogs with diabetes mellitus, hypothyroidism, and hyperadrenocorticism are predisposed to KCS.
- Pigmentary keratitis affects dog breeds with conformational exophthalmos, such as the following:
  - Lhasa apso
  - Shih tzu
  - Pug
  - Pekingese
- Dogs predisposed to pannus include German shepherds and related breeds, greyhounds, and border collies.
- Predispositions to specific types of corneal ulceration are listed under those respective headings.

Defining characteristics
- Refer to the beginning of this chapter for signs of corneal disease.
- *Corneal vascularization*
  - Superficial vessels occur with superficial keratitis (Figures 5.1, 5.4, 5.5, 5.6, 5.7, 5.8).
  - Deep vessels occur with deep keratitis (Figures 5.9, 5.19, 5.21).
- Variable amounts of corneal edema (Figures 5.10, 5.11, 5.12), fibrosis (Figures 5.17, 5.18), and/or melanosis (Figures 5.13, 5.14, 5.15, 5.16, 5.18, 5.30, 5.31, 5.32, 5.33)
- Ocular discharge
  - Serous, mucoid, or mucopurulent
- Conjunctivitis (Chapter 13) is usually also present.

- The combination of corneal and conjunctival inflammation is referred to as keratoconjunctivitis.
- The terms keratitis and keratoconjunctivitis will be used interchangeably in this book.

Clinical significance
- Keratitis is uncomfortable.
- The corneal opacification that occurs with keratitis can lead to visual impairment or blindness.
- The inflamed cornea is unhealthy and at higher risk of developing other ocular diseases (e.g., corneal ulceration).
- Keratitis has underlying causes (e.g., eyelid defects, KCS, immune-mediated inflammation, and intraocular disease) that must be addressed for treatment to be successful.
- In dogs, conformation, eyelid disease, KCS, and trauma are common causes of keratoconjunctivitis.
  - However, sometimes, an obvious cause is not found and keratitis is presumed to be immune-mediated.

Diagnosis
The diagnostic process involves first diagnosing keratitis, then determining the underlying cause of the corneal inflammation.
1 Diagnosis of keratitis
  - Keratitis is diagnosed by visualizing signs of corneal disease (discussed at the beginning of this chapter).
    - Determination of inflammation depth is important as this will help to narrow the potential causes.
2 Determining the cause of keratitis
  - The cause of keratitis is determined by careful ophthalmic examination and ancillary diagnostic testing.
  - Examination of the facial structure will determine if brachycephalic conformation is present.
  - Assessment of palpebral reflex will determine if lagophthalmos is present.
  - Assessment of menace response will determine if the patient can protect the eye by blinking in response to objects moving toward the eye.
  - The STT identifies KCS.
  - The TFBUT identifies qualitative tear film disorders (see Chapter 12).
  - Tonometry helps to identify glaucoma and uveitis.
  - The following are found with careful eyelid examination:
    - Entropion or ectropion
    - Irregularities of the eyelid margin, such as those caused by previous eyelid injuries or surgeries
    - Trichiasis
    - Distichiae
    - Ectopic cilia
    - Eyelid masses or chalazia
  - Careful inspection of the conjunctival fornices and the area between the third eyelid and globe will rule out conjunctival foreign material.
  - Consideration of signalment will also help identify causes of keratitis, due to strong breed predispositions in many cases.

○ In dogs, diagnosis of immune-mediated keratoconjunctivitis should only be made after careful ophthalmic examination and ancillary testing fails to identify a cause.

Treatment

- The goals of treatment are to eliminate inflammation and ocular discomfort.
- Treatment involves (i) treatment of the underlying cause, (ii) anti-inflammatory medications, and (iii) tear film supplementation.
- Treatment for specific syndromes will be discussed later in this chapter under the sections for each specific disease syndrome.
- Nonspecific anti-inflammatory treatment and tear film supplementation, as used for presumed immune-mediated keratoconjunctivitis, are as follows:
  1 Anti-inflammatory therapy: corticosteroids or CsA
    ▪ Corticosteroids
      □ Do not use if corneal ulceration is present.
      □ Not recommended if corneal mineral or lipid deposits are present due to potential for exacerbation of these deposits.
      □ Prednisolone acetate 1% ophthalmic suspension or dexamethasone (0.1% ophthalmic solution or in preparations combined with neomycin and polymyxin B).
      □ Initially, apply one drop of solution/suspension or 1/4″ strip of ointment to the affected eye two to four times daily depending on the severity of disease.
        ◆ Improvement is usually noted within 1–2 weeks of starting therapy.
        ◆ Dose should be gradually tapered as clinical signs improve.
        ◆ The goal is to eventually completely discontinue medications or to taper to the lowest possible dose required to control clinical signs.
        ◆ If indefinite management is required, use no more than one to two times daily.
    ▪ CsA
      □ Cyclosporine 0.2% ophthalmic ointment (Optimmune®).
      □ Dose: 1/4″ strip applied to the affected eye q12h.
      □ Can be used in the presence of corneal ulceration.
      □ Improvement may not be noted before 3 to 4 weeks of treatment.
      □ In addition to anti-inflammatory effects, CsA improves mucin production by the conjunctival goblet cells and therefore also has a stabilizing effect on the precorneal tear film.
      □ For long-term use, CsA is preferred over corticosteroids due to potential for steroid keratopathy and lower risk of complications if corneal ulceration were to develop.
  2 Tear film supplementation
    ▪ See the sections on canine and feline conjunctivitis in Chapter 13 for rationale.
    ▪ In patients with brachycephalic ocular syndrome, long-term or indefinite supplementation of artificial tears

can improve patient comfort and reduce the potential or severity of future surface ocular disease.

Prognosis

- The prognosis for controlling mild or focal keratitis is good provided the underlying cause (e.g., entropion, eyelid mass, and KCS) is treated.
- With more severe inflammation, or keratitis that is chronic or widespread, the potential for permanent corneal opacities (e.g., fibrosis, melanosis) and visual disturbance increases and patients are at elevated risk of developing complications like corneal ulceration.

Keratoconjunctivitis sicca (KCS)

What it is

- Deficiency of the aqueous portion of the tear film resulting in surface ocular inflammation.
- Tear production, as measured by the STT, is below 15 mm/min.
- Also referred to as a quantitative tear film abnormality.

Predisposed individuals

- KCS mainly affects dogs and occurs less often in cats.
  ○ This section will focus on dogs; aqueous tear deficiency in cats will be addressed under "Feline keratitis, nonulcerative and ulcerative."
- Predisposed breeds include the following:
  ○ West Highland white terrier
  ○ Cavalier King Charles spaniel
  ○ English bulldog
  ○ Lhasa apso
  ○ Shih tzu
  ○ Pug

Defining characteristics

- *Copious sticky mucoid discharge* (Figure 5.4).
  ○ Discharge adheres to the ocular surface.
  ○ Discharge is crusted within periocular hairs.
  ○ Discharge is not easily rinsed from the corneal surface.
  ○ Owners report constant buildup of discharge in spite of multiple cleanings per day.
- Dry, roughened corneal surface (Figures 5.1, 5.2, 5.3).
  ○ This can be recognized by seeing that the edges of the reflections on the cornea are indistinct rather than clear.
- *Superficial corneal vascularization* (Figures 5.1, 5.4, 5.5, 5.6, 5.7, 5.8).
  ○ Often accompanied by corneal edema and/or fibrosis.
- *Conjunctival hyperemia* (Figures 4.2, 5.3, 5.7).
- *STT value below 15 mm/min.*

Clinical significance

- KCS is uncomfortable.
  ○ Patients with markedly decreased tear production are usually overtly in pain.

- Adequate precorneal tear film is required for a healthy ocular surface.
  - Functions of the precorneal tear film include nutrition and oxygenation of the cornea, immunologic defense, lubrication of the ocular surface, and removal of debris and metabolic wastes (see Chapter 12).
- Flushing of microorganisms from the conjunctival sac is less efficient with reduced tears; therefore, dogs with KCS are more likely to develop bacterial conjunctivitis.
- Due to frictional irritation of the ocular surface, KCS predisposes to corneal ulceration and delays healing of corneal ulcers.
- Corneal ulcers are at increased risk of infection due to delayed re-epithelialization and accumulation of microbes within the conjunctival sac.
- Chronic corneal irritation leads to corneal opacification.
  - Prolonged duration and severity of irritation can lead to significant visual compromise or even blindness.
- KCS has many potential causes, which must be addressed for effective treatment:
  - Congenital lacrimal gland aplasia or hypoplasia
  - Metabolic disease: hyperadrenocorticism, diabetes mellitus, and hypothyroidism (Williams et al., 2007)
  - Neoplasia of the orbital lacrimal gland or third eyelid gland
  - Infectious disease such as canine distemper
  - Immune-mediated adenitis
    - The most common cause of KCS in dogs
  - Iatrogenic: removal of the third eyelid gland
  - Chronic third eyelid gland prolapse
  - Neurogenic: lesion of the parasympathetic supply to the lacrimal gland.
  - Drugs such as atropine, sulfonamides, etodolac, acetaminophen, and long-acting otic medications (Bercovitz et al., 2021; Kaswan & Salisbury, 1990; Kaswan et al., 1989; Klauss et al., 2007; Mariani & Fulton, 2001).
  - General anesthesia lowers tear production, but this is transient (lasting ~24 hours after anesthesia) and not truly KCS.

Diagnosis

The diagnosis is aimed at (1) diagnosing KCS and (2) diagnosing the cause of KCS.
1 Diagnosing KCS
  - The diagnosis is based on clinical signs and the STT.
2 Diagnosing the underlying cause of KCS
  - KCS in a puppy or very young dog, especially if unilateral, is likely to be congenital lacrimal gland aplasia or hypoplasia.
  - Thorough history will rule out drug-induced KCS.
  - Physical examination and appropriate laboratory testing will rule out metabolic and infectious diseases.
  - Careful ophthalmic examination will detect third eyelid gland prolapse or neoplasia.
  - Thorough history and careful ophthalmic examination will rule out third eyelid gland removal.
  - Physical examination may raise suspicion for lacrimal gland neoplasia if signs of orbital mass are seen (see Chapter 10).
  - Observation of a dry, crusted nare ipsilateral to the affected eye is highly supportive of a neurogenic lesion (due to shared nerve supply) (Matheis et al., 2012).
  - When no obvious cause is identified, KCS is presumed to be immune-mediated.

Treatment

- The goals of KCS treatment are to improve patient comfort, restore normal tear production, and reduce/eliminate surface ocular inflammation.
- Treatment therefore has several components: (1) removal of accumulated discharge, (2) lubrication, (3) lacrimostimulant therapy, and (4) anti-inflammatory therapy.
1 Removal of accumulated discharge
  - Discharge crusted into the periocular hairs should be removed as needed.
  - This will improve patient comfort.
  - The conjunctival sac is rinsed with eyewash to remove accumulated discharge.
  - Performed as needed and immediately prior to medication application to allow medications to reach the ocular surface.
  - Reduces buildup of bacteria that are normally cleared by tears.
2 Lubrication
  - Apply one drop of an artificial tear solution to the affected eye two to four times daily, or more, depending on the severity of KCS.
  - Treat until patient tear production has normalized and signs of keratitis have abated.
  - Many formulations are available.
    - When frequent application is needed, preservative-free tears are preferred due to potential of epithelial toxicity induced by preservatives.
3 Lacrimostimulant therapy
  - Optimmune® (0.2% CsA) is labeled for treatment of canine KCS.
    - Apply 1/4″ strip to the affected eye q12h.
    - For most patients, tear production increases within 1 month of treatment (Kaswan & Salisbury, 1990; Morgan & Abrams, 1991).
    - Occasionally, response to therapy requires more than 1 month (Morgan & Abrams, 1991).
    - CsA suppresses inflammatory response in the lacrimal gland and stimulates lacrimation by influencing hormonal regulation of lacrimation (Kaswan, 1994).
    - CsA also increases mucin stores in the conjunctival goblet cells (Moore et al., 2001).
  - Alternatives exist for patients that do not respond to Optimmune® therapy.

- CsA 1 or 2% ophthalmic solution.
  - Suitable alternative for dogs that partially respond to Optimmune®.
- Tacrolimus 0.02 or 0.03% ophthalmic solution (Berdoulay *et al.,* 2005; Hendrix *et al.,* 2011).
  - Suitable for dogs that do not respond to CsA.
  - Similar mode of action to CsA.
- Both must be compounded by a licensed pharmacist.
- Both are applied to the affected eye q12h.
- Therapy must be applied lifelong; tear production is likely to decrease after medications are discontinued.
- Pilocarpine may be useful for neurogenic KCS.
  - Available as 1 or 2% ophthalmic solution.
    - The ophthalmic solution is applied by mouth or in the food, *not to the eye*, as application of these strengths results in severe ocular irritation.
    - Starting dose is two drops of 2% ophthalmic solution per 10 kg, administered twice daily.
    - Dose is gradually increased by one drop until improvement or until signs of toxicity (vomiting, ptyalism, and diarrhea) are seen.
  - Also may be compounded as a 0.1% ophthalmic solution.
    - This can be applied to the eye, with decreased risk of ocular irritation when compared to the 1 and 2% solutions.
    - Apply up to four times daily (Wegg, 2019).
  - Variable efficacy for improving tear production.
4 Anti-inflammatory therapy
  - CsA and tacrolimus have anti-inflammatory effects.
  - In addition to CsA or tacrolimus, adjunctive ophthalmic corticosteroid therapy is used for patients with moderate to marked surface ocular inflammation.
    - Augments anti-inflammatory action of CsA or tacrolimus.
    - Used in the short term after diagnosis, when inflammation is most severe.
  - Do not use in the presence of corneal ulceration.
  - Prednisolone acetate ophthalmic suspension 1% or dexamethasone (0.1% ophthalmic solution or in combination with neomycin and polymyxin B in both ointment and suspension forms).
  - Apply one drop or 1/4″ strip to the affected eye two to four times daily, depending on the severity of inflammation.
  - Taper dose as inflammation subsides, and eventually discontinue.

First recheck of tear production is recommended within 3–4 weeks of starting therapy. Further rechecks are determined by patient progress and control of tear production. After control of tear production is achieved, once- to twice-yearly rechecks are recommended to ensure continued control of tear production.

Prognosis

- Newly diagnosed cases of KCS have a very good chance of responding to Optimmune® therapy if STT values are greater than 2 mm/min (Kaswan *et al.,* 1989).
- Prognosis is fair to poor for response to Optimmune® if STT is less than 2 mm/min (Kaswan *et al.,* 1989).
- Approximately half of dogs that do not respond to CsA therapy will respond to tacrolimus (Berdoulay *et al.,* 2005).
- Spontaneous resolution may occur in dogs with neurogenic KCS (Matheis *et al.,* 2012).

Additional information

- KCS causes ocular discomfort that cannot be managed with the application of artificial tears alone.
- Cases refractory to treatment should be referred to a veterinary ophthalmologist.
  - If response to medical management is inadequate, parotid duct transposition (PDT) or episcleral cyclosporine implantation may be indicated.
  - With PDT, the parotid duct papilla is transposed from the mouth into the conjunctival sac so that saliva provides moisture to the eye.
  - With episcleral cyclosporine, a sustained-release implant continuously delivers cyclosporine to the eye.
    - This may decrease or eliminate the need for daily medication.
    - The lifespan of the implant is not known and repeat surgery is likely needed (Barachetti *et al.,* 2015).

Pigmentary keratitis

What it is

- Corneal melanosis resulting from chronic corneal irritation.
- The term pigmentary keratitis is often used to specifically describe the pattern of melanin deposition in dogs with brachycephalic ocular syndrome, where melanin is deposited onto the medial corneal quadrants in a bilateral and relatively symmetrical pattern.
- For this discussion, pigmentary keratitis will refer to the specific pattern of corneal melanin seen in dogs with brachycephalic ocular syndrome.

Predisposed individuals

- Brachycephalic dogs are predisposed.

Defining characteristics

- Brachycephalic dogs
  - Exophthalmos
  - Enlarged palpebral fissures
  - Medial trichiasis (due to ventromedial entropion, hairs within medial canthus, and nasal folds).
- Melanin is deposited primarily within the medial corneal quadrant (Figures 5.13, 5.14, 5.15, 5.16).
- See Chapter 10 for further discussion of brachycephalic ocular syndrome.

Clinical significance

- Progressive corneal melanosis can lead to visual compromise or even blindness.
- Chronic corneal inflammation can predispose to development of corneal ulceration.
- Chronic inflammation of the cornea is uncomfortable.

Diagnosis

- The diagnosis is based on the characteristic appearance of bilateral, medially located corneal melanosis in a dog with the anatomic defects of brachycephalic ocular syndrome.

Treatment

- The goal is to decrease surface ocular inflammation and corneal opacification by removing or reducing the underlying cause of chronic irritation.
- It is generally not possible to significantly reduce corneal pigment that is already present; rather, treatment is aimed at reducing further progression.
- See "Brachycephalic ocular syndrome" in Chapter 10 for discussion of medical and surgical therapies for pigmentary keratitis.

Prognosis

- The prognosis is poor for removing corneal melanin that is already present.
- The prognosis is good for at least slowing progression of the melanin, as long as treatment is instituted (as per "Brachycephalic ocular syndrome" in Chapter 10) and the underlying causes are addressed.

Additional information

- Although it is possible to modestly reduce the corneal melanin, it is usually not possible to cause significant regression of corneal melanin.
- Treatment is therefore recommended early in the disease process, rather than waiting until significant corneal melanosis is present.
- Medications are usually required in the long term, even if surgery is elected for brachycephalic ocular syndrome.

Pannus/chronic superficial keratitis

What it is

- Bilateral, chronic, superficial lymphoplasmacytic corneal inflammation.
- The term chronic superficial keratitis is used interchangeably with pannus.

Predisposed individuals

- Predisposed breeds include the following:
  - German shepherd and similar breeds
  - Greyhound
  - Border collie

Defining characteristics

- Bilateral, chronic, superficial keratitis, usually starting at the lateral and ventrolateral corneal quadrants.
  - Other corneal quadrants may be primarily affected or the entire cornea can be affected.
  - May appear predominantly melanotic (Figures 5.30, 5.31), predominantly fibrovascular (Figure 5.32), or a relatively even mixture of the two presentations (Figure 5.33).
  - The third eyelids may be involved (Figures 3.17, 3.18, 3.19, 5.32) in addition to corneal disease, or in absence of corneal disease.
    - When the third eyelids are the only tissue affected, this is sometimes referred to as plasmoma.

Clinical significance

- Pannus is an immune-mediated disease.
- Ultraviolet (UV) light exposure exacerbates signs of pannus.
- Chronic keratitis can be uncomfortable.
- Uncontrolled pannus can be blinding.

Diagnosis

- The diagnosis is made on characteristic appearance.
  - Especially if the patient is of a predisposed breed.
- Other causes of chronic irritation to the lateral cornea should be ruled out.

Treatment

- The goals of treatment are to reduce or eliminate corneal opacification and to decrease surface ocular inflammation.
- Treatment is therefore aimed at immune suppression and reducing UV light exposure.
- Treatment is lifelong, at the lowest effective dose required to control symptoms.

1 Immune suppression.
  - Corticosteroids, CsA, or both in combination
    - This author begins therapy with both classes of drugs, with the goal of weaning completely off corticosteroids but continuing CsA as long-term treatment.
  - Corticosteroids
    - Prednisolone acetate ophthalmic suspension 1% or dexamethasone 0.1% ophthalmic solution.
    - Do not use in the presence of corneal ulceration.
    - Start with one drop applied to the eyes two to four times daily, depending on the severity of keratitis.
    - Gradually taper the dose at 2- to 3-week intervals.
  - CsA
    - Optimmune® is licensed for treatment of pannus.
    - Apply 1/4″ strip to the eyes twice daily.
    - Preferred over corticosteroids for long-term use.
2 Reducing UV light exposure
  - Goggles designed for dogs can be outfitted with lenses that block UV light.
    - To be worn outside under the same conditions in which people wear sunglasses.

- Limit outdoor activity to times of day when UV intensity is less intense.

The first recheck examination is recommended for approximately 4 weeks after initial examination. Further rechecks are determined by patient improvement (i.e., the degree to which the corneal lesions regress). After pannus has been controlled, periodic rechecks are recommended because medication doses will require adjustments over time.

Prognosis

- The prognosis is good for halting progression of keratitis.
- The prognosis is good for reducing the amount of cornea affected.
- However, corneal lesions are rarely eliminated completely.
- The severity of keratitis will vary over time.
  - Due to factors such as seasonal variations in daylight hours and the amount of time spent outdoors.
  - Medication dosage should be adjusted to account for these variations.

Additional information

- Because the severity of keratitis varies with environmental factors, periodic rechecks (e.g., two to three times yearly for well-controlled cases) are recommended so that medication dose adjustments can be made.
- Dogs living at higher altitudes may have more severe keratitis than dogs living at lower altitudes.
- Keratitis often worsens during seasons of increased UV light exposure, and medications will require dose increase.

Corneal ulceration

- Corneal ulceration occurs when there is loss of the corneal epithelium with or without loss of corneal stroma.
- Ulcers are classified as either simple corneal ulcers or complicated corneal ulcers.
  - Simple corneal ulcers are superficial and heal within 1 week.
  - Complicated corneal ulcers include ulcers that do not heal within 1 week due to persistence of an underlying cause and any ulcers with stromal loss. Examples include the following:
    - Indolent ulcers
    - Deep or perforating ulcers
    - Melting corneal ulcers
    - Ulcers where healing is impaired by extraocular disease (e.g., eyelid masses and KCS)
- Because corneal ulceration is a broad topic, it will be discussed under the following separate headings: "Simple corneal ulceration," "Indolent corneal ulceration," "Deep and perforating corneal ulceration," and "Melting corneal ulceration." These sections will focus on canine corneal ulcers.
- Feline corneal ulcers will be discussed in the feline keratitis section, with reference to the sections on aforementioned specific ulcer types when management is similar.

Simple corneal ulceration

What it is

- A loss of corneal epithelium.
- This type of ulcer is not infected.
- The underlying cause of the ulcer has resolved.
- Simple corneal ulcers heal within 1 week.
  - Healing occurs by multiplication and migration of epithelial cells over the defect.

Predisposed individuals

- Individuals that are predisposed to ocular trauma are at higher risk of corneal ulceration:
  - Active dogs
  - Blind animals
  - Animals with brachycephalic ocular syndrome (see Chapter 10).
- Individuals with impaired blinking are predisposed to development of corneal ulceration. Therefore, the following individuals are more susceptible to corneal ulceration:
  - Individuals with lagophthalmos
  - Individuals with facial nerve paralysis
  - Individuals with exophthalmos
- Individuals with eyelid or precorneal tear film disorders are predisposed to development of corneal ulceration.

Defining characteristics

- The reason for presentation to the veterinary clinic is usually ocular pain:
  - *Blepharospasm*
  - *Epiphora* or other ocular discharge
  - Elevation of the third eyelid
  - Rubbing or pawing at the eye
  - The signs were noticed acutely and were of short duration prior to presentation.
- In addition to the clinical signs aforementioned, examination findings may include the following:
  - *Conjunctival hyperemia*
  - Chemosis
  - Mildly roughened or irregular appearance to the corneal surface
    - No obvious divots or craters
- Corneal edema in the roughened cornea
- Miosis
- Superficial corneal vascularization
- *Corneal fluorescein retention* (Figure 5.34)

Clinical significance

- Trauma is presumed to be the cause of many canine simple corneal ulcers.
- Simple corneal ulcers can be quite painful due to the concentration of nerves in the superficial cornea.
- The cornea is at risk of infection while the epithelium is compromised.
  - However, simple ulcers by definition are not infected.

Diagnosis

- As with keratitis, underlying causes are ruled out with careful ophthalmic examination.
- The diagnosis of a corneal ulcer is made by observing corneal fluorescein retention.
  - Fluorescein is water-soluble and does not adhere to the intact, hydrophobic corneal epithelium.
  - Corneal ulceration exposes the hydrophilic corneal stroma, to which fluorescein does adhere.
- The ulcer is diagnosed as superficial based on the following:
  - Absence of visible stromal loss.
  - Any vessels that may be in the cornea are superficial, rather than deep.
- Because simple corneal ulcers are not infected, white cell infiltrate will be absent.
- Short duration is confirmed via
  - history and
  - absence of corneal vessels or superficial corneal vessels no more than a few millimeters in length.

Treatment

Treatment of simple corneal ulcers is aimed at (1) preventing infection, (2) treating ocular pain while the cornea re-epithelializes, and (3) preventing self-trauma.

1 Prevention of infection
  - Opportunistic infections are most likely to arise from conjunctival flora (see Chapter 13 for description of normal flora).
  - Therefore, a broad-spectrum antibiotic with efficacy against Gram-positive anaerobes and Gram-negative bacteria is desired. Examples include
    - Neomycin/polymyxin B/bacitracin ophthalmic ointment or neomycin/polymyxin B/gramicidin ophthalmic solution.
      - Very good prophylaxis for simple corneal ulcers in dogs.
    - Also: oxytetracycline/polymyxin B ophthalmic ointment (Terramycin®), erythromycin 0.5% ophthalmic ointment.
    - Discontinue when re-epithelialization has been documented by negative corneal fluorescein stain.
  - Due to development of resistant bacteria, fluoroquinolones are not recommended for prophylactic use in simple corneal ulcers or other uninfected corneal ulcers.
2 Treatment of ocular pain
  - Atropine ophthalmic 0.5 or 1% solution or ointment.
    - Cycloplegic; paralyzes the ciliary body muscle spasm that contributes to ocular pain.
      - Ciliary body muscle is not visible but can be assumed to be paralyzed if the pupil is dilated and nonresponsive to light.
    - Apply one drop or 1/4″ strip one to two times daily to achieve pupillary dilation, then decrease dose to the lowest possible frequency required to maintain pupillary dilation.

- For simple ulcers, additional doses may not be needed if pupillary dilation from the first 1 to 2 doses persists.
      - If additional doses are needed, they may only be required as infrequently as once every other day.
    - Discontinue when cornea has re-epithelialized.
    - The bitter taste of atropine may induce ptyalism.
      - Occurs shortly after administration, due to exit of medication into the nasolacrimal drainage apparatus.
      - Strategies to decrease this reaction include application of ointment rather than solution and feeding of a treat immediately after administration of medication.
    - Avoid atropine use if KCS is present because this medication can further decrease tear production.
  - Oral analgesics
    - Veterinary NSAIDs can be given at labeled doses.
    - Gabapentin can be administered at a dose of 10–20 mg/kg PO q12h–q8h in dogs.
      - Avoid xylitol-containing preparations due to risk of toxicity.
3 Prevent self-trauma
  - Placement of a hard Elizabethan collar (E-collar).
    - Soft E-collars are not adequate to prevent self-trauma.

The first recheck appointment should be within 5–7 days of initial presentation, at which point the cornea should be re-epithelialized; further rechecks are based on the improvement of the corneal lesions.

Prognosis

- The prognosis for complete resolution is very good.
- Long-term corneal scarring is usually minimal to absent.

Additional information

- Fluorescein stain should be minimally diluted prior to applying to the ocular surface.
- Excessive dilution of fluorescein stain can result in false negatives when the dilute stain is not visibly retained by the cornea.
- Minimal dilution is best achieved by first applying one drop of eyewash to the fluorescein strip, then directly applying the fluorescein strip to the eye.
  - The strip should be applied to the conjunctival, but not the corneal, surface because direct contact of the strip with the cornea can result in a fluorescein-positive lesion.
  - If fluorescein is diluted, use no more than 0.5 ml of diluent (eyewash) per fluorescein strip to avoid excessive dilution.
    - Do not reuse for multiple patients due to risk of cross-contamination.
- Fluorescein should be rinsed thoroughly from the eye following application so that excessive pooling of fluorescein is not mistaken for true corneal retention of stain.
  - Eyewash should run clear.
- Because ophthalmic corticosteroids can impair healing and encourage corneal infection or corneal melting, they should *not* be applied to ulcerated corneas.

Indolent corneal ulceration

What it is

- Corneal ulceration possessing all of the following characteristics:
  - Superficial
  - Chronic
  - Does not heal due to impaired corneal epithelial-stromal attachments
    - Epithelial division and migration over the defect occurs; however, impaired attachments prevent adherence of epithelium to stroma.
  - Not infected
  - Occurs in a dog
- The lack of healing of indolent ulcers is not the result of underlying ophthalmic conditions (e.g., eyelid disease and KCS).
  - The aforementioned conditions cause ulcer chronicity through different mechanisms (i.e., chronic mechanical irritation).
- Indolent ulcers are also referred to as spontaneous chronic corneal epithelial defects (SCCED).

Predisposed individuals

- Boxers
- Corgis
- Middle-aged and older dogs

Defining characteristics

- Presenting clinical signs are similar to those for simple corneal ulceration.
- In contrast to simple corneal ulceration, the ulcer has a history of chronicity.
- The patient is a dog and highly likely to be a boxer, a corgi, or an older dog.
- Nonadherent corneal epithelium is visible at the periphery of the ulcer (Figures 5.35, 5.36a, 5.36b, 5.37, 5.38, 5.39).
- The ulcer is superficial.
- The ulcer is not infected.
- The following signs will be *absent*:
  - Divoting of the cornea (indicative of stromal loss)
  - White cell infiltrate
  - Corneal malacia
  - Other causes of chronicity, such as eyelid masses, entropion, trichiasis, and so on.

Clinical significance

- Corneal ulcers can be quite painful.
- The cornea is at risk of infection while the epithelium is compromised.
  - However, by definition these ulcers are not infected.
- Veterinary intervention is required to encourage attachment between the epithelium and the superficial stroma so that re-epithelialization can occur.

Diagnosis

- An ulcer is diagnosed as indolent if the following are noted:
  - The ulcer is superficial (no signs of stromal loss).
  - The ulcer has a history of chronicity.
    - Usually determined during history-taking.
    - Superficial corneal vascularization is usually present.
  - Nonadherent corneal epithelium.
  - Specific pattern of corneal fluorescein retention.
    - Fluorescein is often visible adhered to exposed stroma and, at the lesion periphery, stroma that is still covered by nonadherent epithelium (Figures 5.35, 5.36 b, 5.38).
  - Absence of other reasons for chronicity, such as the following:
    - White cell infiltrate (indicative of infection)
    - Stromal loss
    - Chronic irritants such as eyelid masses, aberrant hairs, entropion, KCS, and conjunctival foreign body.

Treatment

The goals of treatment are to (1) encourage attachments to form between the epithelium and the stroma, (2) prevent secondary bacterial infection of the cornea, (3) manage ocular pain, and (4) prevent self-trauma.

1 Encouraging attachments between the corneal epithelium and the stroma
  - Corneal debridement followed by either grid keratotomy (GK) or diamond burr keratotomy (DBK).
    - Do not perform if the ulcer does not exhibit all defining characteristics as aforementioned.
    - If you are not comfortable performing these procedures, refer the patient to a veterinary ophthalmologist.
    - These treatments remove nonadherent corneal epithelium and expose healthy stroma.
  - Method:
    - Ensure patient cooperation since unexpected movements during GK could result in needle penetration of the eye.
      - Sedation or general anesthesia may be required.
    - Apply one drop of proparacaine 0.5% ophthalmic solution to the affected eye. After 1 minute, repeat application.
      - Corneal anesthesia in the dog is optimal for the first 25 minutes after application (Herring *et al.*, 2005).
      - Total duration of corneal anesthesia is almost one hour in the dog (Herring *et al.*, 2005).
    - Place a lid speculum to keep the eyelids open.
    - Flush ocular surface with dilute (5%) povidone–iodine solution.
    - Vigorously rub the corneal surface with a dry, sterile cotton swab for the debridement.
      - Continue until all nonadherent epithelium has been removed.
      - This often significantly increases the surface area, but not the depth, of the corneal ulcer.
      - A separate cotton swab may be placed on the third eyelid to prevent it from interfering with debridement and keratotomy.

- Then perform either the GK or DBK.
  - If performing GK: Use a 25- or 27-gauge needle to scratch a grid into the superficial corneal stroma.
    - Place the needle at a 45° angle to the cornea with the bevel facing up.
    - The needle can be grasped halfway along the bevel with a hemostat or needle driver to decrease the chance of inadvertent penetration of the eye.
    - Pull the needle across the superficial corneal stroma.
    - Do not push the needle or move it in a side-to-side direction.
    - The needle should drag through the superficial stroma but no deeper.
    - Create a crosshatching pattern with grid marks no further than 1 mm apart.
    - The final grid should cover the entire surface of exposed stroma and should also extend at least 1 mm beyond the margins of the epithelial defect (the size of the epithelial defect after corneal debridement).
  - If performing DBK: use the diamond burr to "sand" the surface of the cornea.
    - The rotating burr is gently applied to cornea and the entire exposed stroma is treated for approximately 1 minute (Dawson *et al.*, 2017).
    - The risk of puncturing the globe may be less for DBK than for GK.
  - A contact lens can be placed after completion of either GK or DBK.
    - This may shorten time to re-epithelialization (Dees *et al.*, 2017; Grinninger *et al.*, 2015; Wooff & Norman, 2015).
2. Preventing secondary bacterial infection
   - Antibiotic prophylaxis as discussed for simple corneal ulceration.
   - Tetracyclines reduce healing time of indolent corneal ulcers (Chandler *et al.*, 2010).
     - Effect is independent of antimicrobial spectrum.
     - Tetracyclines may therefore be preferred over other antibiotic classes for management of indolent corneal ulcers.
3. Management of ocular pain
   - Atropine use as for simple corneal ulceration.
   - Apply first dose of atropine immediately after completing the GK or DBK.
     - Onset is approximately 30 minutes; this increases the likelihood that cycloplegia is achieved by the time the effect of proparacaine wanes.
   - Use of oral veterinary NSAIDs at labeled doses improves analgesia.
   - Use of gabapentin at a dose of 10–20 mg/kg PO q12h–q8h may also improve analgesia.
     - Avoid preparations containing xylitol due to risk of toxicity.

4. Prevent self-trauma
   - Placement of a hard E-collar.
     - Soft E-collars are not adequate to prevent self-trauma.

The first recheck should occur between 1 and 2 weeks after initial examination, with frequency of further rechecks determined by the results of fluorescein staining and reduction of clinical signs of keratitis.
- Re-epithelialization may not be complete by 1 week, but recheck is recommended so that complications, if present, can be managed.
- Re-epithelialization is usually complete by 2 weeks.

Prognosis

- With appropriate treatment, the prognosis is good for resolution of the ulcer; healing rate can exceed 85% (Dees *et al.*, 2017; Gosling *et al.*, 2013; Stanley *et al.*, 1998).
- Ulcers that persist in spite of corneal debridement and GK or DBK should be referred to a veterinary ophthalmologist for evaluation.
- In an individual that has experienced indolent corneal ulceration, there is potential for the fellow eye to later develop an indolent ulcer (Hung *et al.*, 2020).

Additional information

- A dry cotton swab is more effective at debriding epithelium than a wet cotton swab. During debridement, the swab will become moist. It is recommended to discard the wet swab and start with a fresh swab when this happens. This means that several swabs will be required to complete a corneal debridement.
- Indolent corneal ulceration mainly occurs in dogs.
  - GK should not be performed in cats because this encourages formation of corneal sequestra (La Croix *et al.*, 2001).
  - Chronic corneal ulcers in cats are likely due to FHV-1 infection, rather than a primary epithelial-stromal attachment abnormality.
- Moderate keratitis is present in the short term following treatment, but usually resolves over several weeks after corneal re-epithelialization.
- Because ophthalmic corticosteroids can impair healing and encourage corneal infection or corneal melting, they should *not* be applied to ulcerated corneas.
- If a corneal ulcer does not heal within 1 week, simply switching the ophthalmically applied antibiotic is unlikely to result in healing.
  - Because impaired attachments between the corneal epithelium and the stroma are the cause of impaired healing for indolent corneal ulcers, corneal debridement combined with GK or DBK must be part of the treatment.
- A corneal ulcer that does not heal within 1 week should not automatically be assumed to be indolent; an ulcer is diagnosed as indolent only after criteria listed under "Defining characteristics" are met.

- If corneal white blood cell infiltrate, stromal loss, or melting are seen, the ulcer is not indolent and corneal debridement, GK, and DBK are contraindicated.

Deep and perforating corneal ulceration

What it is
- Loss of corneal stroma in addition to the epithelium.
- Descemetoceles are deep corneal ulcers where the corneal epithelium and all of the stroma have been lost. Only Descemet's membrane and the endothelium remain intact.
- Perforated ulcers are full-thickness defects of the cornea.

Predisposed individuals
- Brachycephalic dogs are at higher risk for complications that change a simple corneal ulcer into a deep corneal ulcer.
- Dogs with KCS are at increased risk of secondary infection of a superficial corneal ulcer, potentially leading to deepening of the ulcer.
- In cats, herpetic ulcers can progress to involve the deep stromal layers.
- When corneal ulcers develop in individuals receiving chronic ophthalmic corticosteroid treatment, the risk of complications leading to stromal loss is higher.

Defining characteristics
- Stromal loss is recognized by a divot in the corneal surface (Figures 5.40, 5.41, 5.42, 5.43, 5.44, 5.45, 5.46, 5.47a, 5.47b, 5.48).
- A descemetocele is recognized by its staining pattern (Figures 5.46, 5.47b).
  - The center of the defect (hydrophobic Descemet's membrane) does not retain fluorescein.
  - The edges of the defect (exposed hydrophilic stroma) retain fluorescein.
- Corneal perforation is recognized by brown or pink tissue (iris) protruding from an irregular corneal surface (Figures 5.49, 5.50, 5.51, 5.52, 5.53, 5.54, 5.55).
  - This is the iris, which moves anteriorly to plug full-thickness corneal defects.
    - Dyscoria and uneven anterior chamber depth, due to iris displacement, are also seen.
  - Fibrin or blood is usually visible within the anterior chamber.
  - Ocular discharge is copious and may be blood-tinged.
  - If corneal perforation is secondary to a penetrating injury, retained foreign body may be visible in the cornea.

Clinical significance
- Corneal ulcers can be quite painful.
- These ulcers are usually infected.
- Eyes with deep corneal ulcers are at high risk of rupture.
- Deep and perforating corneal ulcers carry high rate of visual compromise or blindness.

- Perforated eyes may potentially be salvageable (with permanently decreased vision or blindness) but also may have sufficient damage to necessitate enucleation.
- Rapid veterinary attention and surgical intervention are needed to minimize potential for blindness or loss of the eye.
- Anterior uveitis is present, to varying degrees, and should be treated.
- Healing requires rebuilding of corneal stroma in addition to re-epithelialization.
  - Time course to healing is several weeks, at minimum.

Diagnosis
- The diagnosis is made by ophthalmic examination and recognition of changes as listed under "Defining characteristics."
- Fluorescein stain pattern will identify a descemetocele.
- Corneal cytology and culture and sensitivity are warranted due to high potential of infection.
  - If prompt referral to a veterinary ophthalmologist is possible, this can be performed at the referral center.
  - If prompt referral to a veterinary ophthalmologist is not possible, then cytology and culture and sensitivity should be performed by the primary care veterinarian.
  - Samples should be collected after administration of proparacaine for analgesia, but prior to administering ophthalmic medications.
  - Be cautious and gentle when collecting samples, as it is possible to cause globe rupture during sample collection.
    - Sampling of the ventral conjunctival fornix is an alternative that has a lower risk of damage to the globe and reasonable correlation to results from corneal sampling (Auten *et al.*, 2019).
- Corneal cytology
  - Allows immediate visualization of organisms to guide antimicrobial selection.
  - May be only source of information if culture and sensitivity fails to grow organisms.
- Corneal culture and sensitivity
  - Because corneal samples are small and bacteria are often fastidious, organisms may not grow even when infection is present.

Treatment
- Treatment goals are to (1) control infection, (2) control intraocular inflammation, (3) treat ocular pain, and (4) provide physical support to the eye.
- The patient should be referred on an urgent basis to a veterinary ophthalmologist.
- If referral is not possible or must be delayed, begin medical treatment outlined below.
- When there is risk of rupture, or if rupture has occurred, all ophthalmic medications should be in solution form, not ointment form.
  - Ointment can cause severe uveitis if it enters the eye.

1 Control infection
  ◦ Antibiotic solution applied to the affected eye, one drop at least four times daily.
  ◦ Initial antibiotic selection is based on cytology.
    ▪ If Gram-negative rods are seen, ophthalmic solutions such as gentamicin 0.3%, tobramycin 0.3%, ciprofloxacin 0.3%, and ofloxacin 0.3% are appropriate.
    ▪ If Gram-positive cocci are seen, ophthalmic solutions such as cefazolin 5% (must be compounded from IV formulation), gatifloxacin 0.3%, and moxifloxacin 0.5% are appropriate.
    ▪ Initial treatment with a fluoroquinolone is justified by risk of blindness and loss of the eye.
  ◦ If the globe has already perforated, use of a broad-spectrum antibiotic (e.g., amoxicillin/clavulanic acid, cephalosporins) orally is also indicated.
  ◦ Ultimate antibiotic selection will be dictated by results of culture and sensitivity.
2 Control intraocular inflammation
  ◦ Do not use ophthalmic steroids due to potential to worsen infection and inhibitory effect on tissue healing.
  ◦ Ophthalmic NSAIDs can also inhibit healing and even potentially cause corneal melting (Guidera *et al.*, 2001) and are also not recommended.
  ◦ Use veterinary NSAIDs orally at labeled dose.
3 Treat ocular pain.
  ◦ Atropine 1% ophthalmic solution, one drop to the affected eye one to two times daily.
    ▪ Use as infrequently as needed to maintain mydriasis (and therefore cycloplegia).
  ◦ Analgesia also addressed by oral NSAID use.
  ◦ Oral gabapentin at a dose of 10–20 mg/kg q12h–q8h in dogs can also provide analgesia.
    ▪ Avoid xylitol-containing preparations due to risk of toxicity.
4 Physical support to the eye.
  ◦ A hard E-collar should be worn at all times.
  ◦ Referral for surgical repair, such as a conjunctival graft.
    ▪ Should be performed as soon as possible.
    ▪ If a corneal foreign body is present, this is removed at the same time.
The first recheck examination should be within 1 to 3 days of diagnosis, depending on the depth of the corneal ulcer.
• Further rechecks will depend on progression of healing.
  ◦ In the early stages, rechecks every few days may be required.
  ◦ Thereafter, weekly rechecks may be required.

Prognosis

• For deep corneal ulcers that receive prompt medical and surgical therapy, prognosis is good for retention of the globe.
  ◦ Postoperative corneal scarring may cause vision compromise.
• The prognosis is fair to guarded for deep corneal ulcers that are managed only medically.

  ◦ Due to potential for rupture and loss of the eye.
  ◦ Corneal scarring may limit vision or cause blindness after ulcer resolution.
• The prognosis for perforated ulcers is guarded.
  ◦ Some eyes can successfully be treated with conjunctival grafting.
    ▪ Variable amounts of vision can be retained, depending on the severity of intraocular injury and size of corneal defect.
  ◦ Some eyes may sustain irreversible damage and require enucleation.

Additional information

• When referral is not possible and medical management is the only option, consider placement of a partial, lateral tarsorrhaphy.
  ◦ Improves corneal coverage by the eyelids and therefore protection to the ulcer.
  ◦ Closure of the lateral approximately one-third of the palpebral fissure.
    ▪ Medial opening of the palpebral fissure provides outlet for ocular discharge, allows application of medications, and enables visualization of the ulcer for monitoring.
• If medical management is elected, complete resolution will require at least several weeks, sometimes a couple of months, of treatment.
  ◦ Frequent recheck examinations are needed during this time.
  ◦ Therefore, the cost of medical management may not be significantly different than the cost of surgical treatment.
• Restraint of a patient with a deep or perforating corneal ulcer should be gentle; forceful restraint can result in eye rupture.
• When collecting blood from a patient with a deep or perforating corneal defect, use extreme caution if collecting from the jugular vein.
  ◦ Pressure placed onto the jugular during venipuncture can result in rupture of the eye.
• Reduce exercise and activity levels during treatment to minimize potential for rupture.
• Because ophthalmic corticosteroids can impair healing and encourage corneal infection or corneal melting, they should *not* be applied to ulcerated corneas.

Melting corneal ulceration

What it is

• Corneal ulcers with collagenolysis of corneal stroma
  ◦ Proteinases, produced by both the host and the pathogen, degrade corneal collagen.
  ◦ Stromal collagen loses its rigidity and becomes malacic.

Predisposed individuals

• Predispositions to melting corneal ulcers are similar to those for deep and perforating corneal ulcers (see previous section in this chapter).

- Use of ophthalmic NSAIDs in the presence of corneal ulceration elevates the risk of corneal melting (Guidera *et al.,* 2001).

Defining characteristics

- The cornea becomes opaque and white (Figures 5.56, 5.57, 5.58, 5.59).
- The cornea appears gelatinous rather than solid (Figures 5.56, 5.57, 5.59).
- The corneal curvature becomes altered as the corneal collagen loses its rigidity.
- The corneal surface appears to be "oozing" off the remainder of the eye.
- Moderate to marked signs of keratoconjunctivitis will be present.

Clinical significance

- Corneal ulcers are painful.
- Corneal melting can progress rapidly.
- There is a high risk of loss of vision or the eye if melting is not stopped.
- Melting ulcers are presumed to be infected.
- Melting corneal ulcers are usually accompanied by significant anterior uveitis.

Diagnosis

- The diagnosis is made on characteristic appearance.
- As with deep/perforating corneal ulcers, cytology and culture and sensitivity are recommended.
  - If immediate referral to a veterinary ophthalmologist is possible, these can be performed by the ophthalmologist.
  - If referral is delayed or not possible, samples should be collected by the primary veterinarian after application of proparacaine for analgesia, but prior to application of ophthalmic medications.
    - Be cautious and gentle when collecting samples as it is possible to cause globe rupture during sample collection.
    - Sampling of the ventral conjunctival fornix is an alternative that has a lower risk of damage to the globe and reasonable correlation to results from corneal sampling (Auten *et al.*, 2019).

Treatment

- Treatment goals are to (1) stop collagenolysis, (2) control infection, (3) control intraocular inflammation, (4) treat ocular pain, and (5) provide physical support to the eye.
- The patient should be referred to a veterinary ophthalmologist immediately.
- If referral will be delayed or is not possible, begin medical treatment outlined below.
- Because of the high risk of eye rupture, all ophthalmic medications should be in solution, not ointment, form because ointments can worsen uveitis if they enter the eye.

1 Stop collagenolysis.
  - Application of antiproteinases/anticollagenases.
  - Autologous serum is one readily available anticollagenase.
    - Collect and process patient blood sample to obtain serum.
      - If patient size limits the amount of serum collected, donor serum can be used.
    - Serum can be placed into a sterile dropper bottle for application or can be drawn directly from a red top tube before application.
    - Because serum can encourage bacterial growth, the following guidelines apply:
      - Handle with aseptic technique to minimize contamination.
      - Store in the refrigerator to minimize microbial growth.
      - Discard unused serum within 7 to 10 days.
    - Apply one drop to the affected eye every 1–2 hours for the first 24–48 hours, then decrease to four times daily thereafter.
  - Doxycycline is another option for anticollagenase therapy.
    - A dose of 5–10 mg/kg PO q12h results in detectable levels of drug in the precorneal tear film (Collins *et al.*, 2016).
2 Control infection.
  - Antibiotic selection as discussed for deep/perforating corneal ulcers (see earlier section in this chapter).
  - Apply one drop to the affected eye every 1–2 hours for the first 24–48 hours, then decrease to four times daily thereafter.
3 Control inflammation.
  - Use veterinary NSAIDs orally at labeled dose.
  - Avoid use of ophthalmically-applied NSAIDs due to potential to worsen corneal melting.
4 Treat ocular pain.
  - Atropine 1% ophthalmic solution: one drop to the affected eye one to two times daily to achieve cycloplegia.
  - Oral NSAID therapy also contributes to analgesia.
  - Oral gabapentin at a dose of 10–20 mg/kg q12h–q8h in dogs.
    - Avoid xylitol-containing preparations due to risk of toxicity.
5 Provide physical support to the eye.
  - Hard E-collar to be worn at all times to prevent self-trauma.
  - Referral for surgical repair (e.g., conjunctival graft) or therapies such as corneal collagen cross-linking (Pot *et al.*, 2014) as soon as possible.

Initial recheck examination should be within 1–2 days of diagnosis.

- Timing of further rechecks is dependent on clinical improvement.
- Rechecks may be required every 2–3 days in the early stages, then weekly thereafter.
- Total duration of treatment will depend on the pace of the improvement of corneal lesions.

Prognosis

- The prognosis for maintaining a comfortable eye in the long term is good for melting corneal ulcers that are referred promptly.
  - However, there is high potential for rupture and loss of the eye.
  - Corneal scarring may limit vision after ulcer resolution.

Additional information

- Corneal melting can progress over a matter of hours; melting ulcers are therefore considered to be true ocular emergencies.
- Due to risk of eye perforation, be very cautious if collecting blood from the jugular vein and proceed cautiously if restraint is required.
- If referral is not possible, placement of a partial, lateral tarsorrhaphy is recommended to improve eyelid coverage of the cornea.
- With medical management alone, complete resolution (if achieved) will require at least several weeks, and sometimes a few months, of treatment.
- Because ophthalmic corticosteroids can impair healing and encourage corneal infection or corneal melting, they should *not* be applied to ulcerated corneas.

Feline keratitis, nonulcerative and ulcerative

What it is

- Inflammation of the cornea.
- Superficial keratitis: inflammation of the corneal epithelium and/or superficial stroma.
- Deep or stromal keratitis: inflammation of the deeper stromal layers of the cornea.
- Nonulcerative keratitis refers to keratitis that is not associated with a break in the corneal epithelium.
- Ulcerative keratitis refers to keratitis that is associated with a disruption of the corneal epithelium, that is, a corneal ulcer.

Predisposed individuals

- As with dogs, brachycephalic cats are predisposed to superficial exposure keratitis resulting from their conformational defects and are more prone to trauma-induced keratitis. See Chapter 10 for brachycephalic ocular syndrome.
- Cats experiencing stress or immune suppression are at higher risk of recrudescent disease due to FHV-1.

Defining characteristics

- The clinical signs of keratitis are similar to those in dogs (see the beginning of chapter for signs of corneal disease and the earlier section in this chapter, "Canine keratitis"). These include the following:
  - *Corneal vascularization*, superficial (Figures 5.1, 5.4, 5.5, 5.6, 5.7, 5.8) or deep (Figures 5.9, 5.19, 5.21).
  - Variable amounts of corneal edema (Figures 5.10, 5.11, 5.12) and fibrosis (Figures 5.8, 5.17, 5.18).
  - *Ocular discharge* (serous, mucoid, or mucopurulent).
  - *Conjunctivitis* (Chapter 13) will also be present.
- If the cornea does not retain fluorescein stain, keratitis is nonulcerative.
- If the cornea does retain fluorescein stain, keratitis is ulcerative (Figures 5.60, 5.61).

Clinical significance

- In cats, keratoconjunctivitis is most often assumed to be due to FHV-1 infection.
  - Immune-mediated inflammation, eyelid, and eyelash abnormalities that are common in dogs occur much less often in cats.
  - Presence of dendritic corneal ulcers (Figures 5.60, 5.61) is a pathognomonic sign of FHV-1 infection.
  - However, ulcers do not have to be dendritic to be due to FHV-1, that is, FHV-1 can cause ulcers in any shape.
  - This means that in addition to therapy listed for each type of corneal ulceration, cats should be treated with antiviral medications (see the section on feline conjunctivitis in Chapter 13).
- Although KCS is less commonly recognized in cats than dogs, aqueous deficiency in cats occurs (Uhl *et al.*, 2019) and should be considered when the STT is less than 9 mm/min (Sebbag *et al.*, 2015), especially when keratoconjunctivitis is present.
- As with dogs, keratitis is uncomfortable, the corneal opacification that occurs with keratitis can lead to visual impairment or blindness, and keratitis predisposes to further ocular disease such as corneal sequestrum (see the next section in this chapter).

Diagnosis

- Keratitis is diagnosed on ophthalmic examination.
- Unless overt eyelid or eyelash abnormalities are seen on ophthalmic examination, feline keratitis is presumed to be due to FHV-1 infection.
  - Diagnostic testing for FHV-1 is discussed in the section on feline conjunctivitis in Chapter 13.
- If the STT is less than 9 mm/min, deficiency of the aqueous tear film should be considered (Sebbag *et al.*, 2015).
- Cytology is indicated when plaques are visualized on the cornea, to rule out EK.
- If corneal ulceration is present, diagnosis of deep, perforating, or melting ulcers is based on the same principles as for dogs (see earlier section on deep and perforating corneal ulcers in this chapter).
  - Use of diagnostics such as cytology and culture and sensitivity is also based on the same principles.

Treatment

- The goals of treatment are to control the viral infection, reduce surface ocular inflammation, and treat ocular discomfort.

- When a corneal ulcer is present, then treatment will also involve antibacterial therapy.
1 Antiviral therapy
   - This is administered in the same manner as for feline conjunctivitis. See the section on feline conjunctivitis in Chapter 13 for specifics regarding antiviral therapy.
   - Addressing the viral infection will reduce the corneal and conjunctival inflammation.
2 Tear film supplementation
   - This is administered in the same manner as for conjunctivitis and qualitative tear film deficiency. See the section on feline conjunctivitis in Chapter 13.
   - Tear film supplementation is especially important when STT values are low.
      - It is not clear whether additional therapy with CsA will increase STT in these cats.
   - This is often recommended as a long-term treatment, even after resolution of keratitis, to reduce recurrence of disease.
   - Particularly in cats with brachycephalic ocular syndrome.
3 Treating ocular pain
   - Atropine use as for simple corneal ulceration (see the treatment section within Simple Corneal Ulceration).
   - Use of analgesics like transmucosal buprenorphine (0.01–0.03 mg/kg q8h), gabapentin (5–10 mg/kg PO q12–q8h), or robenacoxib at the labeled dose may be needed depending the degree of discomfort.
4 Antibacterial therapy
   - As for dogs, ophthalmically applied antibiotics should be administered in the presence of a corneal ulceration.
   - Due to lack of efficacy against *Chlamydophila felis* or *Mycoplasma* spp., the combination of neomycin, polymyxin B, and bacitracin (or gramicidin) does not provide complete antimicrobial prophylaxis, and other antibiotics may be more suitable for use in cats.
      - The combination of neomycin, polymyxin B, and bacitracin (or gramicidin) has been associated with the very rare complication of systemic anaphylaxis in cats (Hume-Smith *et al.*, 2011).
   - Antibiotics that offer more complete antimicrobial coverage against feline pathogens include:
      - Oxytetracycline/polymyxin B ophthalmic ointment (Terramycin®).
         - Rarely has been associated with anaphylaxis in cats (Hume-Smith *et al.*, 2011).
      - Erythromycin 0.5% ophthalmic ointment.
   - Apply 1/4″ strip of ointment to the affected eye four times daily.
Additional points for therapy
- For ulcers that are suspected to be infected, deep, or melting, treatment is based on the same principles as for dogs (see earlier sections on deep and perforating corneal ulcers and melting corneal ulcers in this chapter).

Prognosis
- With appropriate antiviral therapy, prognosis for resolution of keratitis is fair to good.
   - There is potential for recurrent disease, especially for patients for which a source of stress can't be managed.
- Cats with extensive or severe ulcerative keratoconjunctivitis may develop permanent adhesions between the cornea and conjunctiva, which are referred to as symblepharon (Figures 5.62, 5.63, 5.64).

Additional information
- Indolent corneal ulceration as it occurs in dogs is not recognized in cats.
   - If an ulcer is chronic, GK is not an appropriate treatment due to the risk of corneal sequestra as a sequela (La Croix *et al.*, 2001).
   - Ulcers nonresponsive to treatment should be referred to a veterinary ophthalmologist.

Feline eosinophilic keratoconjunctivitis (EK)
What it is
- Inflammation of the cornea and conjunctiva with eosinophilic infiltration or plaque formation.

Predisposed individuals
- EK occurs in cats.

Defining characteristics
- Blepharospasm
- *Conjunctival hyperemia*
- Chemosis
- *Superficial corneal vascularization*
- Corneal edema
- *Corneal cellular infiltrates and plaques*
   - Usually white to tan plaques that are raised from the ocular surface (Figures 5.65, 5.66).
   - Can also be diffuse corneal infiltrates rather than discrete plaques (Figures 5.67, 5.68).

Clinical significance
- Presumed to be an immune-mediated disease.
   - FHV-1 DNA has been isolated from cats with EK, but the role of the virus in pathogenesis is unknown.
- Corneal ulceration is often concurrent.
- EK causes discomfort.
- Episodes of EK can be recurrent.

Diagnosis
- EK should be suspected when superficial white cell infiltrate or corneal plaques are seen in the presence of keratitis.
- Corneal scraping with cytology is diagnostic.
   - The diagnosis is confirmed when eosinophils are seen.

- Cytology usually reveals a mixture of epithelial cells, lymphocytes, neutrophils, mast cells, and eosinophils (Allgoewer *et al.*, 2001; Dean & Meunier, 2013; Speiss *et al.*, 2009).

Treatment

- The goals of treatment are to eliminate surface ocular inflammation, prevent secondary bacterial infection, and restore patient comfort.
- Treatment therefore involves (1) suppressing the immune system, (2) tear film supplementation, (3) prophylactic antibiotic therapy, and (4) antiviral therapy.

1 Immune suppression
  - CsA (Optimmune®) or corticosteroids.
  - CsA: Apply 1/4″ strip to the affected eye twice daily.
    - Once clinical signs have resolved, taper the dose at 1- to 2-week intervals.
  - Corticosteroids (prednisolone acetate ophthalmic suspension 1% or dexamethasone 0.1% ophthalmic solution).
    - Apply one drop to the affected eye two to four times daily, depending on the severity of the corneal inflammation.
    - For example, starting dose of twice daily for mild to moderate cases and a starting dose of four times daily for severe cases.
    - As disease improves, gradually taper the dose at 1- to 2-week intervals.
  - The goal is to eventually completely discontinue medications.
    - For some cats, medications cannot be discontinued without recurrence of disease.
      - For these cats, goal is lowest dose that controls symptoms.

2 Tear film supplementation
  - Chronic surface ocular inflammation leads to tear film instability (see section on feline conjunctivitis in Chapter 13).
  - Apply mucinomimetic tear film replacement such as hyaluronan 0.2% or higher (e.g., I-Drop®Vet or an-HyPro) two to four times daily.
  - Continue for 3–4 weeks after resolution of clinical signs.

3 Prophylactic antibiotic therapy
  - Concurrent corneal ulcers are common with EK, and corneal scraping for cytology induces corneal ulceration, even if an ulcer was not present at initial presentation.
  - Antibiotic therapy is recommended to prevent secondary bacterial infection of corneal ulcers.
  - See the treatment section within "Feline keratitis, nonulcerative and ulcerative," for discussion of antibiotic choice and use.
  - Oxytetracycline/polymyxin B (Terramycin®) and erythromycin ophthalmic ointments are suitable for prophylaxis in cats.
  - Apply 1/4″ strip to the affected eye four times daily until the cornea no longer retains fluorescein stain.

4 Antiviral therapy
  - Due to immunosuppressive treatment and potential for FHV-1 infection, antiviral therapy should be considered.
    - Especially when corneal ulcers are present and in cases that do not respond to immunosuppressive and tear film replacement therapies alone.
  - See the section on feline conjunctivitis in Chapter 13 for a discussion of antiviral therapy.
  - Can be discontinued when clinical signs resolve.

5 Patient comfort
  - Atropine use as for simple corneal ulceration (see treatment section within "Simple corneal ulceration").
  - Use of analgesics like transmucosal buprenorphine (0.01–0.03 mg/kg q8h), gabapentin (5–10 mg/kg PO q12–q8h), or robenacoxib at the labeled dose may be needed depending the degree of discomfort.

Initial recheck examination is recommended within 1–2 weeks of initial diagnosis. Further recheck frequencies are determined by the degree of improvement of the corneal lesions and the time frame for these to occur. Recheck examinations should be continued until after medications are completely discontinued (to monitor for recurrence).

Prognosis

- Most cases respond well to ophthalmically applied therapies as aforementioned.
- Recurrence is common.
  - Some cats require medical management only during active disease.
  - Other cats require continuous, low-dose immunosuppressive therapy to prevent recurrence.

Corneal sequestrum

What it is

- Corneal sequestrum refers to an area of necrotic corneal stroma.

Predisposed individuals

- Corneal sequestra mainly affect cats.
- Persians and Himalayans are overrepresented.
- Any cat with chronic corneal trauma (due to conformation or ocular disease such as corneal ulcers) is predisposed to sequestrum formation.

Defining characteristics

- *Brown discoloration of the cornea, usually centrally* (Figures 5.69, 5.70, 5.71, 5.72, 5.73, 5.74).
  - Color can range from light brown to black.
- Discomfort and keratitis are present to varying degrees. Clinical signs include the following:
  - Blepharospasm
  - Epiphora

- *Conjunctival hyperemia*
- Chemosis
- Superficial or deep corneal vascularization
- Corneal edema

Clinical significance

- Corneal sequestra result from chronic corneal irritation.
  - Some sources of chronic corneal irritation include corneal ulceration, lagophthalmos, and tear film instability.
  - If an underlying cause of corneal irritation is present, it must be addressed to adequately treat the sequestrum and to prevent recurrence of new sequestra.
  - FHV-1 may play a role in sequestrum formation by inciting keratitis with or without corneal ulceration (i.e., by inciting chronic corneal irritation).
- Corneal sequestra can be quite painful.
- The cornea is ulcerated and therefore prone to secondary bacterial infection.
- Sequestra can involve deep layers of the cornea.
  - This risks eye rupture if the sequestrum is extruded from the cornea.

Diagnosis

- The diagnosis is made on characteristic appearance.
- The diagnosis of concurrent corneal ulcer is made with fluorescein stain.
  - Fluorescein will be retained at the edges of the sequestrum, but not on the sequestrum itself because the sequestrum is hydrophobic (Figure 5.71).

Treatment

- The goals of treatment are to prevent secondary bacterial infection, to restore patient comfort, and to eliminate surface ocular inflammation.
  - Treatment is therefore aimed at (1) prophylactic antibiotic therapy, (2) treating ocular pain, (3) tear film replacement, and (4) sequestrum removal.
1 Prophylactic antibiotic therapy
  - The presence of corneal ulceration leaves the cornea at risk of infection.
  - See treatment section within "Feline keratitis, nonulcerative and ulcerative," for a discussion of appropriate antibiotic prophylaxis.
2 Treating ocular pain
  - Atropine use as for simple corneal ulceration (see the treatment section within "Simple corneal ulceration)".
  - Use of analgesics like transmucosal buprenorphine (0.01–0.03 mg/kg q8h), gabapentin (5–10 mg/kg PO q12–q8h), or robenacoxib at the labeled dose may be needed depending the degree of discomfort.
3 Tear film replacements
  - Because most sequestra are associated with keratoconjunctivitis, the tear film is likely to be unstable (see the treatment section within Feline conjunctivitis in Chapter 13).

- Use of lubricants can reduce the corneal drying that results from conformational lagophthalmos and chronic central corneal exposure.
  - One drop of hyaluronan ophthalmic solution 0.2% (e.g., I-Drop®Vet, an-HyPro) applied to the affected eye three to four times daily.
4 Sequestrum removal
  - Referral to a veterinary ophthalmologist for removal of a sequestrum is recommended at the time of diagnosis.
  - The sequestrum is removed via DBK or excised via surgical keratectomy.
    - With keratectomy, a conjunctival or corneoconjunctival graft may be placed over the surgical site.
    - Corneal inflammation should subside following sequestrum removal.

Prognosis

- The DBK can be effective for removal of superficial sequestra, but for dense or deep sequestra, it is often not possible to remove a sequestrum in its entirety.
- The prognosis is good for removal of a corneal sequestrum via keratectomy.
- Recurrence is possible and can occur in as many as 20% of cases (Featherstone & Sansom, 2004; Multari *et al.*, 2021) because predisposing factors (e.g., conformation) are often still present.

Additional information

- Waiting for a sequestrum to extrude on its own is not recommended.
  - This prolongs patient discomfort since the time course to sloughing is unknown (and it may not occur at all).
  - The risk of secondary bacterial infection is present for as long as the cornea is ulcerated.
  - If the sequestrum does extrude on its own, and the sequestrum involved the deeper layers of the cornea, the resulting defect is a deep corneal ulcer, which is also very serious (see Deep and perforating corneal ulceration).
- Attempts to remove the corneal sequestrum by individuals other than veterinary ophthalmologists are not recommended.
  - Inadvertent penetration into the anterior chamber is a potential consequence.
- For brachycephalic cats (see Brachycephalic ocular syndrome within Chapter 10 for conformational abnormalities), indefinite treatment with tear film replacements may decrease corneal irritation and potentially discourage future sequestrum formation.

Further reading

Corneal ulcers

Belknap, EB. 2015. Corneal emergencies. *Topics in Companion Animal Medicine*. 30(3):74–80.

References

Allgoewer, I, *et al.* 2001. Feline eosinophilic conjunctivitis. *Veterinary Ophthalmology.* 4(1):69–74.

Armor, MD, *et al.* 2019. Endothelial keratoplasty for corneal endothelial dystrophy in a dog. *Veterinary Ophthalmology.* 22(4):545–551.

Auten, CR, *et al.* 2019. Comparison of bacterial culture results collected via direct corneal ulcer vs conjunctival fornix sampling in canine eyes with presumed bacterial ulcerative keratitis. *Veterinary Ophthalmology.* 23(1):135–140.

Barachetti, L, *et al.* 2015. Use of episcleral cyclosporine implants in dogs with keratoconjunctivitis sicca: pilot study. *Veterinary Ophthalmology.* 18(3):234–241.

Bercovitz, GR, *et al.* 2021. A retrospective investigation of neurogenic keratoconjunctivitis sicca after administration of the long lasting otic medications Claro, Neptra and Osurnia. *Proceedings of the 52nd Annual ACVO Scientific Conference*, Indianapolis, IN, USA, September 29 October 2, 2021.

Berdoulay, A, *et al.* 2005. Effect of topical 0.02% tacrolimus aqueous suspension on tear production in dogs with keratoconjunctivitis sicca. *Veterinary Ophthalmology.* 8(4):225–232.

Chandler, HL, *et al.* 2010. In vivo effects of adjunctive tetracycline treatment on refractory corneal ulcers in dogs. *Journal of the American Veterinary Medical Association.* 237(4):378–386.

Collins, SP, *et al.* 2016. Tear film concentrations of doxycycline following oral administration in ophthalmologically normal dogs. *Journal of the American Veterinary Medical Association.* 249(5):508–514.

Crispin, SM. 2002. Ocular lipid deposition and hyperlipoproteinaemia. *Progress in Retinal and Eye Research.* 21(2):169–224.

Dawson, C, *et al.* 2017. Immediate effects of diamond burr debridement in patients with spontaneous chronic corneal epithelial defects, light and electron microscopic evaluation. *Veterinary Ophthalmology.* 20(1):11–15.

Dean, E & Meunier, V. 2013. Feline eosinophilic keratoconjunctivitis: a retrospective study of 45 cases (56 eyes). *Journal of Feline Medicine and Surgery.* 15(8):661–666.

Dees, DD, *et al.* 2017. Effect of bandage contact lens wear and postoperative medical therapies on corneal healing rate after diamond burr debridement in dogs. *Veterinary Ophthalmology.* 20(5): 382–389.

Featherstone, HJ & Sansom, J. 2004. Feline corneal sequestra: a review of 64 cases (80 eyes). *Veterinary Ophthalmology.* 7(4):213–227.

Giannikaki, S, *et al.* 2020. A modified technique of keratoleptynsis ("letter-box") for treatment of canine corneal edema associated with endothelial dysfunction. *Veterinary Ophthalmology.* 23(6):930–942.

Gosling, AA, *et al.* 2013. Management of spontaneous chronic corneal epithelial defects (SCCEDs) in dogs with diamond burr debridement and placement of a bandage contact lens. *Veterinary Ophthalmology.* 16(2):83–88.

Grinninger, P, *et al.* 2015. Use of bandage contact lenses for treatment of spontaneous chronic corneal epithelial defects in dogs. *Journal of Small Animal Practice.* 56(7):446–449.

Guidera, AC, *et al.* 2001. Keratitis, ulceration, and perforation associated with topical nonsteroidal anti-inflammatory drugs. *Ophthalmology.* 108(5):936–944.

Hendrix, DV, *et al.* 2011. An investigation comparing the efficacy of topical ocular application of tacrolimus and cyclosporine in dogs. *Veterinary Medicine International.* 2011(2011):487592.

Herring, IR, *et al.* 2005. Duration of effect and effect of multiple doses of topical ophthalmic 0.5% proparacaine hydrochloride in clinically normal dogs. *American Journal of Veterinary Research.* 66(1): 77–80.

Hume-Smith, *et al.*, 2011. Anaphylactic events observed within 4 h of ocular application of an antibiotic-containing ophthalmic preparation: 61 cats (1993–2010). *Journal of Feline Medicine and Surgery.* 13(10):744–751.

Hung, JH, *et al.* 2020. Clinical characteristics and treatment of spontaneous chronic corneal epithelial defects (SCCEDs) with diamond burr debridement. *Veterinary Ophthalmology.* 23(4):764–769.

Kaswan, RL. 1994. Characteristics of a canine model of KCS: effective treatment with topical cyclosporine. In: *Lacrimal Gland, Tear Film, and Dry Eye Syndromes.* (ed DA Sullivan), p. 583–593. Plenum Press, New York.

Kaswan, RL & Salisbury, MA. 1990. A new perspective on canine keratoconjunctivitis sicca. *Veterinary Clinics of North America Small Animal Practice.* 20(3):583–613.

Kaswan, RL, *et al.* 1989. Spontaneous canine keratoconjunctivitis sicca, a useful model for human KCS. *Archives of Ophthalmology.* 107(8):1210–1216.

Klauss, G, *et al.* 2007. Keratoconjunctivitis sicca associated with administration of etodolac in dogs: 211 cases (1992–2002). *Journal of the American Veterinary Medical Association.* 230(4): 541–547.

La Croix, NC, *et al.* 2001. Nonhealing corneal ulcers in cats: 29 cases (1991–1999). *Journal of the American Veterinary Medical Association.* 218(5):733–735.

Mariani, CL & Fulton, RB. 2001. Atypical reaction to acetaminophen intoxication in a dog. *Journal of Veterinary Emergency and Critical Care.* 11(2):123–126.

Matheis, FL, *et al.* 2012. Canine neurogenic keratoconjunctivitis sicca: 11 cases (2006–2010). *Veterinary Ophthalmology.* 15(4):288–290.

Miller, T, *et al.* 2003. Use of thermokeratoplasty for treatment of ulcerative keratitis and bullous keratopathy secondary to corneal endothelial disease in dogs: 13 cases (1994–2001). *Journal of the American Veterinary Medical Association.* 222(5):607–612.

Moore, CP, *et al.* 2001. Effect of cyclosporine on conjunctival mucin in a canine keratoconjunctivitis sicca model. *Investigative Ophthalmology and Visual Science.* 42(3):653–659.

Morgan, RV & Abrams, KJ. 1991. Topical administration of cyclosporine for treatment of keratoconjunctivitis sicca in dogs. *Journal of the American Veterinary Medical Association.* 199(8):1043–1046.

Multari, D, *et al.* 2021. Corneal sequestra in cats: 175 eyes from 172 cases (2000–2016). *Journal of Small Animal Practice.* doi: 10.1111/jsap.13303.

Pot, SA, *et al.* 2014. Corneal collagen cross-linking as treatment for infectious and noninfectious corneal melting in cats and dogs: results of a prospective, nonrandomized, controlled trial. *Veterinary Ophthalmology.* 17(4):250–260.

Samuel, M, *et al.* 2019. Effects of 5% sodium chloride ophthalmic ointment on thickness and morphology of the normal canine cornea. *Veterinary Ophthalmology.* 22(3):229–237.

Sebbag, L, *et al.* 2015. Reference values, intertest correlations, and test-retest repeatability of selected tear film tests in healthy cats. *Journal of the American Veterinary Medical Association.* 246(4):426–435.

Speiss, AK, *et al.* 2009. Treatment of proliferative feline eosinophilic keratitis with topical 1.5% cyclosporine: 35 cases. *Veterinary Ophthalmology.* 12(2):132–137.

Stanley, RG, *et al.* 1998. Results of grid keratotomy, superficial keratectomy and debridement for the management of persistent corneal erosions in 92 dogs. *Veterinary Ophthalmology.* 1(4):233–238.

Uhl, LK, *et al.* 2019. Clinical features of cats with aqueous tear deficiency: a retrospective case series of 10 patients (17 eyes). *Journal of Feline Medicine and Surgery.* 21(10):944–950.

Wegg, ML. 2019. A retrospective evaluation of systemic and/or topical pilocarpine treatment for canine neurogenic dry eye: 11 cases. *Veterinary Ophthalmology.* 23(2):341–346.

Williams, DL. 1999. Histological and immunohistochemical evaluation of canine chronic superficial keratitis. *Research in Veterinary Science.* 67(2):189–193.

Williams, DL, *et al.* 2007. Reduced tear production in three canine endocrinopathies. *Journal of Small Animal Practice.* 48(5):252–256.

Wooff, PJ and Norman, JC. 2015. Effect of corneal contact lens wear on healing time and comfort post LGK for treatment of SCCEDs in boxers. *Veterinary Ophthalmology.* 18 (5):364–370.

CHAPTER 14

15 Anterior uvea

Please see Chapter 6 for images of the anterior uvea.

The uveal tract consists of the iris, ciliary body, and choroid. The iris and ciliary body comprise the anterior uvea. The choroid, which is the posterior uvea, will be discussed in Chapter 17.

When viewed during the ophthalmic examination, only the anterior iris is visible (Figures 6.1, 6.2). The ciliary body cannot be seen due to its location posterior to the iris. Terminologies used to describe areas of the anterior iris are as follows:
- Pupillary zone
  - This is the region of the iris that is adjacent to the pupil.
- Iris collarette
  - This is the zone that transitions between the pupillary and ciliary zones.
- Ciliary zone
  - This is the peripheral region of the iris, the area that is nearest the sclera.

The iris is located anterior to the lens. Components are as follows:
- Anterior border of the iris
  - This is a discontinuous layer of cells that allows communication between the anterior chamber and the iris stroma.
- Iris stroma
  - This is composed of connective tissue, melanocytes, nerves, blood vessels, and smooth muscle (listed later).
  - The vascular endothelium contributes to the blood–aqueous barrier.
  - Variations in the melanin content determine the eye color.
- Iris sphincter muscle
  - These muscle fibers are found in the pupillary zone of the iris only (not the collarette or peripheral zones).
  - The muscle fibers are arranged circumferentially such that constriction leads to miosis.
- Iris dilator muscle
  - The muscle fibers extend through the pupillary zone, iris collarette, and peripheral zone.
  - The muscle fibers are radially arranged such that constriction leads to mydriasis.
- Posterior pigmented epithelium
  - This is the densely melanotic portion of the iris.
  - It is the most posterior layer of the iris.

Anteriorly, the ciliary body is plicated; each of these plications is referred to as a ciliary body process. It is in this area that lens zonules insert. The ciliary body flattens out posteriorly as it approaches its junction with the retina. Components of the ciliary body include the following:
- Bilayered epithelium
  - Inner nonpigmented epithelium and outer pigmented epithelium.
  - The epithelium is involved in aqueous humor production and also forms a portion of the blood–aqueous barrier.
- Stroma
  - Connective tissue, blood vessels, and nerves
- Smooth muscle
  - Constriction and relaxation of this muscle affects accommodation and aqueous humor outflow.

Functions of the anterior uvea include the following:
- Provision of vascular supply to the eye
- Regulation of entrance of light into the eye
- Control of accommodation
- Formation of the blood–aqueous barrier
- Production of aqueous humor

Anterior uveal diseases

Persistent pupillary membranes (PPMs)

What they are
- PPMs are congenital, nonprogressive remnants of embryonic vasculature in the anterior chamber.

Predisposed individuals
- Cats with eyelid agenesis
- Overrepresented dog breeds include the following:
  - Basenji
  - Pembroke Welsh Corgi
  - Mastiff
  - Chow chow

Small Animal Ophthalmic Atlas and Guide, Second Edition. Christine C. Lim.
© 2023 John Wiley & Sons, Inc. Published 2023 by John Wiley & Sons, Inc.
Companion website: www.wiley.com/go/lim/atlas

Defining characteristics

- Strands of uveal tissue that arise from the iris collarette and insert on the cornea, iris, or lens
- Iris-to-cornea PPMs
  - Uveal tissue extends from the iris collarette to the corneal endothelium (Figures 6.3, 6.4).
  - Corneal fibrosis is present where the PPM contacts the cornea.
- Iris-to-iris PPMs
  - Uveal strands lay flat across the anterior iris or across the pupil (Figures 6.5, 6.6).
  - Rarely interfere with pupil movement.
- Iris-to-lens PPMs
  - Strands of uveal tissue extend from the iris collarette to the anterior lens capsule (Figure 6.7).
  - Opacification of the lens (cataract) is present where the PPMs insert onto the lens.

Clinical significance

- PPMs are not associated with ocular discomfort.
- Iris-to-iris PPMs are rarely of clinical significance.
  - Except in Basenjis, where PPM formation can be extensive and associated with visual compromise.
- Corneal opacification accompanying iris-to-cornea PPMs can limit vision.
- Cataract associated with iris-to-lens PPMs can interfere with vision.
- PPMs are considered heritable in the Basenji, mastiff, chow chow, and Pembroke Welsh Corgi.
  - Breeding is discouraged.

Diagnosis

- The diagnosis is based on clinical appearance.
- PPMs always arise from the iris collarette, not the pupillary or ciliary zones.
  - Noting the origin point of PPMs can help to differentiate PPMs from anterior or posterior synechiae, which can resemble PPMs.

Treatment

- PPMs are rarely treated.
  - Extensive PPMs should be referred to a veterinary ophthalmologist.

Prognosis

- For most cases, the prognosis is good as there is no overt visual compromise, patients are comfortable, and PPMs do not progress.
- For cases with mild corneal or lenticular opacification, the prognosis for maintaining a comfortable eye with functional vision is good.

- Evaluation by a veterinary ophthalmologist is recommended.
- If corneal or lenticular opacities are extensive, the prognosis for comfort is good, but vision may be limited.
  - Evaluation by a veterinary ophthalmologist is recommended.

Additional information

- Due to similar appearance, it may be difficult to differentiate anterior synechiae from iris-to-cornea PPMs and posterior synechiae from iris-to-lens PPMs.
  - Differentiation is made by visualizing the location of the affected iris.
  - The iris attachments of the PPMs are at the iris collarette.
  - Anterior synechiae arise from the pupillary zone (Figure 6.50) or, less commonly, the ciliary zone of the iris.
  - Posterior synechiae arise from the pupillary zone of the iris (Figures 6.51, 6.52, 6.53, 6.54).
  - Differentiation is important because PPMs are usually clinically insignificant, while synechiae indicate previous or current intraocular inflammation (which warrants further investigation due to potential impact on comfort and vision).

Uveal cysts

What they are

- Fluid-filled structures lined by secretory epithelium of the iris or ciliary body.

Predisposed individuals

- Uveal cysts are seen more often in dogs than cats.
- In cats, Burmese may be overrepresented (Blacklock *et al.*, 2016).

Defining characteristics

- Round, pigmented structures, either free-floating in the anterior chamber (Figures 6.8, 6.9, 6.10) or adhered to the iris or ciliary body (Figures 6.11, 6.12, 6.13).
- In cats, cysts are often adhered to the pupillary margin (Blacklock *et al.*, 2016) (Figures 6.11, 6.12).
- Cysts may be present in the posterior chamber (between the iris and the lens) (Figure 6.13).
- Cysts tend to be rounded with smooth edges.
- Degree of pigmentation varies from a translucent light brown to opaque black.
- Anterior uveal melanoma/melanocytoma is the main rule-out.
- Transillumination can differentiate between a cyst and neoplasm in most cases.
  - Due to the thin wall of the cyst, the examiner should be able to see light pass through the cyst wall during transillumination (Figures 6.9, 6.13).
  - Light does not pass through a solid neoplasm.

Clinical significance

- In most cases, cysts are incidental, benign findings.
- Uncommonly, cysts can be associated with visual disturbance (for example, when they obstruct the pupil) or behavior abnormalities (for example, biting at the air as if trying to catch an object).
- Uncommonly, if cysts are large and/or numerous, they may obstruct aqueous outflow and cause IOP elevation.
- In golden retrievers, great Danes, and American bulldogs, cysts can occur as part of a uveitic syndrome that may also include changes such as cataracts and glaucoma (Pumphrey *et al.*, 2013; Sapienza *et al.*, 2000; Speiss *et al.*, 1998).

Diagnosis

- The diagnosis is based on characteristic appearance and transillumination.

Treatment

- Treatment is rarely required.
- Cysts are only treated if they are suspected to cause visual compromise, behavior problems, or elevated IOP.
  - Referral to a veterinary ophthalmologist is needed (for laser deflation, cyst aspiration, or removal from anterior chamber).

Prognosis

- Because most cysts are incidental findings, the prognosis for a comfortable, visual eye is good.
- Development of more cysts is possible.
- American bulldogs, great Danes, and golden retrievers with cysts as part of uveitic syndromes are at risk of vision loss and/or ocular discomfort from sequelae such as cataract or glaucoma. (See the uveitis section for discussion of sequelae to uveitis.)

Additional information

- Rarely, cyst walls are too thick to allow transillumination.
  - This is often noted in cats (Fragola *et al.*, 2018).
  - If the objects are free-floating, then they are cysts and not neoplasms.
  - If they are not free-floating, ultrasound can be used to differentiate the fluid-filled cyst from a solid neoplasm.
  - Referral to a veterinary ophthalmologist is recommended if the diagnosis is not clear.
- Observation of cysts alone in American bulldogs, great Danes, and golden retrievers does not necessarily indicate uveitis.
  - However, since cysts can be early signs of uveitic syndromes, periodic monitoring is recommended.
  - Observation over time will determine if uveitis develops or if cysts are clinically insignificant.
  - Referral to a veterinary ophthalmologist is recommended in these breeds, or in other breeds if there is suspicion for concurrent uveitis.

Iris atrophy

What it is

- Iris atrophy refers to degeneration of the iris tissue.

Predisposed individuals

- Iris atrophy is a normal aging change.
- The iris can also atrophy as a result of anterior uveitis.

Defining characteristics

- The pupillary margin may look irregular (often described as "scalloped") (Figures 6.14, 6.15).
- The iris surface may look thinned (often described as "moth-eaten") (Figures 6.16, 6.17).
  - The iris in these areas may look black; as the iris stroma atrophies, the posterior pigmented epithelium becomes more visible.
- Large, full-thickness defects can also appear (Figures 6.15, 6.18).

Clinical significance

- Iris atrophy does not cause clinical problems.
- Severe iris atrophy may cause the following ophthalmic examination abnormalities:
  - Anisocoria
  - Dyscoria
  - Reduced pupillary constriction

Diagnosis

- The diagnosis is based on clinical appearance.

Treatment

- Iris atrophy is not treated.

Prognosis

- With age-related iris atrophy, the prognosis for a comfortable, visual eye is very good.
- For iris atrophy secondary to uveitis, the prognosis for retaining vision and comfort is related to the uveitis (the severity and chronicity of uveitis and response to therapy) rather than the atrophy itself.

Feline diffuse iris melanoma

What it is

- Primary, melanocytic neoplasia of the feline iris and/or ciliary body.

Predisposed individuals

- Cats 11 years of age or older are overrepresented (Bellhorn & Henkind, 1970; Patnaik & Mooney, 1988).

Defining characteristics

- *Iridal hyperpigmentation*
  - Benign melanosis is also characterized by iridal hyperpigmentation and is the main differential consideration.
  - Differentiating early melanoma from benign melanosis is challenging and sometimes impossible with clinical examination alone.
- In early stages, hyperpigmentation can be focal (Figures 6.19, 6.20), but as melanoma progresses, the color change becomes diffuse (Figures 6.21, 6.22, 6.23, 6.24).
  - Early, focal melanoma can be indistinguishable from benign melanosis.
  - Progression can occur slowly over years, or as rapidly as over weeks.
    - Benign lesions that remain static for years can undergo neoplastic transformation later in life.
- Early lesions are flat.
  - With progression, the normal surface texture of the iris is altered, becoming thicker or raised (Figure 6.24).
- Dyscoria (Figures 6.21, 6.24) and altered pupillary function can be present (Edwards *et al.*, 2015).
  - Due to neoplastic infiltration of iris stroma and muscles.
  - Often accompanied by increased visibility of the posterior pigmented epithelium at the pupillary margin (Figure 6.21).
  - Benign melanosis should not cause distortion of the iris or pupil.
- Signs of uveitis (see "Anterior uveitis" later in this chapter) may be present with advanced lesions (Figure 6.25).
  - Benign melanosis does not cause uveitis.
- IOP can be elevated, if the iridocorneal angle is involved.
  - Benign melanosis does not cause glaucoma.

Clinical significance

- This is the most common primary intraocular tumor of cats.
- Reported metastatic rates vary, ranging from under 20% to over 60% (Patnaik & Mooney, 1988; Wiggans *et al.*, 2016).
  - Metastasis most often affects the liver and lungs, but can also affect lymph nodes, bone, and other locations (Bellhorn & Henkind, 1970; Duncan & Peiffer, 1991; Patnaik & Mooney, 1988; Planellas, 2010).
- Risk of metastatic disease is higher if neoplastic cells extend further into ocular structures than the anterior iris stroma (Kalishman *et al.*, 1998; Wiggans *et al.*, 2016).
  - Neoplastic cells may leave the eye through the iridocorneal angle or vasculature of the uvea or sclera.
- Time period to clinical evidence of metastatic disease can be prolonged.
  - Metastatic disease requiring euthanasia may not emerge until several years after enucleation (Duncan & Peiffer, 1991; Patnaik & Mooney, 1988).

Diagnosis

- There is no one pathognomonic clinical finding; tentative diagnosis is based on clinical suspicion, which is based on clinical appearance.
- Signs that are more suggestive of melanoma than of benign melanosis are as follows:
  - Rapid progression of size
  - Diffuse iridal hyperpigmentation
  - Thickening of hyperpigmented areas of iris
  - Dyscoria
  - Altered pupil movement
  - Anterior uveitis
  - Elevated IOP
- Definitive diagnosis (and therefore differentiation from benign melanosis) requires histopathology.
  - Globe is submitted following enucleation.
  - Iris biopsy, without enucleation, is uncommonly performed due to potential for causing ocular damage.
- Tumor staging, especially if lesions do not appear confined to the anterior iris.
  - Physical examination
  - CBC, serum biochemical profile, and urinalysis
  - Thoracic radiographs or CT
  - Abdominal ultrasound or CT
  - Fine-needle aspirates of any enlarged lymph nodes

Treatment

- The goals of treatment are to remove the tumor, reduce potential for metastasis, and manage patient discomfort.
- Referral to a veterinary ophthalmologist for evaluation is recommended.
- Small, discrete hyperpigmented lesions like the lesions shown in Figures 6.19 and 6.20 can be monitored with serial photographs.
  - To determine if the lesion is enlarging and the rate of growth.
  - Photographs are more objective than drawings for documenting presence or absence of progression.
- Laser ablation of small, discrete lesions is sometimes performed (Cook & Wilkie, 1999).
  - Success rate of this procedure is not known.
- Enucleation is warranted for
  - larger lesions or those showing size progression,
  - lesions with associated uveitis or glaucoma, and
  - lesions that alter iris structure or function.
- Tumor staging prior to enucleation is recommended.
- Following enucleation, the eye must be submitted for histopathology.
  - Aids in prognostication by determining cellular characteristics, extent of tumor, and if cells have reached ocular exit pathways.

Prognosis

- Prognosis for survival is best when the eye is enucleated at a stage when iris hyperpigmentation is the only abnormality detected on ophthalmic examination.
  - This means the prognosis for survival is best when the eye is removed while still comfortable and visual.
- When tumors do not extend beyond the anterior iris stroma, survival time is not diminished (Kalishman *et al.*, 1998).
- Factors associated with reduced survival time include:
  - tumor extension into the posterior pigmented epithelium of the iris or ciliary body (Kalishman *et al.*, 1998),
  - neoplastic cells within the choroid (Wiggans *et al.*, 2016),
  - neoplastic cells within the scleral venous plexus (Kalishman *et al.*, 1998) or extrascleral extension of neoplastic cells (Wiggans *et al.*, 2016),
  - histological evidence of increased pigmentation and moderate cellular differentiation, and
  - presence of glaucoma (Kalishman *et al.*, 1998).

Additional information

- Histopathology should always be performed after enucleation.
  - Definitive diagnosis is obtained.
  - Assists in prognostication.
- Routine clinical examination cannot determine if melanotic cells extend into the iridocorneal angle.
  - Gonioscopy, performed by a veterinary ophthalmologist, is recommended to rule this out, especially when hyperpigmentation approaches the peripheral iris (ciliary zone).
- Because it is not always possible to definitively diagnose melanoma prior to enucleation, clients should be informed that histopathology may reveal benign melanosis.

Canine anterior uveal melanocytic neoplasia

What it is

- Melanocytic neoplasia arising from the canine iris and/or ciliary body.
- Melanocytoma, a benign tumor, is the most common.
  - Malignant melanocytic neoplasia is rare.
  - Therefore, further discussion is focused on melanocytoma.

Predisposed individuals

- Middle-aged to older dogs are most commonly affected.

Defining characteristics

- The appearance of anterior uveal melanocytoma can vary slightly.
  - Focal, flat, hyperpigmented lesion of the iris (Figure 6.26)
  - A diffuse, melanotic thickening of the iris.
  - A raised, melanotic mass of the iris or the ciliary body (Figures 6.27, 6.28, 6.29).

- During transillumination, light cannot be seen passing through the mass.
  - This is in contrast to uveal cysts, which usually have thin walls that allow the passage of light.
- Lesions with irregular edges are unlikely to be uveal cysts, which tend to have smooth, rounded borders.
- Dyscoria is often present (Figures 6.27, 6.28, 6.29).

Clinical significance

- This is the most common primary intraocular tumor of dogs.
- Canine uveal melanocytoma is benign, but enlargement of the tumor can compromise adjacent ocular structures in addition to the anterior uvea:
  - Dyscoria (Figures 6.27, 6.28, 6.29)
  - Altered pupil function
  - Displacement of the iris
  - Displacement of the lens
  - Uveitis
  - Glaucoma
- These must be differentiated from uveal cysts, which can also appear mass-like.
  - Transillumination allows for differentiation in most cases.
- Malignant melanoma often occurs in eyes with melanocytoma (Dubielzig *et al.*, 2010), but this tumor is rare in dogs.

Diagnosis

- Tentative diagnosis is based on clinical appearance (see aforementioned).
- Definitive diagnosis requires histopathologic evaluation.
  - Iris biopsy, without enucleation, is generally not performed due to potential for damage caused by such a procedure.
- Tumor staging.
  - Physical examination
  - CBC, serum biochemical profile, and urinalysis
  - Thoracic radiographs or CT
  - Abdominal ultrasound or CT
  - Fine-needle aspirates of any enlarged lymph nodes

Treatment

- The goals of treatment are to manage any patient discomfort, minimize potential for metastasis, and, when necessary, remove the tumor.
- Focal lesions can be monitored with serial photographs.
  - To objectively determine if the lesion is progressing.
  - Lesions that remain static in size, without concurrent uveitis or displacement of intraocular structures, may not require definitive treatment.
  - These should be monitored for enlargement and/or development of the aforementioned complications.
- Focal melanotic lesions can be referred to a veterinary ophthalmologist for laser ablation (Cook & Wilkie, 1999).

- In rare cases, small lesions referred to veterinary ophthalmologists may be excised (Davis *et al.*, 2020).
- Eyes with more extensive lesions, especially with impingement on other ocular structures, concurrent uveitis, or glaucoma, should be enucleated.

Prognosis
- Prognosis for survival is excellent following enucleation.
  - Survival time is not diminished (Giuliano *et al.*, 1999).
- Recurrence following enucleation is uncommon (Dieters *et al.*, 1983; Giuliano *et al.*, 1999).
- Metastasis is rare (Dieters *et al.*, 1983; Giuliano *et al.*, 1999).

Additional information
- Malignant uveal melanoma is very uncommon in dogs.
  - However, histopathology after enucleation is required to rule this out.

Iridociliary neoplasia

What it is
- Neoplasms arising from the epithelium of the iris or ciliary body.
- Adenoma is much more common than adenocarcinoma.

Predisposed individuals
- Iridociliary neoplasia is more common in dogs than cats.
  - The discussion therefore focuses on dogs.
- Middle-aged to older individuals are overrepresented.
- Labrador and golden retrievers are overrepresented (Dubielzig *et al.*, 1998).

Defining characteristics
- A mass arising from the iris or from posterior to the iris (Figures 6.30, 6.31).
- The mass may displace the iris and/or the lens.
- The mass can be pigmented or nonpigmented.

Clinical significance
- Iridociliary neoplasms are the second-most common primary intraocular tumor of dogs.
- Malignancy is uncommon.
- Although usually benign, enlargement of the tumor can cause the following:
  - Displacement of the iris
  - Displacement of the lens
  - Uveitis
  - Glaucoma

Diagnosis
- Tentative diagnosis is based on visualization of a mass arising from the posterior chamber (behind the iris).
- Definitive diagnosis is achieved with histopathology.
- Tumor staging

- Physical examination
- CBC, serum biochemical profile, and urinalysis
- Thoracic radiographs or CT
- Abdominal ultrasound or CT
- Fine-needle aspirates of any enlarged lymph nodes

Treatment
- The goals of treatment are to manage any patient discomfort, minimize potential for metastasis, and remove the tumor.
- Although most cases are benign, enucleation is warranted when iridociliary neoplasia displaces intraocular structures or incites uveitis and/or glaucoma.
- It is possible for small lesions to be resected when referred to a veterinary ophthalmologist.
  - However, this treatment is uncommon due to the potential for damage to the eye and the high potential for incomplete resection and recurrence (Beckwith-Cohen *et al.*, 2015).

Prognosis
- The prognosis is excellent following enucleation.
  - Recurrence is uncommon.
  - Metastasis is rare.
    - Can occur in advanced disease (Peiffer, 1983).

Anterior uveitis

What it is
- Inflammation of the iris, ciliary body, or both.
- Anterior uveitis can be further categorized by specific structures that are inflamed:
  - Iritis: inflammation of the iris
  - Cyclitis: inflammation of the ciliary body
  - Iridocyclitis: inflammation of the iris and ciliary body
  - However, in practice, it is not possible to differentiate to this level, so the broader term of anterior uveitis is generally used.
- Results from breakdown of the blood–aqueous barrier.

Predisposed individuals
- Dogs and cats of any age can develop anterior uveitis.
- Predispositions to specific uveitic syndromes exist:
  - LIU
    - Dogs with cataracts
  - Pigmentary uveitis
    - Golden retriever
    - Great Dane
  - Uveodermatologic syndrome (Vogt–Koyanagi–Harada–like syndrome)
    - Akita
    - Samoyed
    - Siberian husky
  - Uveitis secondary to infectious disease
    - Younger to middle-aged animals
  - Uveitis as a consequence of primary or secondary neoplastic disease
    - Middle-aged to older individuals

Defining characteristics

- Potential ophthalmic examination findings (Figures 6.32, 6.33, 6.34):
  - *Blepharospasm*
  - *Epiphora*
  - Elevated third eyelid
  - *Episcleral congestion*
  - *Corneal edema*
  - Deep corneal vessels
  - *Hypotony*
    - IOP below 10–12 mm Hg with clinical signs is suggestive of anterior uveitis.
    - A difference of more than 20% between eyes, even if both measure within the normal range, can also be suggestive of anterior uveitis (Maggs, 2009).
  - *Aqueous flare* (Figure 6.36)
    - Pathognomonic for anterior uveitis.
    - Severity of flare correlates with severity of uveitis.
    - Absence of flare (Figure 6.35), however, does not necessarily mean absence of uveitis.
  - *Miosis*
  - Keratic precipitates (Figures 6.37, 6.38, 6.39, 6.47, 6.48)
  - Fibrin in the anterior chamber (Figure 6.48)
  - Hypopyon (Figures 5.2, 5.58, 6.34, 6.38)
  - Hyphema (Figures 6.40, 6.41, 6.42, 6.43)
  - Lipid within the aqueous (Figure 6.33)
  - Rubeosis iridis (Figures 6.44, 6.45, 6.46, 6.47, 6.48)
  - Iridal hemorrhage (Figure 6.49)
  - Iris thickening (Figure 6.45)
  - Iris nodule formation
  - Anterior synechiae (Figure 6.50)
  - Posterior synechiae (Figures 6.51, 6.52, 6.53, 6.54)
  - Photophobia

Clinical significance

- Anterior uveitis is painful.
- Anterior uveitis can lead to secondary complications that are blinding and painful (see "Prognosis").
- Posterior uveitis may be present concurrently (see Chorioretinitis in Chapter 17).
  - It is imperative to perform a complete ophthalmic examination, which includes the fundic examination.
- Anterior uveitis may have an underlying cause, which must be treated for effective treatment of uveitis.
- Anterior uveitis may be a symptom of an underlying systemic disease, some of which are life-threatening.
- Select causes of uveitis include:
  - Neoplastic disease
    - This is one of the three most common cause of uveitis in dogs and cats (Bergstrom *et al.,* 2017; Davidson *et al.,* 1991; Massa *et al.,* 2000; Peiffer & Wilcock, 1991; Wegg *et al.,* 2021).
    - Melanocytic and iridociliary neoplasms (discussed earlier) are common primary intraocular tumors.

- Lymphoma is the most common metastatic tumor to the eye.
- Any systemic neoplasm has the potential to metastasize to the eye.
  - Infectious disease
    - Infectious disease is one of the three most common causes of nontraumatic uveitis in dogs and cats (Bergstrom *et al.,* 2017; Davidson *et al.,* 1991; Massa *et al.,* 2000; Peiffer & Wilcock, 1991; Wegg *et al.,* 2021).
    - Bacterial disease, for example, *Leptospira* spp., and *Brucella canis.*
    - Viral disease, for example, FIV, FeLV, FIP, and canine distemper virus.
    - Fungal disease, for example, *Blastomyces dermatitidis, Cryptococcus neoformans, Histoplasma capsulatum,* and *Coccidioides immitis.*
    - Tick-borne disease, for example, *Ehrlichia canis, Rickettsia rickettsii,* and *Anaplasma caninum.*
    - Protozoal disease, for example, *Toxoplasma gondii* and *Neospora caninum.*
    - Parasitic disease, for example, *Leishmania* spp., onchocerciasis, and aberrant migration of parasite larvae.
    - Algal disease, for example, *Prototheca* spp.
  - Immune-mediated disease
    - LIU
    - Uveodermatologic syndrome
  - Trauma
    - Corneal ulceration
    - Blunt or penetrating trauma to the eye
    - Intraocular surgery
  - Others
    - Breed-related uveitic syndromes, such as those affecting great Danes, American bulldogs, and golden retrievers
    - Systemic hypertension
    - Coagulopathy
  - Uveitis can also be idiopathic.
    - This category represents the majority of uveitis cases in cats and dogs.
    - This may account for approximately 60–70% of cases in dogs (Bergstrom *et al.,* 2017; Massa *et al.,* 2000).
    - In cats, this may account for 40–70% of cases (Davidson *et al.,* 1991; Jinks *et al.,* 2016; Wegg *et al.,* 2021).

Diagnosis

- The diagnostic process is divided into (1) diagnosing uveitis and (2) determining its underlying cause.
1. Diagnosing uveitis
   - The diagnosis is based on clinical signs. (See "Defining characteristics.")
   - Episcleral congestion with corneal edema, aqueous flare, miosis, and hypotony is the most common combination of clinical signs.
   - Severity of clinical signs generally correlates with severity of inflammation.

◦ Fundic examination should also be performed to rule in/rule out concurrent posterior uveitis (see "Chorioretinitis" in Chapter 17).

  ▪ If fundic examination is not possible due to anterior segment opacification, referral to a veterinary ophthalmologist for further diagnostics (e.g., ocular ultrasound) is recommended.

2 Determining the underlying cause

Although idiopathic uveitis is the most common "cause" of uveitis, diagnostics to rule out systemic disease should be performed.

- Idiopathic uveitis is a diagnosis of exclusion.
- Treatment is less effective if an underlying disease is present but not addressed.
- Underlying systemic disease can cause significant morbidity and mortality.

Testing for an underlying disease involves the following:

- Physical examination.
- CBC, serum biochemical profile, and urinalysis.
- Infectious disease testing as dictated by clinical suspicion, lifestyle, geographic location, and travel history
- Fine-needle aspirates of any enlarged lymph nodes, cutaneous or subcutaneous masses.
- Following referral to a veterinary ophthalmologist, select cases may undergo aqueous humor aspirates.
  ◦ This test yields a diagnosis in a minority of canine cases, and is not considered helpful in cats (Wiggans *et al.,* 2014).
- Thoracic radiographs or CT.
- Abdominal radiographs, ultrasound, or CT.
- Histopathology of enucleated eyes.

Treatment

The goals of treatment are to remove the underlying cause of uveitis, eliminate inflammation, manage patient discomfort, and minimize development of sequelae. Treatment therefore involves the following: (1) treatment of the underlying disease, (2) anti-inflammatory therapy, (3) atropine therapy, and (4) other analgesic therapy.

1 Treatment of the underlying cause
  ◦ An underlying cause, if present, must be treated for treatment of anterior uveitis to be effective.
  ◦ Only possible if an underlying cause can be identified.

2 Anti-inflammatory therapy
  ◦ Whether treatment is administered to the eye or systemically, initial treatment involves either corticosteroids or NSAIDs.
    ▪ The goal is to wean the dose of medications and completely discontinue medications after resolution of clinical signs.
    ▪ However, some individuals require a low dose in the long term to prevent recurrence of inflammation.
      ▫ Use the lowest possible dose to achieve this.

◦ Ophthalmically applied medications:
  ▪ If inflammation is limited to the anterior segment of the eye (i.e., absence of posterior uveitis), then ophthalmic therapy alone may be sufficient to treat inflammation.
  ▪ Ophthalmic administration is preferred to minimize side effects of systemically administered drugs.
  ▪ Corticosteroids: prednisolone acetate 1% ophthalmic suspension or dexamethasone 0.1% ophthalmic solution.
    ▫ Prednisolone has superior intraocular penetration to dexamethasone (McGhee *et al.,* 1990).
    ▫ Initially apply one drop two to four times daily, depending on the severity of uveitis.
    ▫ As clinical signs improve, taper the dose gradually.
    ▫ Do not use in the presence of corneal ulceration.
  ▪ NSAIDs: diclofenac 0.1% ophthalmic solution, flurbiprofen 0.03% ophthalmic solution, or ketorolac tromethamine 0.5% ophthalmic solution; many others are available.
    ▫ Initially apply one drop two to four times daily, depending on the severity of uveitis.
    ▫ As clinical signs improve, taper the dose gradually.
    ▫ Not recommended for use in the presence of corneal ulceration.
    ▫ Not recommended for use with active intraocular hemorrhage.

◦ Systemic medications:
  ▪ If concurrent posterior uveitis is present, systemic administration is required.
    ▫ Ophthalmically administered medications generally do not reach therapeutic concentrations in the posterior segment.
  ▪ Systemic therapy can be used for anterior uveitis without concurrent posterior uveitis, usually in the following situations:
    ▫ Instead of ophthalmic medications when patients do not tolerate administration of medications to the eye.
    ▫ Instead of ophthalmic medications in the presence of corneal ulceration.
    ▫ To augment ophthalmic medications when they cannot be administered as often as required.
  ▪ Corticosteroids: prednisone/prednisolone.
    ▫ Initially administer 0.5–1 mg/kg PO q24h–q12h.
    ▫ Gradually taper the dose as clinical signs improve.
    ▫ Do not use if infectious disease is suspected.
    ▫ Not recommended for use if lymphoma is suspected, as this can alter results of diagnostics or influence efficacy of chemotherapeutic protocols.
    ▫ Do not use in patients with systemic disease where corticosteroid use is contraindicated (e.g., hepatic dysfunction).
    ▫ Do not use concurrently with systemically administered NSAIDs.

- NSAIDs: veterinary-labeled products such as carprofen (Rimadyl®), meloxicam (Metacam®), and robenacoxib (Onsior®), as well as others.
  - Use at labeled dose.
  - Do not use concurrently with systemically administered corticosteroids.
  - Not recommended for use in patients with systemic conditions for which NSAIDs are contraindicated (e.g., those with renal compromise).
3 Atropine therapy
  - Atropine stabilizes the blood–aqueous barrier (van Alphen & Macri, 1966).
  - Atropine also provides analgesia.
    - Uveitis pain arises from spasm of the ciliary body muscle.
    - This muscle is not visible on ophthalmic examination; however, its spasm is inferred if spasm of the iris sphincter muscle (resulting in miosis) is observed.
    - Atropine causes cycloplegia (paralysis of the ciliary body muscle).
      - Cycloplegia is inferred when paralysis of the iris sphincter muscle is seen (mydriasis).
  - Minimizes posterior synechiae formation.
    - Mydriasis decreases the surface area of contact between the iris and the lens and therefore the potential for adhesions (synechiae) between these structures.
  - Guidelines for use:
    - Atropine 1% ophthalmic solution or ointment.
    - Initially apply one drop (or ¼" strip) q24h–q12h to maintain pupillary dilation.
      - The higher dose is required for severe inflammation.
      - After mydriasis is achieved, the dose can be decreased to the lowest possible dose needed to maintain dilation (e.g., even q48h).
  - Do not use if IOP is elevated (see Chapter 18) because mydriasis can exacerbate glaucoma.
4 Other analgesic therapy
  - Consider analgesics like transmucosal buprenorphine (in cats; 0.01–0.03 mg/kg q8h) or oral gabapentin (5–10 mg/kg q12–q8h in cats; 10–20 mg/kg PO q12h–q8h in dogs) if anti-inflammatory therapy does not provide sufficient pain management.

In many cases, painful, blinding sequelae occur in spite of treatment. For eyes that are blind and painful, enucleation is recommended to relieve pain. Histopathology of the enucleated globe also provides valuable diagnostic information.

Prognosis

- The prognosis for a comfortable, visual eye is extremely variable.
  - For mild uveitis that responds to therapy, prognosis is very good.
  - For eyes with chronic inflammation, severe inflammation, or inflammation that does not improve with treatment, the prognosis is guarded due to development of sequelae (see below-mentioned information).

- Sequelae can lead to visual impairment or blindness:
  - Synechiae
  - Iris atrophy
  - Cataract (see Chapter 16)
  - Lens luxation (see Chapter 16)
  - Glaucoma (see Chapter 18)
    - With or without iris bombé (Figures 6.42, 6.54)
  - Retinal detachment
  - Phthisis bulbi
- Some patients require indefinite treatment to prevent recurrence of uveitis.
  - Breed-related uveitic syndromes (such as those seen in the golden retriever, great Dane, and American bulldog) and immune-mediated syndromes (such as uveodermatologic syndrome) usually require lifelong therapy.
- Patients with a history of uveitis are more susceptible to future episodes of inflammation.
- Any underlying systemic disease will influence prognosis for the eye as well as the entire patient.

Additional information

- Uveitis of any cause can be unilateral or bilateral.
  - Unilateral cases are more likely to be idiopathic or due to causes such as trauma or corneal ulceration.
  - Bilateral cases are more likely to be due to an underlying systemic disease.
- Development of secondary glaucoma can be insidious.
  - Monitor trend of IOP over time so that secondary glaucoma is caught early.
  - Since IOP in anterior uveitis is usually low, normal IOP in the presence of inflammation can be an early indicator of secondary glaucoma.
- As inflammation subsides, severity of clinical signs should decrease.
  - If IOP remains low after clinically visible abnormalities has resolved, this may indicate persistent, low-grade inflammation requiring continued treatment.
- Recheck examination after complete cessation of medications is recommended to monitor for recurrence of inflammation.
- Periodic monitoring after resolution of anterior uveitis is warranted, as patients may be more susceptible to future episodes of inflammation.
- Geriatric dogs and cats can have low IOP without concurrent ocular disease (Gelatt & MacKay, 1998; Kroll et al., 2001).
  - Therefore, in a patient with no history of intraocular inflammation, low IOP as the only abnormality on ophthalmic examination is unlikely to be significant.

Further reading

Uveitis
Maggs, DJ. 2009. Feline uveitis. An "intraocular lymphadenopathy." *Journal of Feline Medicine and Surgery.* 11(3):167–182.
Telle, MR & Betbeze, C. 2015. Hyphema: considerations in the small animal patient. *Topics in Companion Animal Medicine.* 30(3):97–106.

References

Beckwith-Cohen, B, et al. 2015. Outcome of iridociliary epithelial tumour biopsies in dogs: a retrospective study. *Veterinary Record.* 176(6):147–151.

Bellhorn, RR & Henkind, P. 1970. Intraocular malignant melanoma in domestic cats. *Journal of Small Animal Practice.* 10(11): 631–637.

Bergstrom, BE, et al. 2017. Canine panuveitis: a retrospective evaluation of 55 cases (2000–2015). *Veterinary Ophthalmology.* 20(5):390–397.

Blacklock, BT, et al. 2016. Uveal cysts in domestic cats: a retrospective evaluation of thirty-six cases. *Veterinary Ophthalmology.* 19(S1):56–60.

Cook, CS & Wilkie, DA. 1999. Treatment of presumed iris melanoma in dogs by diode laser photocoagulation: 23 cases. *Veterinary Ophthalmology.* 2(3):217–225.

Davidson, MG, et al. 1991. Feline anterior uveitis: a study of 53 cases. *Journal of the American Animal Hospital Association.* 27(1):77–83.

Davis, RL, et al. 2020. Surgical excision of iridociliary tumors using a postero-anterior cyclo-iridectomy and thermocautery in two dogs. *Veterinary Ophthalmology.* 23(3):579–587.

Dieters, RW, et al. 1983. Primary ocular melanoma in dogs. *Veterinary Pathology.* 20(4):379–395.

Dubielzig, RR, et al. 1998. Iridociliary epithelial tumors in 100 dogs and 17 cats: a morphological study. *Veterinary Ophthalmology.* 1(4):223–231.

Dubielzig, RR, et al. 2010. The uvea. In: Veterinary Ocular Pathology, p. 245–322. Saunders Elsevier, New York.

Duncan, DE & Peiffer, RL. 1991. Morphology and prognostic indicators of anterior uveal melanomas in cats. *Progress in Veterinary & Comparative Ophthalmology.* 1(1):25–32.

Edwards, S, et al. 2015. Abstract no. 066: Feline diffuse iris melanoma vs. melanosis: a retrospective case series. *Veterinary Ophthalmology.* 18(6):E27.

Fragola, JA, et al. 2018. Iridociliary cysts masquerading as neoplasia in cats: a morphologic review of 14 cases. *Veterinary Ophthalmology.* 21(2):125–131.

Gelatt, KN & MacKay, EO. 1998. Distribution of intraocular pressure in dogs. *Veterinary Ophthalmology.* 1(2–3):109–114.

Giuliano, EA, et al. 1999. A matched observational study of canine survival with primary intraocular melanocytic neoplasia. *Veterinary Ophthalmology.* 2(3):185–190.

Jinks, MR, et al. 2016. Causes of endogenous uveitis in cats presented to referral clinics in North Carolina. *Veterinary Ophthalmology.* 19(S1):30–37.

Kalishman, JB, et al. 1998. A matched observational study of survival in cats with enucleation due to diffuse iris melanoma. *Veterinary Ophthalmology.* 1(1):25–29.

Kroll, MM, et al. 2001. Intraocular pressure measurements obtained as part of a comprehensive geriatric health examination from cats seven years of age or older. *Journal of the American Veterinary Medical Association.* 219(10):1406–1410.

Maggs, DJ. 2009. Feline uveitis. An "intraocular lymphadenopathy." *Journal of Feline Medicine and Surgery.* 11(3):167–182.

Massa, KL, et al. 2000. Causes of uveitis in dogs: 102 cases. *Veterinary Ophthalmology.* 5(2):93–98.

McGhee, DNJ, et al. 1990. Penetration of synthetic corticosteroids into human aqueous humour. *Eye.* 4(3):526–530.

Patnaik, A & Mooney, S. 1988. Feline melanoma: a comparative study of ocular, oral, and dermal neoplasms. *Veterinary Pathology.* 25(2):105–112.

Peiffer, RL. 1983. Ciliary body epithelial tumors in the dog and cat; a report of thirteen cases. *Journal of Small Animal Practice.* 24(6):347–370.

Peiffer, RL & Wilcock, BP. 1991. Histopathologic study of uveitis in cats: 139 cases (1978–1988). *Journal of the American Veterinary Medical Association.* 198(1):135–138.

Planellas, M, et al. 2010. Unusual presentation of a metastatic uveal melanoma in a cat. *Veterinary Ophthalmology.* 13(6):391–394.

Pumphrey, SA, et al. 2013. Glaucoma associated with uveal cysts and goniodysgenesis in American bulldogs: a case series. *Veterinary Ophthalmology.* 16(5):377–385.

Sapienza, JS, et al. 2000. Golden Retriever uveitis: 75 cases (1994–1999). *Veterinary Ophthalmology.* 3(4):241–246.

Speiss, BM, et al. 1998. Multiple ciliary body cysts and secondary glaucoma in the Great Dane: a report of nine cases. *Veterinary Ophthalmology.* 1(1): 41–45.

Van Alphen, GWHM & Macri, FJ. 1966. Entrance of fluorescein into aqueous humor of cat eye. *Archives of Ophthalmology.* 75(2):247–253.

Wegg, ML, et al. 2021. A multicenter retrospective study into endogenous causes of uveitis in cats in the United Kingdom: Ninety two cases. *Veterinary Ophthalmology.* doi:10.1111/vop.12898

Wiggans, KT, et al. 2014. Diagnostic utility of aqueocentesis and aqueous humor analysis in dogs and cats with anterior uveitis. *Veterinary Ophthalmology.* 17(3):212–220.

Wiggans, KT, et al. 2016. Histologic and immunohistochemical predictors of clinical behavior for feline diffuse iris melanoma. *Veterinary Ophthalmology.* 19(S1):44–55.

CHAPTER 15

16 Lens

Please see Chapter 7 for images of the lens.

The crystalline lens is a biconvex structure positioned posterior to the iris and anterior to the vitreous. By being clear and colorless, it provides an unobstructed visual axis. It facilitates light transmission into the eye and helps to focus light that enters the eye.

Anatomy and physiology of the lens:
- The lens is suspended within the eye via zonules, which attach to the peripheral lens (referred to as the lens equator) and the ciliary body.
- The lens capsule is the outermost component of the lens.
- A layer of epithelium lines the interior anterior lens capsule.
  - The source of lens fibers, which make up the contents internal to the capsule (cortex and nucleus).
- As lens fibers grow, they elongate and become U-shaped as they run underneath the anterior capsule, equatorial capsule, and posterior capsule.
- Areas where tips of lens fibers contact one another are referred to as Y sutures.
- Lens fibers form and elongate throughout life.
  - Newest fibers deposit in the outermost portions of the lens (lens cortex), nearest the capsule.
  - Older lens fibers are pushed toward the center of the lens (lens nucleus), further from the capsule.
  - Since this process continues throughout life, the lens density increases with age (nuclear sclerosis).

Similar to the cornea, the lens is clear and colorless. Factors contributing to the clarity of the lens include the following:
- Relative dehydration
- Orderly alignment of lens fibers and tight packing of fibers within the capsule
- Lack of blood vessels
- Lack of pigment

Because the lens lacks a blood supply, it is heavily reliant on the aqueous humor for nutrition and waste removal.
- Diseases that interfere with aqueous humor dynamics (e.g., uveitis and glaucoma) therefore have the potential to cause lens pathology.

- This becomes visible to the clinician as partial or complete opacification of the lens (cataract).

The main pathologies of the lens are cataract, lens subluxation, and lens luxation. These will be the focus of this chapter.

Diseases of the lens

Nuclear sclerosis

What it is
- Increased density of the lens, particularly its nucleus.
  - Older lens fibers are increasingly compacted into the nucleus as new lens fibers are deposited in the outer lens cortices.
- Also referred to as lenticular sclerosis.

Predisposed individuals
- Nuclear sclerosis occurs as the lens ages.
  - Usually visible as early as 6–7 years of age in dogs, while in cats usually not visible until after 10 years of age.
  - Can be seen in at least half of dogs near 10 years of age (Williams *et al.,* 2004).
  - Can be seen in at least half of cats near 15 years of age (Williams & Heath, 2006).

Defining characteristics
- Cloudy appearance of the central lens (Figures 7.1, 7.2).
- The cloudy change is circular.
- The cloudiness of the lens will vary with the angle of light entering the eye and the angle from which the lens is viewed.
  - The appearance of the same lens nucleus can vary from only mild cloudiness (Figures 7.3, 7.4) to markedly white (Figures 7.1, 7.2).
- Although the sclerotic lens can appear opaque, changing the direction of light entering the eye and the angle from which the lens is viewed will reveal that light passes through this opacity unobstructed.

Small Animal Ophthalmic Atlas and Guide, Second Edition. Christine C. Lim.
© 2023 John Wiley & Sons, Inc. Published 2023 by John Wiley & Sons, Inc.
Companion website: www.wiley.com/go/lim/atlas

- Compare Figures 7.1 and 7.2 to Figures 7.3 and 7.4.
- *The ability to see the full tapetal reflection indicates that light passes unimpeded through the sclerotic nucleus. This differentiates nuclear sclerosis from cataract.*
- A true cataract would appear cloudy from all angles and would attenuate the tapetal reflection.

Clinical significance

- Nuclear sclerosis is usually not associated with noticeable visual disturbances in dogs and cats.
  - Except in very aged dogs, where extremely dense nuclear sclerosis can cause observable vision decline.
- Unlike cataracts, nuclear sclerosis is not associated with other ocular pathologies.

Diagnosis

- The diagnosis is based on ophthalmic examination.
- Differentiation between nuclear sclerosis and cataract is more easily achieved when the pupil is dilated.

Treatment

- Nuclear sclerosis is not usually treated.

Prognosis

- The prognosis is excellent for maintenance of a comfortable, visual eye.

Cataract

What it is

- A cataract refers to an opacity within the lens.
- Cataracts may be classified in several ways (age of onset, size, cause, etc.).
- The most useful classification schemes address size and chronicity of cataract. One such scheme is described as follows:
  - Incipient cataract (Figures 7.5, 7.6, 7.7a, 7.7b, 7.25)
    - Refers to a small cataract, one in which less than 10–15% of the lens is opaque.
  - Incomplete cataract (Figures 7.8, 7.9, 7.10, 7.11, 7.12, 7.13a, 7.13b, 7.14a, 7.14b)
    - Describes a large range of lens opacification; more than 10–15% lens involvement but less than 100% opacification.
    - The tapetal reflection, although attenuated, is still visible.
    - Also referred to as immature cataract.
  - Complete cataract (Figures 7.15, 7.16, 7.17)
    - The entire lens is opaque.
    - The tapetal reflection is not visible.
    - Also referred to as mature cataract.
  - Resorbing cataract (Figures 7.18, 7.19, 7.20, 7.21, 7.22, 7.23, 7.24)
    - This term refers to the chronicity, but not size, of the cataract.

- A resorbing cataract is chronic and one in which signs of lens fiber degeneration are visible (see "Defining characteristics").
- Size of cataract varies and is usually either incomplete (tapetal reflection visible) or complete (tapetal reflection obscured completely).
- Signs of anterior uveitis may also present (see Chapter 15).
- Also referred to as hypermature cataract.

Predisposed individuals

- Cataracts are presumed to be heritable in many canine breeds.
  - The total number of breeds is too numerous to list.
  - Some breeds more commonly noted in retrospective studies include cocker spaniels, toy and miniature poodles, miniature schnauzers, Boston terriers, and bichon frises (Adkins & Hendrix, 2005; Gelatt & MacKay, 2005).
  - Also common in mixed breed dogs.
- Increased age is associated with higher prevalence of cataract (Gelatt & MacKay, 2005).
- Most dogs with diabetes mellitus develop cataract.
  - Approximately 80% within 16 months of diabetes diagnosis (Beam *et al.*, 1999).
- Ocular diseases that can increase potential for cataract development are as follows:
  - Uveitis
  - Glaucoma
  - Progressive retinal atrophy

Defining characteristics

- Varying degrees of lens opacification, as per definitions listed earlier.
- Tapetal reflection will be altered by the lens opacity because the cataract scatters light passing through the lens (Figures 7.7b, 7.8, 7.9, 7.10, 7.12, 7.13b, 7.14b).
  - Degree of tapetal reflection attenuation directly correlates with size and density of the cataract.
- Resorbing cataracts exhibit at least some of the following:
  - *Sparkly areas within the lens cortex* (Figures 7.19, 7.20, 7.21, 7.22, 7.23, 7.24)
  - *Lens capsule wrinkling* (Figures 7.18, 7.19, 7.23)
  - Liquefaction of the lens cortex
  - Subcapsular plaques
  - Brown discoloration of the lens, referred to as brunescence (Figure 7.20)

Clinical significance

Causes of cataract may have implications for ocular and/or systemic health of the individual or for progeny.

- Genetics
  - Most common cause of cataracts in dogs.
  - Breeding of dogs with suspected heritable cataracts is not recommended.

- Uveitis
  - This is the most common cause of cataracts in cats.
  - Various ocular and systemic diseases can incite uveitis (see Chapter 15).
- Age
  - Older dogs are more likely to have cataracts (Williams *et al.*, 2004).
- Diabetes mellitus
  - This is an extremely common cause of cataracts in dogs.
  - Byproducts of glucose metabolism in the lens create osmotic forces that pull fluid into the lens.
  - This disrupts the normally orderly arrangement of lens fibers.
  - Diabetic cataracts occur rarely in cats.
- Nutrition
  - Cataract development has been associated with the use of milk replacers in puppies and kittens (Remillard *et al.*, 1993).
- Others
  - Penetrating ocular injury
  - PRA (see Chapter 17)
  - Radiation therapy
  - Electric shock
  - Various drug toxicities

Cataracts can impair vision and cause LIU, which predisposes to further ocular disease.

Visual impairment
- Incipient cataracts are unlikely to have detectable effects on vision.
- Visual impairment from incomplete cataracts correlates directly with the size and density of lens opacification.
  - Although some degree of impairment must be present, clinical signs of impairment range from none to overt blindness.
- Complete cataracts are blinding.
  - Diabetic cataracts almost always become complete.

LIU
- Leakage of lens protein into the anterior chamber incites uveitis.
- LIU is present in all stages of cataract, even if clinical signs of uveitis are not visible (Dziezyc *et al.*, 1997).
  - Mild inflammation may not be clinically visible, while more severe inflammation may be accompanied by clinical signs of uveitis as listed in Chapter 15 (Krohne *et al.*, 1995) (see "Anterior uveitis").
  - The amount of intraocular inflammation varies with the stage of cataract.
  - Less inflammation accompanies incipient and incomplete cataracts when compared with complete and resorbing cataracts (Dziezyc *et al.*, 1997).
  - Diabetic cataracts tend to have more severe uveitis than cataracts of other causes.
- Untreated LIU leads to painful complications and decreased surgical success rates.

- Complications of uveitis include secondary glaucoma, lens luxation, and retinal detachment.
  - Chronicity of uveitis decreases success following surgical cataract extraction (Biros *et al.*, 2000; Davidson *et al.*, 1991; Sigle & Nasisse, 2006).

Cataract progression is not predictable.
- While some incipient cataracts may remain stable for years, others may progress to complete cataracts in short periods of time (weeks or months).
  - Owners of diabetic dogs often report progression to complete cataracts and blindness overnight.

Diagnosis
- Cataracts are diagnosed during ophthalmic examination.
  - Pupillary dilation is necessary to visualize the entire lens on examination.
- Stage of cataract is diagnosed by determining the amount of lens involved and if signs of resorption are present.
- LIU is assumed to be present even if obvious signs of inflammation are not seen.
  - Clinical signs may not be visible for smaller cataracts.
  - Severity of uveitis correlates with the stage of the cataract (Dziezyc *et al.*, 1997).

Treatment
- Goals of treatment are to improve patient comfort, minimize sequelae to LIU, and retain vision.
- *Early referral to a veterinary ophthalmologist is essential for maximizing outcomes.*
  - Recommended when cataracts are first diagnosed, whether or not surgery is pursued.
  - Surgical treatment of cataract is most successful when performed early in the course of the disease.
    - That is, complication rate increases with increasing stage of cataract (Biros *et al.*, 2000; Davidson *et al.*, 1991; Lim *et al.*, 2011; Sigle & Nasisse, 2006; van der Woerdt *et al.*, 1992).
- For incipient cataracts that do not enlarge, monitoring at routine intervals may be the only treatment.
  - Although overt enlargement may not be seen over the long term, periodic monitoring is recommended because progression is not predictable.
- Routine monitoring with long-term topical anti-inflammatory therapy is the minimum recommendation for incomplete, complete, and resorbing cataracts.
  - To lower risks of complications secondary to LIU (see "Clinical significance").
  - Prednisolone acetate 1% ophthalmic suspension, dexamethasone 0.1% ophthalmic solution, flurbiprofen 0.03%, diclofenac 0.01%, or other ophthalmic NSAIDs, one drop applied one to four times daily.
  - Severity of LIU determines the frequency of dosing.
  - Untreated dogs may be at higher risk of complications when compared to dogs undergoing medical management of LIU (Lim *et al.*, 2011).

- Surgical removal of the cataract is the only treatment that has the potential to improve vision.
  - Phacoemulsification, with intraocular lens implantation whenever possible.
  - Retention/restoration of vision improves quality of life.

Prognosis

- Prognosis for maintaining a comfortable, visual eye is variable and depends on factors such as cataract progression, concurrent ocular disease, and the cause of cataract.
- Complications are more likely as the stage of cataract advances.
- For age-related incipient cataracts with little progression, prognosis for a comfortable, visual eye is excellent.
- For incomplete, complete, and resorbing cataracts, prognosis for a comfortable eye is fair to good.
  - With progression of cataract, vision will be reduced.
  - Complications are more likely than with incipient cataracts, but medical management can reduce their likelihood (Lim *et al.*, 2011).
- For canine eyes undergoing phacoemulsification, long-term surgical success rates average around 80% (Boss *et al.*, 2019; Klein *et al.*, 2011; Lim *et al.*, 2011; Newbold *et al.*, 2018).
  - Potential for surgical success varies inversely with stage of cataract.
- For feline eyes undergoing phacoemulsification, the success rate appears to be over 90% (Braus *et al.*, 2017; Fenollosa-Romero *et al.*, 2019).
- Complications are more likely for cataracts that occur secondary to ocular trauma or other ocular disease (Fischer & Meyer-Lindenberg, 2018).
- Complications leading to loss of the eye may not occur until several years after surgery (Lannek & Miller, 2001; Lim *et al.*, 2011).
  - Due to shortened life span, older patients may avoid complications.
- Because diabetic cataracts tend to progress more rapidly and have more severe LIU than hereditary cataracts, they are at higher risk for complications.
  - Prompt referral is especially crucial for diabetic cataracts.

Additional information

- Referral to a veterinary ophthalmologist should occur early; it should not be delayed until after a cataract visibly progresses.
- Following the initial ophthalmic examination, candidacy for cataract surgery is determined by preoperative diagnostics such as ERG, ocular ultrasound, and gonioscopy.
- Because the most common cause of feline cataracts is uveitis, cats are more often treated medically than surgically.
  - Management of uveitis (see "Anterior uveitis" in Chapter 15).
- Because postoperative complications can develop years after surgery, patients undergoing phacoemulsification should be monitored routinely by a veterinary ophthalmologist in the long term after surgery.
- Because diabetic cataracts develop from fluid influx into the lens, lens rupture (and severe uveitis) is a potential complication; early referral is therefore especially important for diabetic patients.

Lens subluxation and luxation

What it is

- Lens subluxation is a partial dislocation of the lens.
  - It is associated with breakdown of the zonules.
  - Severity of subluxation correlates directly with percentage of zonular fibers that have broken.
  - Subluxation is a precursor to lens luxation.
- Lens luxation is a complete dislocation of the lens.
  - All zonules have degenerated.
  - Anterior lens luxation: lens is in the anterior chamber.
  - Posterior lens luxation: lens is in the vitreous cavity.

Predisposed individuals

- Breed predispositions for primary lens luxation:
  - Terrier breeds, such as Jack Russell terrier, rat terrier, and fox terrier.
  - Shar pei
  - Chinese crested dog
  - Tibetan terrier
- Predispositions to lens luxation of other causes:
  - Chronic uveitis (for example, LIU)
  - Glaucoma
  - Advanced age

Defining characteristics

Lens subluxation
- *Aphakic crescent* (Figures 7.25, 7.26)
- Anterior chamber narrower or deeper than normal
- Irregular anterior chamber depth
- Vitreous in the anterior chamber
- Phacodonesis
- Iridodonesis

Anterior lens luxation
- Signs of ocular pain: *blepharospasm, epiphora,* and *third eyelid elevation*
- *Episcleral congestion*
- *Corneal edema*
- *Lens in the anterior chamber* (Figures 7.27, 7.28, 7.29, 7.30)
  - Because the lens is in front of the iris, the iris isn't seen clearly.
- Vitreous in the anterior chamber
- Aphakic crescent (Figure 7.27)

Posterior lens luxation (Figures 7.31, 7.32, 7.33, 7.34)
- Signs may be minimal.
- Episcleral congestion.
- Deep anterior chamber.

- Vitreous in the anterior chamber.
- Lens may be visible in vitreous cavity.

Clinical significance

Lens subluxation and luxation can be primary or secondary.

- Primary lens luxation
  - The luxation is caused by hereditary zonular dysplasia.
  - Zonules break down over time, without an inciting ocular disease.
- Secondary lens luxation
  - Zonular breakdown occurs secondary to another ocular disease. Examples of diseases causing lens luxation include the following:
    - *Chronic uveitis*
      - Inflammation causes zonular degeneration.
      - Underlying cause of uveitis may have implications for ocular or systemic health.
    - *Glaucoma*
      - Zonules stretch and break as the eye becomes buphthalmic.
    - Trauma
      - Causes zonular tearing.
      - Other signs of ocular trauma will also be present.
- Zonules can also degenerate as a result of aging (age-related zonular degeneration).

Complications resulting from lens instability can lead to blindness or loss of the eye.

- Lens subluxation
  - Allows movement of the lens during head and eye movement.
  - More stress is placed on remaining zonules, encouraging further breakdown.
  - Extraneous motion incites intraocular inflammation.
  - Uveitis can promote further zonular degeneration.
  - Complications of chronic uveitis may develop (e.g., glaucoma and cataract).
- Anterior lens luxation
  - This is painful.
  - Anterior lens luxation causes anterior uveitis.
  - Complications of chronic uveitis may develop.
  - Anterior lens luxation may increase IOP.
  - The presence of a lens in the anterior chamber can impair aqueous humor outflow.
- Posterior lens luxation
  - This incites posterior uveitis.
  - Complications of posterior uveitis (e.g., retinal detachment and retinal degeneration) may occur.

Diagnosis

The diagnosis of lens subluxation or luxation is made on ophthalmic examination, by visualizing abnormalities as listed in "Defining characteristics."

To differentiate between primary and secondary lens subluxation/luxation, consider the following:

- Breed
  - Is the affected patient from a breed predisposed to primary lens instability?
- Age
  - Primary lens luxation tends to occur between 3 and 7 years of age (Curtis, 1983; Foster *et al.*, 1986).
  - Age-related zonular degeneration is usually seen in individuals of advanced age.
- The presence or absence of concurrent ophthalmic abnormalities, especially if chronic or severe
  - Uveitis
  - Glaucoma
- History of trauma

Treatment

- The goal of treatment is to retain vision and the eye.
- Patients should be referred to a veterinary ophthalmologist for evaluation.
  - For luxations, immediate referral is warranted.
- Treatment for lens subluxation depends on the degree of instability.
  - Mild lens subluxation (majority of zonules intact and no obvious phacodonesis or iridodonesis) may be treated with long-term topical anti-inflammatory medications and routine monitoring only.
  - For example, prednisolone acetate 1% ophthalmic suspension, dexamethasone 0.1% ophthalmic solution, flurbiprofen 0.03%, diclofenac 0.01%, or other ophthalmic NSAIDs, one drop applied one to four times daily.
  - Long-term topical miotics such as prostaglandin analogs or demecarium bromide have also been used with the intent of delaying lens luxation in an eye with primary lens instability (Binder *et al.*, 2007).
  - More advanced lens subluxation can be treated surgically by a veterinary ophthalmologist.
    - Phacoemulsification.
    - Intracapsular lens extraction.
- Treatment for lens luxation depends on the location of the lens and concurrent ophthalmic disease.
  - If IOP is elevated, start dorzolamide 2% ophthalmic solution (see Chapter 18).
    - Dogs: one drop into the affected eye q8h.
    - Cats: one drop into the affected eye q12h to q8h.
  - Start topical anti-inflammatory medications as listed for lens subluxation.
  - Anteriorly luxated lenses are referred immediately for surgical removal of the lens (intracapsular lens extraction).
    - Transcorneal reduction of the lens is sometimes attempted when surgery is not an option (Montgomery *et al.*, 2014).
  - Posteriorly luxated lenses are often treated medically.

- Long-term administration of a miotic in combination with anti-inflammatory medications.
  - Prostaglandin analogs or demecarium bromide, in an attempt to trap the lens in the vitreous.
  - Topical anti-inflammatory medications as listed earlier.
- Eyes that are blind and painful should be enucleated.

Prognosis

- For subluxated lenses with minimal displacement or lens movement, the prognosis for maintenance of a comfortable, visual eye is generally good with therapy.
  - Patients should be monitored for progression of lens instability and concurrent uveitis.
- For severe subluxation or luxation, the prognosis is poor to fair with treatment (Binder *et al.*, 2007; Glover *et al.*, 1995).
  - Due to progression of subluxation and/or development of complications such as glaucoma and retinal detachment.
- In the author's experience, complications, including recurrence of anterior lens luxation, are common after transcorneal reduction.
  - Transcorneal reduction is less likely to be successful when synechiae are present.
  - In some cases, attempts to move the lens into the posterior segment are unsuccessful.

Additional information

- Mild lens subluxation can be missed if the pupil is not dilated for examination.
  - Aphakic crescent can be hidden behind the iris when the pupil is not dilated.
- Because primary lens instability affects both eyes, diagnosis of lens subluxation or luxation in one eye warrants careful examination of the fellow eye.
- Affected cats should be tested for FIV due to its potential as an underlying cause of uveitis (Olivero *et al.*, 1991).

Further reading

Colitz, CM. 2015. Lens emergencies: not always so clear. *Topics in Companion Animal Medicine.* 30(3): 81–85.

La Croix, N. 2008. Cataracts: when to refer. *Topics in Companion Animal Medicine.* 23(1):46–50.

References

Adkins, EA & Hendrix, DVH. 2005. Outcomes of dogs presented for cataract evaluation: a retrospective study. *Journal of the American Animal Hospital Association.* 41(4):235–240.

Beam, S, *et al.* 1999. A retrospective-cohort study on the development of cataracts in dogs with diabetes mellitus. *Veterinary Ophthalmology.* 2(3):169–172.

Binder, DR, *et al.* 2007. Outcomes of nonsurgical management and efficacy of demecarium bromide treatment for primary lens instability in dogs: 34 cases (1990–2004). *Journal of the American Veterinary Medical Association.* 231(1):89–93.

Biros, DJ, *et al.* 2000. Development of glaucoma after cataract surgery in dogs. *Journal of the American Veterinary Medical Association.* 216(11):1780–1786.

Boss, C, *et al.* 2019. Preliminary report of postoperative complications of phacoemulsification in Pugs: A multicenter retrospective study of 32 cases. *Veterinary Ophthalmology.* 23(3):442–449.

Braus, BK, *et al.* 2017. Outcome of phacoemulsification following corneal and lens laceration in cats and dogs (2000–2010). *Veterinary Ophthalmology.* 20(1):4–10.

Curtis, R. 1983. Aetiopathological aspects of inherited lens dislocation in the Tibetan terrier. *Journal of Comparative Pathology.* 93(1):151–163.

Davidson, MG, *et al.* 1991. Phacoemulsification and intraocular lens implantation: a study of surgical results in 182 dogs. *Progress in Veterinary and Comparative Ophthalmology.* 1(4):233–238.

Dziezyc, J, *et al.* 1997. Fluorescein concentrations in the aqueous of dogs with cataracts. *Veterinary & Comparative Ophthalmology.* 7(4):267–270.

Fenollosa-Romero, E, *et al.* 2020. Outcome of phacoemulsification in 71 cats: A multicenter retrospective study (2006–2017). *Veterinary Ophthalmology.* 23(1):141–147.

Fischer, MC & Meyer-Lindenberg, A. 2018. Progression and complications of canine cataracts for different stages of development and aetiologies. *Journal of Small Animal Practice.* 59(10):616–624.

Foster, SJ, *et al.* 1986. Primary lens luxation in the border collie. *Journal of Small Animal Practice.* 27(1):1–6.

Gelatt, KN & MacKay EO. 2005. Prevalence of primary breed-related cataracts in the dog in North America. *Veterinary Ophthalmology.* 8(2):101–111.

Glover, TL, *et al.* 1995. The intracapsular extraction of displaced lenses in dogs: a retrospective study of 57 cases (1984–1990). *Journal of the American Animal Hospital Association.* 31(1):77–81.

Klein, HE, *et al.* 2011. Postoperative complications and visual outcomes of phacoemulsification in 103 dogs (179 eyes): 2006–2008. *Veterinary Ophthalmology.* 14(2):114–120.

Krohne, SG, *et al.* 1995. Use of laser flaremetry to measure aqueous humor protein concentration in dogs. *Journal of the American Veterinary Medical Association.* 206(8):1167–1172.

Lannek, EB & Miller, PE. 2001. Development of glaucoma after phacoemulsification for removal of cataracts in dogs: 22 cases (1987–1997). *Journal of the American Animal Hospital Association.* 218(1):70–76.

Lim, CC, *et al.* 2011. Cataracts in 44 dogs (77 eyes): a comparison of outcomes for no treatment, topical medical management, or phacoemulsification with intraocular lens implantation. *Canadian Veterinary Journal.* 52(3):583–588.

Montgomery, KW, *et al.* 2014. Trans-corneal reduction of anterior lens luxation in dogs with lens instability: a retrospective study of 19 dogs (2010–2013). *Veterinary Ophthalmology.* 17(2):275–279.

Newbold, GM, *et al.* 2018. Phacoemulsification outcomes in Boston terriers as compared to non-Boston terriers: a retrospective study (2002–2015). *Veterinary Ophthalmology.* 21(4):353–361.

Olivero, DK, *et al.* 1991. Feline lens displacement. *Progress in Veterinary and Comparative Ophthalmology.* 1(4):239–244.

Remillard, RL, *et al.* 1993. Comparison of kittens fed queen's milk with those fed milk replacers. *American Journal of Veterinary Research.* 54(6):901–907.

Sigle, KJ & Nasisse, MP. 2006. Long-term complications after phacoemulsification for cataract removal in dogs. *Journal of the American Veterinary Medical Association.* 228(1):74–79.

van der Woerdt, A, *et al.* 1992. Lens-induced uveitis in dogs: 151 cases (1985–1990). *Journal of the American Veterinary Medical Association.* 201(6):921–926.

Williams, DL & Heath, MF. 2006. Prevalence of feline cataract: results of a cross-sectional study of 2000 normal animals, 50 cats with diabetes and one hundred cats following dehydrational crises. *Veterinary Ophthalmology.* 9(5):341–349.

Williams, DL, *et al.* 2004. Prevalence of canine cataract: preliminary results of a cross-sectional study. *Veterinary Ophthalmology.* 7(1):29–35.

17 Posterior segment

Please see Chapter 8 for images of the posterior segment.
- The posterior segment of the eye includes the vitreous, retina, optic nerve, choroid, and posterior sclera.
- From innermost to outermost of the eye, the sequence of structures is the vitreous, retina and optic nerve, choroid, and then sclera.

1 Vitreous
- This is a clear, colorless jelly mainly composed of water that inhabits most of the space in the posterior portion of the eye.
- Vitreous assists in focusing of light that enters the eye, maintenance of eye shape, and provides nutrition to the ocular structures.

2 Retina and optic nerve
- The retina and optic nerve are situated between the vitreous and the choroid (external to the vitreous and internal to the choroid).
- The retina is broadly divided into the anterior neurosensory retina and the posterior RPE.
- Layers of the neurosensory retina, from innermost to outermost (from vitreous toward choroid) are as follows:
  - Internal limiting membrane
  - Nerve fiber layer
  - Ganglion cell layer
  - Inner plexiform layer
  - Inner nuclear layer
  - Outer plexiform layer
  - Outer nuclear layer
  - Outer limiting membrane
  - Photoreceptors
- RPE
  - This is the outermost (closest to choroid) layer of retina.
  - This is the layer of the retina that contains melanin.
    - RPE melanin content is decreased in the dorsal half of fundus.
- The retina generates electrical signals in response to light entering the eye and transmits this information via the optic nerve to the subcortical visual pathways and visual cortex.
  - Photoreceptors hyperpolarize in response to light.
  - The generated signal moves inward (anteriorly) through the layers of the neurosensory retina to the retinal ganglion cells.
  - Retinal ganglion cells generate action potentials that are transmitted along the nerve fiber layer to the optic nerve.
    - This is the afferent arm for pupillary light reflexes and for vision.

3 Choroid
- The choroid lies between the retina and the sclera (external to the retina and internal to the sclera).
- It is composed mainly of blood vessels and melanin.
  - The choroid provides the blood supply to photoreceptors.
- The tapetum lucidum is present in the dorsal half of the innermost (closest to the retina) choroid.
  - The function of the tapetum is to increase light within the eye (acting as a mirror, reflecting light within the eye).
  - The tapetum is reflective, usually green, orange, or yellow in color.
  - The tapetum is blue in individuals younger than 3–4 months of age.

4 Sclera
- This is the outermost (most posterior) layer of the fundus.
- With the cornea, the sclera forms the outer fibrous tunic of the eye. Some of its functions include the following:
  - Maintenance of ocular shape
  - Insertion site for extraocular muscles
- Compared with surrounding sclera, it is structurally weaker where the optic nerve exits the eye.

Fundus
- This term refers to the image obtained when the posterior segment is viewed through the pupil with an ophthalmoscope.
- It is an image of the retina, choroid, and sclera *in situ*, viewed through the clear ocular media (cornea, aqueous humor, lens, and vitreous humor) (Figures 8.1, 8.2, 8.3, 8.4, 8.5, 8.6, 8.7).
  - The retina is seen most clearly because it is the innermost, or most anterior, layer.
  - Because the choroid is immediately posterior (external) to the retina, portions of it are seen through the retina only where the RPE is less pigmented.
    - For example, the tapetum in the dorsal fundus (also referred to as the tapetal fundus).
- Sclera, which is posterior (external) to the choroid, is rarely seen due to overlying retina and choroid.

Small Animal Ophthalmic Atlas and Guide, Second Edition. Christine C. Lim.
© 2023 John Wiley & Sons, Inc. Published 2023 by John Wiley & Sons, Inc.
Companion website: www.wiley.com/go/lim/atlas

Viewing the fundus:

- The fundus is best viewed after pharmacologic dilation.
  - Dilation sufficient to perform a good examination of the fundus is achieved 15–20 minutes after application of one drop of tropicamide 1% ophthalmic solution.
- Indirect ophthalmoscopy offers the best overall view of the fundus.
  - This method provides the best balance between field of view and magnification.
  - More areas of the fundus can be viewed at once, making it easier to examine the entire fundus.
    - The ability to see a large overview quickly is advantageous when working with a patient that is not cooperative for examination.
  - Remember that the image seen by the examiner is inverted when compared with true orientation of the fundic structures.
- The direct ophthalmoscope, which is widely available in most general practices, offers higher magnification than indirect ophthalmoscopy.
  - This comes at the expense of field of view, making it much more difficult to examine the entire fundus.
  - The direct ophthalmoscope is better used for detailed examination of a specific structure at higher magnification, rather than for an overall fundic examination.
  - The image obtained by this method shows fundic structures in their true orientation.
- The PanOptic™ ophthalmoscope is a "middle ground" between direct and indirect ophthalmoscopy.
  - The field of view is narrower than with indirect ophthalmoscopy but wider than for direct ophthalmoscopy.
  - Similarly, the level of magnification is higher than with indirect ophthalmoscopy but less than for direct ophthalmoscopy.
  - The image obtained by this method shows fundic structures in their true orientation.
- All regions and structures of the fundus should be viewed during each fundic examination.
  - That is, central, dorsal, ventral, medial, and lateral regions, ensuring that peripheral extent of these regions is viewed.
  - This will ensure that all of the important structures/regions are examined: tapetal fundus, nontapetal fundus, optic nerve, and blood vessels.
  - Because structures are located on the same plane, all portions of the image should be in focus at the same time.

1 Tapetal fundus
  - The dorsal half of the fundus.
  - Appears green, orange, or yellow and visibly reflects light.
  - Although the retina lies anterior to the tapetum, the RPE in this region contains minimal amounts of melanin and is thus almost transparent. This allows the tapetum to be seen through the retina.

2 Nontapetal fundus
  - The ventral half of the fundus.
  - Appears brown due to melanin within RPE. The melanin makes the retina opaque and therefore prevents visualization of underlying choroid and sclera.
    - Exceptions exist; see normal variants.

3 Optic nerve
  - Dog
    - White in color due to myelin.
    - Circular to triangular shape, depending on the degree of myelination.
    - Blood vessels should be visible crossing the optic nerve head.
    - Located approximately central in the fundus, near tapetal/nontapetal junction.
  - Cat
    - Dark color due to lack of myelin.
    - Circular shape.
    - Blood vessels reach edges of the nerve but do not cross over top of the nerve.
    - Located approximately central in the fundus, within the tapetal fundus near the tapetal/nontapetal junction.

4 Retinal vessels
  - Three to four larger vessels spanning from the optic nerve to the peripheral fundus.
  - Several very narrow vessels are also visible.

Normal variants of this typical appearance exist.

- Subalbinotic fundus (Figures 8.8 and 8.9)
  - This variant is seen in lightly pigmented animals (light coat colors and/or blue irides).
  - The appearance is due to decreased amounts of melanin in the retina and choroid.
  - Because melanin is lacking in the retina, it is almost transparent, enabling visualization of the underlying choroidal vessels.
  - Choroidal vessels are recognized because they are thicker and more numerous than retinal vessels and because they are aligned with one another in a relatively organized fashion.
  - Underlying sclera may also be visible between the choroidal vessels if choroid also lacks melanin.
  - Individuals with subalbinotic fundi are often also atapetal.
- Atapetal fundus (Figure 8.8)
  - This describes a fundus where the tapetum is absent.
  - The fundus is otherwise normal.

Pathologic changes to the fundus

- Hyperreflectivity (Figures 8.10, 8.11, 8.12, 8.13, 8.14, 8.15, 8.16, 8.17, 8.18)
  - This occurs in the tapetal fundus.
  - The term describes a tapetal reflection that is brighter than normal due to thinning of overlying retina.
    - The tapetal reflection appears brighter because it is viewed through less tissue than normal.
  - This indicates an inactive lesion, that is, retinal degeneration/retinal scar.

- Hyporeflectivity (Figures 8.19, 8.20, 8.21, 8.22, 8.23, 8.24, 8.25, 8.26)
  - This occurs in the tapetal fundus.
  - The term describes a tapetal reflection that is duller than normal due to thickening of overlying retina.
    - The tapetum is viewed through increased amount of tissue, which blunts its reflection.
  - Hyporeflectivity almost always indicates active inflammation (e.g., cellular infiltrate or edema will thicken the retina), that is, chorioretinitis.
- Increased pigmentation of the nontapetal fundus (Figure 8.27).
  - The affected area is darker brown than normal (than the surrounding, nonaffected nontapetal fundus).
  - This is most commonly seen with retinal degeneration, as a result of melanocyte clumping.
  - This is less commonly seen as a result of neoplasia (e.g., melanocytic neoplasia).
- Decreased pigmentation of the nontapetal fundus (Figures 8.27, 8.28, 8.29).
  - The affected area is paler than normal (than the surrounding, nonaffected nontapetal fundus).
  - This can be due to addition of lightly colored material: fluid or white cell infiltrate obscuring the view of normally melanotic retina and choroid (active inflammation/chorioretinitis).
  - This can be due to removal of melanin: post-inflammatory retinal and choroidal depigmentation, which allows visualization of the white sclera (retinal degeneration/chorioretinal scar).
- Bleeding (Figures 8.30, 8.31, 8.32, 8.33, 8.34, 8.35, 8.36)
  - Red discoloration of variable sizes and shapes, not contained within vessels.
  - Some common causes include diabetes, systemic hypertension, inflammation, neoplasia, bleeding disorders, and trauma.
- Retinal detachment (Figures 8.34, 8.35, 8.37, 8.38, 8.39, 8.40a, 8.40b, 8.41, 8.42, 8.43).
  - Variable appearance depending on the amount of retina detached, distance of detachment, and presence or absence of retinal tears.
  - Because the detached retina is at a different plane than other structures (and is not all in the same plane itself), a portion of the fundic image will always be defocused.
  - Because concurrent subretinal fluid and/or cellular accumulation is often present, the tapetal fundus tends to be hyporeflective (Figures 8.34, 8.35, 8.40b, 8.41).
- Vascular attenuation (Figures 8.10, 8.11, 8.12, 8.13, 8.14, 8.15)
  - This describes narrowing and shortening of retinal vessels such that they no longer reach the peripheral fundus.
  - Depending on severity of attenuation, vessels may be more difficult to visualize, or not visible at all.
  - Vascular attenuation occurs with retinal degeneration.

- Vascular tortuosity
  - Vessels become engorged and increasingly twisted.
  - Accompanies inflammation, hypertension, and conditions in which blood becomes more viscous.
- Optic nerve atrophy (Figures 8.44, 8.45)
  - Demyelinization causes the nerve to become smaller and darker.
  - Commonly occurs after inflammation or glaucoma.
- Optic disc cupping (Figures 8.46, 8.47, 9.11)
  - This refers to atrophy and posterior displacement of the optic nerve.
  - Optic disc cupping is caused by glaucoma.
    - Because sclera in the area of the optic nerve is weaker than surrounding sclera, it is pushed more posteriorly than the rest of the sclera when the IOP is elevated.
- Optic nerve swelling (Figures 8.48, 8.49)
  - Nerve is enlarged, raised, and edges are indistinct.
  - Accompanies inflammation, neoplasia, and increased intracranial pressure.

The most common posterior segment diseases encountered in general practice involve the retina and choroid. Therefore, retinal and choroidal diseases comprise most of this chapter.

Diseases of the posterior segment

Asteroid hyalosis

What it is

- Asteroid hyalosis describes calcium and phospholipid accumulations within the vitreous.

Predisposed individuals

- Asteroid hyalosis affects older dogs.

Defining characteristics

- Multiple, small, white, round, refractile particles suspended within the vitreous (Figures 8.50, 8.51).
  - These round particles have a sparkly appearance.
- Asteroid hyalosis is visible through the pupil and on fundic examination.

Clinical significance

- Asteroid hyalosis is usually an incidental finding during ophthalmic examination.
  - It is uncommonly associated with signs of visual compromise.
  - Occasionally, it is associated with other intraocular diseases such as ciliary body neoplasia (Dubielzig *et al.*, 1998).

Diagnosis

- The diagnosis is based on ophthalmic examination.

Treatment

- Asteroid hyalosis is not treated.

Prognosis
- The prognosis for maintaining a comfortable eye is excellent.
- The prognosis for maintaining vision is good.
  - Severe asteroid hyalosis may mildly impair vision in the same manner as floaters in people.

Collie eye anomaly

What it is
- Collie eye anomaly (CEA) describes a set of congenital, hereditary posterior segment defects found mainly in herding breeds.

Predisposed individuals
- Rough and smooth collies
- Shetland sheepdog
- Australian shepherd

Defining characteristics
- The clinical presentation of CEA varies widely.
- CEA is bilateral but not necessarily symmetrical.
- The posterior segment anomalies associated with CEA are as follows:
  - *Choroidal hypoplasia* (Figures 8.52, 8.53)
    - This occurs lateral to the optic disc.
    - It is recognized by bizarre distribution of choroidal vessels and/or hypopigmentation of the choroid.
    - It is present in all cases of CEA, but to variable degrees.
    - Choroidal hypoplasia can be difficult to detect when the overlying, melanotic RPE obscures visualization of the choroid.
  - Posterior polar coloboma (Figure 8.53)
    - This is a congenital absence of tissue within or around the optic nerve.
    - When present, it varies in severity.

Clinical significance
- CEA is an inherited defect (Parker *et al.*, 2007).
  - Severity of defects in offspring is not predictable and can vary widely within a litter.
  - Although widespread, selective breeding can reduce the incidence of this disease (Wallin-Hakanson *et al.*, 2000).
- The effects of CEA on vision range from no detectable visual deficits to complete blindness.
  - Choroidal hypoplasia is not typically associated with visual deficits.
  - Posterior polar colobomas, at minimum, cause visual compromise, and can also be blinding.
  - Retinal detachment and intraocular hemorrhage can occur secondary to CEA and can be blinding.

Diagnosis
- The diagnosis is based on funduscopy.
- Choroidal hypoplasia, the consistent abnormality of CEA, can be masked by a melanotic RPE that obscures the choroid.
  - Examination by 6–8 weeks of age, prior to full pigmentation of the RPE, can identify choroidal hypoplasia.

Treatment
- Choroidal hypoplasia and posterior polar colobomas cannot be treated; therefore, treatment goals are to limit ocular sequelae and to reduce the syndrome in the population.
  - Retinal detachment and intraocular hemorrhage, if present, can sometimes be treated (see the Treatment section in "Retinal detachment").
  - Breeding programs to reduce CEA prevalence.

Prognosis
- The lesions of CEA are nonprogressive.
- However, more severely affected dogs are at risk of developing retinal detachment or intraocular bleeding.
  - These complications result in visual compromise or blindness.

Additional information
- Puppies from predisposed breeds should be examined by a veterinary ophthalmologist by 6–8 weeks of age so that affected individuals can be identified before RPE becomes fully pigmented.

Progressive retinal atrophy (PRA)

What it is
- Bilateral, progressive, inherited photoreceptor degeneration.
  - Many causal genes have been identified and vary between breeds.

Predisposed individuals
Many breeds are predisposed to PRA. A small list is as follows:
- Canine: Labrador retriever, golden retriever, toy poodle, miniature poodle, cocker spaniel, Dachshund, Norwegian elkhound, papillon, and Irish setter
- Feline: Abyssinian, Persian, and Siamese

Defining characteristics
- Most individuals are affected as young adults; however, the onset of some forms of PRA begins before 1 year of age.
- Clinical history and ophthalmic examination findings for PRA are characteristic.

Clinical history
- Visual deficits noticed over several months.
  - Mild signs initially, noticed only in *dim light* settings (e.g., evenings).
  - Initial deficits may be thought of as behavioral and only attributed to visual compromise in retrospect; for example, reluctance to go outside before bedtime or reluctance to use staircases and change in behavior during walks.
- Over time, visual deficits become more pronounced and occur in both dim-light and bright-light situations.
  - Overt inability to navigate familiar surroundings.

- Owners may also report that the eyes appear more shiny or bright.
  - Result of mydriasis and increased visibility of tapetal reflection.

Ophthalmic examination abnormalities are *bilateral and symmetrical*:

- *Difficulty navigating.*
- *Mydriasis at rest.*
- *Abnormal PLRs.*
  - Sluggish, incomplete, or absent
- *Abnormal menace response.*
  - Intermittent or absent
- Some degree of cataract development may be present.
- *Diffuse tapetal hyperreflectivity* (Figures 8.10, 8.11, 8.12, 8.13, 8.14, 8.15).
  - In cats, hyperreflectivity begins in an oval area dorsal and lateral to the optic nerve but becomes diffuse with disease progression.
- *Retinal vascular attenuation* (Figures 8.10, 8.11, 8.12, 8.13, 8.14, 8.15).
  - Vessels become narrower and shorter, then completely invisible with disease progression.

Clinical significance

- PRA eventually leads to complete blindness.
- PRA in dogs is associated with cataract development.
  - Although phacoemulsification is rarely pursued, cataracts should still be managed medically as per Chapter 16 to minimize painful complications of LIU.
- PRA is a hereditary disease.
  - Most forms are recessively inherited.
  - Affected individuals are not recommended for breeding.

Diagnosis

- A diagnosis of PRA is based on a history of progressive visual loss combined with aforementioned examination findings.
- Breed-specific genetic tests exist and can help to determine carrier status.
  - Because the genetic mutations responsible for PRA vary between breeds, the test used must be specific for the breed.

Treatment

- Treatments to stop or reverse retinal atrophy are not currently available.
- Therefore, the goals are to assist adjustment to blindness and maintain quality of life.
  - Use night lights in the evenings to help patients navigate the home.
  - Minimize change to the home environment so that pets can memorize the layout of the house and navigate more easily.
  - Place items, textures, or scents as markers around the home to help with orientation.
    - If a pet has been carried into a room, consistently set him/her down near a specific item or scent so that the pet knows its location.

- Rugs or mats with different textures placed throughout the home can help pets know where they are.
- Use auditory cues, such as bells on other pets or people, or toys that emit sounds.
- Teach verbal commands so that pets know what to expect when out walking (e.g., teaching right and left and to step up or down).
- Limit access to staircases, pools, and other potentially hazardous situations.
- Companion pets can help blind pets navigate.

Prognosis

- All patients progress to complete blindness.
- The prognosis for maintaining a comfortable eye is very good, provided that cataracts and LIU are managed.
  - Sequela to chronic LIU as discussed in Chapter 16 may occur.

Additional information

- Cataracts may be present at the time of a PRA diagnosis.
  - Even if not yet large enough to preclude fundic examination, the diagnosis of PRA is sometimes missed because the cataracts are presumed to be the cause of visual deficits.
- In many cases, cataracts may not develop until years after a PRA diagnosis.
  - Patients should be routinely monitored following a diagnosis of PRA so that medical treatment for LIU is initiated when cataracts develop.
- Blind dogs are at higher risk of corneal ulceration because they walk into objects.
  - Products to reduce the risk of this, such as goggles designed for dogs or harnesses with attachments to act as a front bumper (sometimes referred to as "halos"), can minimize ocular trauma.
- Although blindness is irreversible, dogs and cats with PRA can maintain a good quality of life.

Sudden acquired retinal degeneration syndrome (SARDS)

What it is

- Bilateral, acute photoreceptor degeneration of undetermined etiology

Predisposed individuals

- SARDS affects dogs, not cats.
- Some overrepresented characteristics/breeds are as follows:
  - Overweight
  - Small breed
  - Middle-aged
  - Female
  - Dachshund
  - Miniature schnauzer

Defining characteristics

Clinical history:

- *Acute* blindness.
- Often, signs very similar to those of hyperadrenocorticism are present:
  - Polyuria
  - Polydipsia
  - Polyphagia
  - Weight gain

Ophthalmic examination abnormalities are *bilateral and symmetrical*:

- *Difficulty navigating.*
- *Mydriasis at rest.*
- PLRs may be normal, sluggish, incomplete, or absent.
- *Abnormal menace response.*
  - Intermittent or absent.
- *Normal fundic examination* (Figures 8.1, 8.2, 8.3, 8.4).
  - In most cases, when hyperreflectivity and vascular attenuation are present at the time of diagnosis, they are subtle.
  - Overt ophthalmoscopic evidence of retinal degeneration usually does not appear for several weeks after blindness.

Clinical significance

- The etiopathogenesis of SARDS is not understood.
  - Immune-mediated mechanisms appear likely (Grozdanic *et al.*, 2019; Mowat *et al.*, 2020).
  - SARDS may truly represent a collection of diseases, of differing etiologies, rather than one disease syndrome.
- Although clinical signs compatible with hyperadrenocorticism are often present, this condition has not been definitively linked with SARDS.

Diagnosis

- Clinical history (see "Defining characteristics"), signalment, and ophthalmic examination findings should raise the suspicion for SARDS.
- Referral for an ERG is required to diagnose SARDS.
  - An ERG showing absence of retinal function confirms SARDS.
  - An ERG showing presence of retinal function means neurologic causes of blindness, rather than SARDS, are likely.

Treatment

- Although research is ongoing, an effective therapy for SARDS has not yet been identified.
- As with PRA (see aforementioned), pet owners should help their pets adapt to blindness.

Prognosis

- Blindness is irreversible.
- The prognosis for maintaining a comfortable eye is excellent.
- The prognosis for maintaining quality of life is very good (Stuckey *et al.*, 2013).
  - Systemic clinical signs may persist throughout life or may resolve (Mattson *et al.*, 1992; Stuckey *et al.*, 2013).

Additional information

- Some systemic illnesses may be found in a higher proportion of dogs with SARDS when compared to dogs unaffected by SARDS (Washington *et al.*, 2020).
- Cancer-associated retinopathy is rare, but can mimic SARDS (Grozdanic *et al.*, 2021).
- Consider diagnostic testing to rule out concurrent systemic disease.

Retinal degeneration (excluding PRA and SARDS)

What it is

- Loss of any or all of the 10 layers of the retina.

Predisposed individuals

- Predispositions are not for retinal degeneration per se but for the various underlying etiologies (see individual sections).

Defining characteristics

- Retinal degeneration may be focal or diffuse, depending on the cause.
- Changes within tapetal fundus that support retinal degeneration are as follows:
  - *Tapetal hyperreflectivity*
    - Focal areas of hyperreflectivity may have a central, darkly pigmented core (Figures 8.16, 8.17, 8.18).
  - Retinal vascular attenuation
    - This may not be present if degeneration is focal and does not affect an area of retina through which the vessels cross.
- Within the nontapetal fundus, decreased pigmentation can be an indicator of retinal degeneration.
  - Due to loss of melanotic RPE and choroid (Figures 8.28, 8.29).
  - This allows the underlying choroidal vessels and white sclera to become visible.

Clinical significance

Significance of retinal degeneration relates to the underlying cause and to effects on vision.

1 Significance relating to underlying cause:

Causes of retinal degeneration commonly seen in practice (excluding PRA and SARDS, mentioned earlier) include the following:

- Posterior uveitis
  - Underlying causes of uveitis are many (see "Anterior uveitis" in Chapter 15).
  - Every attempt should be made to find the underlying cause of uveitis, as this has implications for systemic health and prognosis for vision.
  - Degeneration is focal or diffuse, depending on the extent of inflammation.
- Retinal detachment
  - Photoreceptor death due to separation from blood supply.

○ Degeneration is focal or diffuse, depending on the amount of retina detached.

Causes of retinal degeneration that have become less common, but are discussed due to their importance, include the following:

- Dietary taurine deficiency in cats.
  ○ This rarely affects cats eating commercial cat foods, but homemade diets may not be balanced.
  ○ In early stages of disease, only an oval area dorsal and lateral to the optic disc is degenerate, but degeneration becomes diffuse with prolonged taurine deficiency.
  ○ Taurine deficiency is also associated with dilated cardiomyopathy.
- Enrofloxacin toxicity in cats
  ○ Due to a functional defect in the feline retina (Ramirez *et al.*, 2011).
  ○ Risk of degeneration is high when doses exceed manufacturer recommendation, but can occur even when used according to drug label (Wiebe & Hamilton, 2002).
    ▪ Geriatric cats
    ▪ Renal or hepatic impairment
  ○ This causes diffuse retinal degeneration.

2 Significance for vision:
  ○ Degenerate retina is nonfunctional; therefore, degenerate areas are blind spots.
  ○ Retinal degeneration is irreversible.
    ▪ Degenerate areas do not regain function.
    ▪ Progression of degeneration can be limited if the underlying etiology is addressed (see "Treatment").
  ○ Severity of visual deficits depends on the amount and location of retina affected.
    ▪ Small, focal areas of degeneration may not result in detectable visual deficits, while vision loss is usually noticeable with widespread retinal degeneration.
    ▪ Visual impact is higher when degeneration affects the retina closer to the optic nerve, rather than the peripheral retina.

Diagnosis
- The diagnosis of retinal degeneration is based on funduscopy.
- Diagnosis of the underlying cause is based on ophthalmic examination, physical examination, thorough history, and labwork.

Treatment
- Treatments to regenerate the retina are not available.
- The goal is therefore to limit progression of retinal degeneration.
  ○ Address the underlying cause of degeneration.
  ○ For example, treat uveitis, treat retinal detachment, provide a balanced diet without nutritional deficiencies, and discontinue enrofloxacin.

Prognosis
- Retinal degeneration and visual compromise cannot be reversed.
- If the underlying cause is adequately addressed, it may be possible to limit further degeneration and maintain function of nondegenerate retina.
  ○ The amount of vision retained is influenced by the amount of retina that has degenerated before the underlying etiology is addressed.

Additional information
- Avoid iatrogenic retinal degeneration by avoiding enrofloxacin use in cats.
  ○ Use only when culture and sensitivity indicates that this drug is appropriate and no alternatives are available.
  ○ Use only at labeled doses.

Chorioretinitis
What it is
- Inflammation of the choroid and the retina.
- Also referred to as posterior uveitis.

Predisposed individuals
- Dogs and cats of any age can develop chorioretinitis.
- Predispositions to specific uveitic syndromes exist (see "Anterior uveitis" in Chapter 15).

Defining characteristics
- *Hyporeflectivity* in the tapetal fundus (Figures 8.19, 8.20, 8.21, 8.22, 8.25, 8.26, 8.41).
- *White to gray infiltrates in the nontapetal fundus* (Figures 8.27, 8.28).
- Affected areas may appear to be raised.
- Affected areas may be out of focus relative to the remainder of the fundus.
- Chorioretinal hemorrhage (Figures 8.30, 8.31, 8.32, 8.33, 8.34, 8.35, 8.36).
- May be accompanied by neuro-ophthalmic abnormalities.
  ○ Mydriasis
  ○ Incomplete, sluggish, or absent direct PLR
  ○ Intermittent or absent menace response in the affected eye

Clinical significance
Significance of chorioretinitis relates to both the underlying cause as well as its effect on vision.

1 Underlying causes of chorioretinitis
  ○ As for anterior uveitis, underlying causes may be systemic diseases, which can have serious implications for overall health.
  ○ A diagnostic workup to rule out systemic disease should therefore be performed following every diagnosis of chorioretinitis (see "Anterior uveitis" in Chapter 15).

- The list for potential causes of posterior uveitis is similar to that for potential causes of anterior uveitis (see "Anterior uveitis" in Chapter 15).
  - Fungal organisms have a predilection for the posterior uvea.
2 Chorioretinitis has a higher potential for causing blindness than anterior uveitis does.
  - Unless treated promptly, inflamed choroid and retina will likely degenerate.
  - Inflammation can lead to retinal detachment, which can also lead to retinal degeneration.
  - Severe or prolonged inflammation can incite other potentially blinding ocular diseases:
    - Cataract
    - Vitreous opacities
    - Optic nerve atrophy
    - Phthisis bulbi

Diagnosis

The diagnostic process is divided into (1) making a diagnosis of chorioretinitis and (2) determining its underlying cause.
1 Diagnosing chorioretinitis
  - The diagnosis is made when the aforementioned abnormalities are seen on fundic examination.
    - Anterior segment abnormalities may not be present if concurrent anterior uveitis is absent.
2 Determining the underlying cause
  - Similar underlying causes as for anterior uveitis (see "Anterior uveitis" in Chapter 15).
  - A diagnostic workup (see "Anterior uveitis" in Chapter 15) is crucial to rule out systemic disease, which can cause significant morbidity and even mortality).

Treatment

The goal of treatment is to stop inflammation so that vision loss is minimized. Treatment is therefore aimed at both the underlying cause of uveitis and anti-inflammatory therapy.
1 Treatment of the underlying cause
  - If found, the underlying cause must be treated for treatment of chorioretinitis to be effective.
2 Anti-inflammatory therapy
  - Medications must be administered systemically.
    - Ophthalmically applied medications do not reach therapeutic concentrations in the posterior segment.
  - Corticosteroids or veterinary-labeled NSAIDs.
    - Corticosteroids: prednisone/prednisolone
      - Initially administer 0.5–1 mg/kg PO q24h–q12h.
      - Gradually taper the dose as clinical signs improve.
      - Do not use if infectious disease is suspected.
      - Not recommended for use if lymphoma is suspected, as this can alter results of diagnostics or influence the efficacy of chemotherapeutic protocols.

      - Do not use in patients with systemic disease where corticosteroid use is contraindicated (e.g., hepatic dysfunction).
      - Do not use concurrently with systemically administered NSAIDs.
    - NSAIDs: veterinary-labeled products such as carprofen (Rimadyl®), meloxicam (Metacam®), and robenacoxib (Onsior®), as well as others.
      - Use at labeled dose.
      - Decrease the dose or discontinue as clinical signs improve.
      - Do not use concurrently with systemically administered corticosteroids.
      - Not recommended for use in patients with systemic conditions for which NSAIDs are contraindicated (e.g., those with renal compromise).
      - As inflammation improves, taper doses.
- The goal is complete cessation of medication, but there is potential to require long-term, low-dose treatment to control signs.

As with anterior uveitis, painful, blinding sequelae may still occur despite diligent treatment. For eyes that have become blind and painful, enucleation is recommended. In addition to improving patient comfort, histopathology of the eye can assist with identifying an underlying cause of the inflammation.

Prognosis

- If a relatively small portion of the fundus is affected and inflammation is controlled quickly, vision and comfort can be maintained.
- The prognosis for vision is poor with widespread or prolonged inflammation.
  - Increased likelihood and extent of retinal degeneration.
  - Increased likelihood of blinding complications such as glaucoma, cataract, retinal detachment, optic nerve atrophy, or phthisis bulbi.

Additional information

- Due to high potential for vision loss, referral to a veterinary ophthalmologist at the time of diagnosis is recommended.
- An individual with chorioretinitis may not show outward abnormalities if that is the only ocular disease.
  - Performing a fundic examination as a part of every ophthalmic examination is therefore crucial so that chorioretinitis is not missed.
  - Fundic examination as a routine part of a physical examination is also highly recommended.

Retinal detachment

What it is

- Separation of the neurosensory retina from the RPE.

- Types of retinal detachments can be classified by mode of detachment:
  - Serous retinal detachment (Figures 8.19, 8.20, 8.34, 8.35, 8.37, 8.39, 8.40a, 8.40b, 8.41)
    - Also referred to as exudative or bullous detachment.
    - This occurs as a result of fluid and/or inflammatory cell accumulation between the RPE and the neurosensory retina (the subretinal space), which pushes the neurosensory retina off its normal position.
  - Tractional retinal detachment
    - Contraction of vitreous traction bands, caused by inflammation, pulls the neurosensory retina off its normal position.
  - Rhegmatogenous (Figures 8.42, 8.43)
    - This refers to detachment associated with tears or holes in the retina.
    - The breaks in the retina allow vitreous to enter the subretinal space.
    - Vitreous in subretinal space forces neurosensory retina and RPE further apart.

Predisposed individuals

- Individuals with specific ocular diseases are predisposed to retinal detachments.
  - Congenital abnormalities
    - Vitreous and retinal dysplasias
      - Shih tzu
      - Labrador retriever
      - English springer spaniel
      - Miniature schnauzer
    - CEA (see earlier in chapter)
  - American bichon frise with cataract (Braus *et al.*, 2012; Gelatt *et al.*, 2003)
  - Previous intraocular surgery
  - Lens luxation
  - Systemic hypertension
  - Posterior uveitis
  - Intraocular neoplasia

Defining characteristics

- Although appearance varies widely (depending on the type of retinal detachment, amount of detached retina, and distance of separation), all retinal detachments will reveal areas of crisp focus interspersed with areas of defocus (Figures 8.34, 8.35, 8.40a, 8.40b, 8.41).
- With focal detachments, outward abnormalities may not be detectable.
- If detached area is large, or if both eyes are affected, visual deficits or blindness are usually noticed.
- With larger areas of detachment, neuro-ophthalmic abnormalities may be present.
  - Mydriasis
  - Incomplete, sluggish, or absent direct PLR
  - Intermittent or absent menace response in the affected eye

- Pet owners may report a change in the appearance of the eye.
1 Serous retinal detachment
   - Focal detachments appear raised (Figures 8.19, 8.20).
     - Vessels crossing over detached areas bend more acutely.
   - With large detachments, the retina can billow forward (Figures 8.35, 8.37, 8.38, 8.39, 8.40a, 8.40b, 8.41).
     - Retina is seen in many different planes.
     - Usually visible on gross examination by transillumination (Figures 8.37, 8.38, 8.39, 8.40a).
2 Tractional retinal detachment
   - On fundic examination, vitreous traction bands may be seen adherent to the detached retina.
3 Rhegmatogenous retinal detachment
   - The edge of the tear may be visible.
   - With large, dorsally located tears, gravity pulls the retina ventrally.
     - Retina drapes over the optic nerve, giving an appearance of a veil (Figures 8.42, 8.43).

Clinical significance

- The significance of retinal detachments relates to the underlying cause, their effect on vision, and their effect on overall ocular health.
1 Causes of retinal detachments
   - Retinal detachments are often secondary to inflammation.
     - The original cause of chorioretinitis (see "Anterior uveitis" in Chapter 15 for a list of potential causes of uveitis) may have implications for overall health.
   - Some underlying causes can affect the fellow eye.
     - For example, bilateral congenital anomalies, chorioretinitis as a result of systemic disease, and systemic hypertension.
2 Effects on vision
   - Degree of vision loss varies from no detectable deficits to complete blindness, correlating directly with the following:
     - Amount of retina detached
       - Larger detachments result in a larger number of compromised photoreceptors.
     - Duration of detachment
       - Photoreceptor die-off begins shortly after a detachment (Anderson *et al.*, 1983), and this does not stop until after reattachment occurs.
       - With very short duration of detachment, limited photoreceptor recovery can occur (Lewis *et al.*, 2002).
3 Effects on the eye
   - Retinal detachments often lead to complications such as chronic uveitis, intraocular hemorrhage, and secondary glaucoma.

Diagnosis

- Retinal detachment is diagnosed with funduscopy.
  - Large serous detachments can be seen with transillumination.

- The cause of retinal detachment is determined through careful history-taking, ophthalmic examination, physical examination, and further diagnostics.
  - History of intraocular surgery
  - Ophthalmic examination to rule in/rule out intraocular disease such as congenital ocular abnormalities, cataract, and concurrent uveitis
  - Blood pressure measurement
  - Diagnostics to rule out underlying systemic disease as a cause of chorioretinitis
    - See "Anterior uveitis" in Chapter 15 for diagnostic tests that should be considered.
- Similar to uveitis, a cause for retinal detachment is sometimes not identified in spite of diagnostics.

Treatment

- The goal of treatment is to limit photoreceptor degeneration by encouraging reattachment of the retina.
- Referral to a veterinary ophthalmologist at the time of diagnosis is advised.
- Prompt therapy is crucial to preserve photoreceptor function and vision.
  - Reattachment within 24 hours can halt or even reverse retinal damage (Lewis et al., 2002).
  - Cellular recovery is best if reattachment occurs within 1 week and poor if after 1 month (Anderson et al., 1986).
- Serous retinal detachments are usually treated medically.
  - Treat the underlying disease, if identified, to encourage fluid resorption and return of retina to its anatomic position.
  - If an underlying disease is not identified, treat with systemic anti-inflammatories as for chorioretinitis.
    - Corticosteroids preferred over NSAIDs, provided contraindications for their use are absent.
  - Laser retinopexy is sometimes performed by veterinary ophthalmologists to discourage enlargement.
    - Adhesions created around borders of detachment.
- Tractional and rhegmatogenous detachments should be referred for surgical treatment.
  - In addition to anti-inflammatory therapy as for serous detachments.
  - Surgical removal of traction bands.
  - The retina is returned to anatomic position and pexied in place with a laser.

Prognosis

- Photoreceptor degeneration begins shortly after detachment (Anderson et al., 1983); therefore, the duration and amount of affected retina are important determinants of future vision.
  - For example, the prognosis for recovery or maintenance of vision is better for focal than for diffuse detachments and better for acute than for chronic detachments.
  - Because visual deficits are not always obvious, the duration of retinal detachment at the time of presentation is often unknown in veterinary patients.

- Height of detachment also affects retinal damage (Anderson et al., 1983).
  - That is, the distance of separation between neurosensory retina and RPE correlates with cellular degeneration.
- Prognosis also depends on the underlying cause of detachment.
  - For example, the prognosis for successfully managing systemic hypertension is better than for treating neoplastic chorioretinitis.
- Treatment is always indicated because even for chronic detachments, the potential to preserve some useful vision exists (Grahn et al., 2007).
  - Even a small amount of vision can improve quality of life.
- Resolution of serous detachments is possible if the underlying cause is managed.
- Prognosis for tractional and rhegmatogenous detachments is grave unless surgery is pursued.
  - These will not reattach with medical therapy alone.
  - High risk of development of uveitis and secondary glaucoma (Grahn et al., 2007).
- Prognosis for tractional and rhegmatogenous detachment undergoing surgery is fair (Grahn et al., 2007; Spatola et al., 2015; Steele et al., 2012).
  - Surgery should be performed as soon as possible to minimize vision loss.

Hypertensive chorioretinopathy

What it is

- Hypertensive chorioretinopathy refers to lesions to the retina, choroid, and optic nerve as a result of systemic hypertension.
- The syndrome results from ischemic injury to vessel walls.
  - Chronic hypertension leads to constriction of vessels supplying the retina and optic nerve.
  - Prolonged vasoconstriction results in vessel wall ischemia, necrosis, and fluid leakage.

Predisposed individuals

- The higher the level of blood pressure elevation, the more likely ocular lesions are to develop.
  - In hypertensive dogs, retinal hemorrhages are associated with higher levels of blood pressure elevation when compared to dogs without retinal hemorrhages (LeBlanc et al., 2011).
  - Cats with ocular lesions tend to have blood pressures above 200 mm Hg (Littman, 1994; Morgan, 1986; Sansom et al., 1994; Turner et al., 1990).
- Ocular lesions are more likely to develop if hypertension is severe and prolonged (Morgan, 1986).

Defining characteristics

- Lesions are usually bilateral but not symmetrical (Maggio et al., 2000).
- *Retinal hemorrhage* (Figures 8.30, 8.31, 8.32, 8.33, 8.34, 8.35, 8.36)

- Small hemorrhages are often found incidentally on ophthalmic examination and can be the first indicator of hypertension.
  - In dogs, hemorrhage is the most common lesion associated with high blood pressure (LeBlanc *et al.,* 2011).
- *Retinal detachment*
  - In cats, this is the most common lesion at presentation and is usually accompanied by hemorrhage (Maggio *et al.,* 2000).
  - Severity of detachment can range from focal (Figures 8.19, 8.20) to complete (Figures 8.34, 8.35) detachment.
  - Often, acute blindness due to complete, bilateral retinal detachment is the reason for presentation and the first indication of hypertension in cats.
- Retinal edema (Figure 8.19, 8.20)
- Hyphema (Figures 6.40, 6.41, 6.42, 6.43)
- Tortuous retinal vessels
- More advanced lesions may be accompanied by mydriasis, incomplete/absent PLRs, and intermittent/absent menace response.

Clinical significance

Hypertensive chorioretinopathy is significant for its effects on vision as well as overall health.

1. Significance for systemic health
   - In addition to idiopathic hypertension, several systemic diseases can be associated with hypertension (Acierno *et al.,* 2018).
     - Acute or chronic kidney disease (Kobayashi *et al.,* 1990; Littman, 1994; Maggio *et al.,* 2000; Morgan, 1986)
       - Chronic kidney disease is the most common concurrent disease in cats with ocular lesions.
     - Feline hyperthyroidism (Kobayashi *et al.,* 1990)
     - Diabetes mellitus
     - Canine hyperadrenocorticism
     - Primary hyperaldosteronism
     - Pheochromocytoma
   - Uncontrolled hypertension leads to further morbidity.
     - Progression of renal disease
     - Left ventricular hypertrophy
     - Cerebral vascular hemorrhage
2. Significance for vision
   - Uncontrolled hypertension can lead to blindness.
     - When lesions are still mild (e.g., small hemorrhages and mild retinal edema), evidence of visual impairment may not be present.
     - Overt vision loss is usually associated with retinal detachment.
     - Retinal degeneration limits return to vision even if retinas reattach.

Diagnosis

- Lesions are identified during funduscopy.
  - Lesions listed under "Defining characteristics" should raise suspicion for systemic hypertension.

- Diagnosis of systemic hypertension is based on guidelines published elsewhere (Acierno *et al.,* 2018; Taylor *et al.,* 2017).

Treatment

- The goals of treatment are to limit ocular pathology and to normalize blood pressure.
- Treat concurrent systemic disease, if identified.
- Treat hypertension.
  - Ocular lesions improve with normalization of blood pressure.
  - Guidelines for treatment are published elsewhere (Acierno *et al.,* 2018).
    - In dogs, angiotensin-converting enzyme inhibitors such as benazepril or enalapril are usually first-line therapy.
    - In cats, the calcium channel blocker amlodipine is usually first-line therapy.
      - Amlodipine treatment is associated with blood pressure reduction and improvement of ocular lesions (Cirla *et al.,* 2021; Maggio *et al.,* 2000).
- If anterior segment disease is present, treat with topical anti-inflammatory medications as per Chapter 15.

Prognosis

- The prognosis for maintenance of vision is good if lesions are mild (e.g., focal retinal hemorrhages and mild retinal edema) and blood pressure is controlled.
- The prognosis declines if retinal detachment is present.
  - Reported rates of retinal reattachment and return to vision vary, but tend to be low (Cirla *et al.,* 2021; Maggio *et al.,* 2000; Young *et al.,* 2019).
- Presence of hyphema increases the risk of secondary glaucoma (Sansom *et al.,* 1994).

Additional information

- A very typical presentation is a geriatric cat presented for acute blindness and bilateral retinal detachment as the major ophthalmic abnormality.
- To increase early detection of hypertension and its ophthalmic lesions, fundic examination is recommended:
  - During routine physical examination in cats older than 8 years (Carter *et al.,* 2013; Crispin & Mould, 2001).
  - When hypertension is diagnosed.
  - When a systemic disease associated with hypertension is diagnosed.

Optic neuritis

What it is

- Inflammation of the optic nerve.

Predisposed individuals

- Optic neuritis affects dogs more often than cats.

Defining characteristics

- History
  - Waxing and waning visual deficits.
  - Acute blindness.
  - Behavior change may or may not be reported.
  - Neurologic abnormalities may or may not be reported.
- Ophthalmic examination
  - *Enlarged optic nerve* protruding into the vitreous (Figure 8.48).
  - *Blurry, indistinct nerve edges* (Figures 8.48, 8.49).
  - Retina immediately around nerve may be detached.
  - Fluid, cells, and/or hemorrhage may be present around the optic nerve (Figures 8.21, 8.22, 8.49).

Clinical significance

- Optic neuritis causes vision impairment and blindness.
- Optic neuritis may affect only the optic nerves or may signify more widespread central nervous system disease.
  - The optic nerves are considered extensions of the brain.
  - Central nervous system disease can cause severe morbidity or mortality.

Potential causes of optic neuritis are as follows:

- Neoplasia
  - Meningioma and lymphoma among the most common affecting the optic nerve (Grahn *et al.*, 2012; Mauldin *et al.*, 2000).
- Idiopathic
- Inflammatory
  - Meningoencephalitides such as granulomatous meningoencephalitis, necrotizing meningoencephalitis, meningoencephalitis of unknown etiology
  - Orbital cellulitis/abscess
- Infectious
  - For example, systemic mycoses, tick-borne disease, bacterial, protozoal, and viral disease
- Traumatic
  - Inadvertent penetration of orbit during dental procedures.
  - If due to other external trauma, additional signs of trauma will be present.

Diagnosis

- The diagnostic process is divided into (1) diagnosing optic neuritis, (2) determining the extent of disease, and (3) determining its underlying cause.
1 Diagnosis of optic neuritis
  - Optic neuritis is diagnosed when optic nerve changes are seen on funduscopy (see "Defining characteristics").
  - Referral to a veterinary ophthalmologist is recommended promptly after diagnosis.
2 Determining the extent of disease
  - Determine if disease is limited to optic nerves or if there is central nervous system involvement.
    - Neurologic examination
    - MRI or CT scan

3 Determining the underlying cause
  - Diagnostic workup to rule out systemic disease, similar to that for anterior uveitis (see "Anterior uveitis" in Chapter 15).
  - Collection of cerebrospinal fluid for cytology, culture and sensitivity, and infectious disease titers.

Treatment

- The treatment goal is to halt inflammation of the optic nerve. It must therefore address both the underlying cause of optic neuritis and anti-inflammatory therapy.
1 Treatment of the underlying cause, if identified
  - Necessary for effective treatment
2 Systemic anti-inflammatory therapy
  - Crucial, often the only component of therapy when the underlying cause is not identified.
  - Corticosteroids are first line.
    - Prednisone or prednisolone 1–2 mg/kg PO per day initial dose.
    - Do not use if infectious disease is suspected.
    - As inflammation improves, taper the dose at 1- to 3-week intervals.
      - Improvement is judged by the appearance of optic nerve and improvement of visual and neurologic deficits.
      - Repeat MRI or CT scan may also be used to evaluate clinical progression.
      - Long-term, low-dose treatment to prevent recurrence may be required.
- If there is inadequate control of disease or side effects of steroids are excessive, alternative immunosuppressives (e.g., CsA, leflunomide, azathioprine, mycophenolate, and others) may be required.

Prognosis

- There is potential for return of vision if inflammation and underlying cause (if identified) are controlled promptly; however, many patients do not regain vision (Bedos *et al.*, 2020; Smith *et al.*, 2018).
- The underlying cause of optic neuritis influences prognosis.
  - For example, prognosis for vision and for life for fungal meningoencephalitis is worse than for idiopathic optic neuritis.
- With increased duration or severity of inflammation, there is increased potential for optic nerve atrophy and permanent blindness, regardless of the underlying cause or ultimate control of inflammation.

Additional information

- Central nervous system disease should always be considered when optic neuritis is diagnosed.
  - Central nervous system disease can be present even if obvious neurologic deficits do not accompany blindness.
  - Knowledge of the extent of central nervous system involvement is important for prognostication.

○ Advanced imaging should therefore always be recommended.

○ Prompt referral for diagnostics is recommended.

Further reading

General posterior segment disease

Meekins, JM. 2015. Acute blindness. *Topics in Companion Animal Medicine*. 30(3):118–125.

www.blindtails.com

SARDS

Komáromy, AM, *et al.* 2016. Sudden acquired retinal degeneration syndrome (SARDS)—a review and proposed strategies toward a better understanding of pathogenesis, early diagnosis, and therapy. *Veterinary Ophthalmology*. 19(4):319–331.

Stuckey, JA, *et al.* 2013. Long-term outcome of sudden acquired retinal degeneration syndrome in dogs. *Journal of the American Veterinary Medical Association*. 243(1):1426–1431.

Retinal degeneration

Wiebe, V & Hamilton, P. 2002. Fluoroquinolone-induced retinal degeneration in cats. *Journal of the American Veterinary Medical Association*. 221(11):1568–1571.

Hypertensive chorioretinopathy

Acierno, MJ, *et al.* 2018. ACVIM consensus statement: guidelines for the identification, evaluation, and management of systemic hypertension in dogs and cats. *Journal of Veterinary Internal Medicine*. 32(6):1803–1833.

Carter, J. 2019. Hypertension in cats: a guide to fundic lesions to facilitate early diagnosis. *Journal of Feline Medicine and Surgery*. 21(1):35–45.

LeBlanc, NL, *et al.* 2011. Ocular lesions associated with systemic hypertension in dogs: 65 cases (2005–2007). *Journal of the American Veterinary Medical Association*. 238(7):915–921.

References

Acierno, MJ, *et al.* 2018. ACVIM consensus statement: guidelines for the identification, evaluation, and management of systemic hypertension in dogs and cats. *Journal of Veterinary Internal Medicine*. 32(6):1803–1833.

Anderson, DH, *et al.* 1983. Retinal detachment in the cat: the pigment epithelial-photoreceptor interface. *Investigative Ophthalmology and Visual Science*. 24(7):906–926.

Anderson, DH, *et al.* 1986. Morphological recovery in the reattached retina. *Investigative Ophthalmology and Visual Science*. 27(2):168–183.

Bedos, L, *et al.* 2020. Presumed optic neuritis of non-infectious origin in dogs treated with immunosuppressive medication: 28 dogs (2000–2015). *Journal of Small Animal Practice*. 61(11):676–683.

Braus, BK, *et al.* 2012. Cataracts are not associated with retinal detachment in the Bichon Frise in the UK—a retrospective study of preoperative findings and outcomes in 40 eyes. *Veterinary Ophthalmology*. 15(2):98–101.

Carter, JM, *et al.* 2013. The prevalence of ocular lesions associated with hypertension in a population of geriatric cats in Auckland, New Zealand. *New Zealand Veterinary Journal*. 62(1):21–29.

Cirla, A, *et al.* 2021. Ocular fundus abnormalities in cats affected by systemic hypertension: Prevalence, characterization, and outcome of treatment. *Veterinary Ophthalmology*. 24(2):185–194.

Crispin, SM & Mould, JRB. 2001. Systemic hypertensive disease and the feline fundus. *Veterinary Ophthalmology*. 4(2):131–140.

Dubielzig RR, *et al.* 1998. Iridociliary epithelial tumors in 100 dogs and 17 cats: a morphological study. *Veterinary Ophthalmology*. 1(4):223–231.

Gelatt, KN, *et al.* 2003. Cataracts in the Bichon Frise. *Veterinary Ophthalmology*. 6(1):3–9.

Grahn, BH, *et al.* 2007. Chronic retinal detachment and giant retinal tears in 34 dogs: outcome comparison of no treatment, topical medical therapy, and retinal reattachment after vitrectomy. *Canadian Veterinary Journal*. 48(10):1031–1039.

Grahn, BH, *et al.* 2012. Diagnostic ophthalmology. *Canadian Veterinary Journal*. 53(11):1223–1224.

Grozdanic, SD, *et al.* 2019. Optical coherence tomography and molecular analysis of sudden acquired retinal degeneration syndrome (SARDS) eyes suggests the immune-mediated nature of retinal damage. *Veterinary Ophthalmology*. 22(3):305–327.

Grozdanic, SD, *et al.* 2021. Presumed cancer-associated retinopathy (CAR) mimicking Sudden Acquired Retinal Degeneration Syndrome (SARDS) in canines. *Veterinary Ophthalmology*. 24(2):125–155.

Kobayashi, DL, *et al.* 1990. Hypertension in cats with chronic renal failure or hyperthyroidism. *Journal of Veterinary Internal Medicine*. 4(2):58–62.

LeBlanc, NL, *et al.* 2011. Ocular lesions associated with systemic hypertension in dogs: 65 cases (2005–2007). *Journal of the American Veterinary Medical Association*. 238(7):915–921.

Lewis, GP, *et al.* 2002. The ability of rapid retinal reattachment to stop or reverse the cellular and molecular events initiated by detachment. *Investigative Ophthalmology and Visual Science*. 43(7):2412–2420.

Littman, MP. 1994. Spontaneous systemic hypertension in 24 cats. *Journal of Veterinary Internal Medicine*. 8(2):79–86.

Maggio, F, *et al.* 2000. Ocular lesions associated with systemic hypertension in cats: 69 cases (1985–1998). *Journal of the American Veterinary Medical Association*. 217(5):695–702.

Mattson, A, *et al.* 1992. Clinical features suggesting hyperadrenocorticism associated with sudden acquired retinal degeneration syndrome in a dog. *Journal of the American Animal Hospital Association*. 28(3):199–202.

Mauldin, EA, *et al.* 2000. Canine orbital meningiomas: a review of 22 cases. *Veterinary Ophthalmology*. 3(1):11–16.

Morgan, RV. 1986. Systemic hypertension in four cats: ocular and medical findings. *Journal of the American Animal Hospital Association*. 22(5):615–621.

Mowat, FM, *et al.* 2020. Detection of circulating anti-retinal antibodies in dogs with sudden acquired retinal degeneration syndrome using indirect immunofluorescence: a case-control study. *Experimental Eye Research*. doi:10.1016/j.exer.2020.107989.

Parker, HG, *et al.* 2007. Breed relationships facilitate fine-mapping studies: a 7.8-kb deletion cosegregates with collie eye anomaly across multiple dog breeds. *Genome Research*. 17(11):1562–1571.

Ramirez, CJ, *et al.* 2011. Molecular genetic basis for fluoroquinolone-induced retinal degeneration in cats. *Pharmacogenetics and Genomics*. 21(2):66–75.

Sansom, J, *et al.* 1994. Ocular disease associated with hypertension in 16 cats. *Journal of Small Animal Practice*. 35(12):604–611.

Smith, SM, *et al.*, 2018. Optic neuritis in dogs: 96 cases (1983–2016). *Veterinary Ophthalmology*. 21(5):442–451.

Spatola, RA, *et al.* 2015. Preoperative findings and visual outcome associated with retinal reattachment surgery in dogs: 217 cases (275 eyes). *Veterinary Ophthalmology.* 18(6):485–496.

Steele, KA, *et al.* 2012. Outcome of retinal reattachment surgery in dogs: a retrospective study of 145 cases. *Veterinary Ophthalmology.* 15(S2):35–40.

Stuckey, JA, *et al.* 2013. Long-term outcome of sudden acquired retinal degeneration syndrome in dogs. *Journal of the American Veterinary Medical Association.* 243(10):1426–1431.

Taylor, SS, *et al.* 2017. ISFM consensus guidelines on the diagnosis and management of hypertension in cats. *Journal of Feline Medicine and Surgery.* 19(3):288–303.

Turner, JL, *et al.* 1990. Idiopathic hypertension in a cat with secondary hypertensive retinopathy associated with a high-salt diet. *Journal of the American Animal Hospital Association.* 26(6):647–651.

Wallin-Hakanson, B, *et al.* 2000. Influence of selective breeding on the prevalence of chorioretinal dysplasia and coloboma in the rough collie in Sweden. *Journal of Small Animal Practice.* 41(2):56–59.

Washington, DR, *et al.* 2021. Canine sudden acquired retinal degeneration syndrome: Owner perceptions on the time to vision loss, treatment outcomes, and prognosis for life. *Veterinary Ophthalmology.* 24(2):156–168.

Wiebe, V & Hamilton, P. 2002. Fluoroquinolone-induced retinal degeneration in cats. *Journal of the American Veterinary Medical Association.* 221(11):1568–1571.

Young, WM, *et al.* 2019. Visual outcome in cats with hypertensive chorioretinopathy. *Veterinary Ophthalmology.* 22(2):161–167.

18 Glaucoma

Please see Chapter 9 for images of eyes with glaucoma.

Normal IOP in the dog and cat ranges from 10 to 25 mm Hg. Pressure is maintained within this range by a balance of aqueous humor production and drainage.

Aqueous humor production

- Aqueous humor is formed at the ciliary body, in the posterior chamber (between the iris and the lens), via passive and active mechanisms.
- Passive mechanisms: diffusion and ultrafiltration.
- Active production: formation of bicarbonate and hydrogen ion by combination of carbon dioxide and water.
  ∘ Production of bicarbonate results in entry of water into the posterior chamber.
  ∘ Carbonic anhydrase catalyzes this reaction.

Aqueous humor circulation and drainage

- From the posterior chamber, aqueous humor circulates through the pupil, into the anterior chamber, then into the exit pathways from the eye.
- The main pathway for aqueous humor to leave the eye is through the iridocorneal angle (conventional outflow).
- A smaller proportion of aqueous humor leaves the eye by diffusion through the iris root (unconventional or uveoscleral outflow).
- Elevations of IOP result from impaired aqueous humor drainage.

Glaucoma

What it is

- Glaucoma is damage to the optic nerve and retina associated with elevated IOP.
  ∘ IOP > 25 mm Hg
- Glaucoma is classified as either primary or secondary.
- Primary glaucoma:
  ∘ Is believed to be an inherited condition,
  ∘ Is not the result of other ophthalmic or systemic diseases, and
  ∘ Is often associated with goniodysgenesis (also referred to as pectinate ligament dysplasia), a congenital malformation of the iridocorneal angle.

∘ There are two forms of primary glaucoma: primary open-angle glaucoma (POAG) and primary angle-closure glaucoma (PACG).
∘ PACG is much more common than POAG.
- Secondary glaucoma:
  ∘ Results from concurrent ophthalmic disease.

Predisposed individuals

- Primary glaucoma
  ∘ Dogs
    ▪ Beagle, Norwegian elkhound, cocker spaniel, Labrador retriever, Siberian husky, Shiba Inu, Boston terrier, chow chow, Samoyed, and many others
    ▪ Female
  ∘ Rare in cats but Burmese and Siamese are overrepresented.
- Secondary glaucoma
  ∘ Individuals with uveitis, cataract, lens subluxation or luxation, intraocular neoplasia, and retinal detachment

Defining characteristics

- Glaucoma may have a sudden onset or develop insidiously.
  ∘ POAG develops insidiously and bilaterally.
  ∘ PACG develops acutely and unilaterally.
  ∘ Secondary glaucomas do not have a typical pattern of development.
- Clinical signs are more obvious with higher magnitude or more rapid development of IOP elevation.
- Clinical signs evolve with chronicity.

Clinical signs of acute glaucoma include the following (Figures 9.1, 9.2):
- *Episcleral congestion*
- *Diffuse corneal edema*
- *Mydriasis*
- *Blindness in the affected eye*
- Signs of ocular pain, such as epiphora and blepharospasm

Clinical signs of chronic glaucoma include the following:
- Signs as listed earlier for acute glaucoma

Small Animal Ophthalmic Atlas and Guide, Second Edition. Christine C. Lim.
© 2023 John Wiley & Sons, Inc. Published 2023 by John Wiley & Sons, Inc.
Companion website: www.wiley.com/go/lim/atlas

- *Buphthalmos* (Figures 9.3, 9.4)
  - Chronically elevated IOP stretches and enlarges the eye.
  - May be accompanied by keratitis or corneal ulceration secondary to lagophthalmos (complete eyelid closure is difficult over enlarged eye, causing the central cornea to be exposed).
  - Do not confuse buphthalmos with exophthalmos (the latter indicating orbital pathology). The horizontal corneal diameter of the buphthalmic eye is greater than the measurement for the fellow eye, whereas diameters are equal if an eye is exophthalmic.
- Haab's striae (Figures 9.5, 9.6, 9.7, 9.8)
  - Ocular stretching causes breaks within Descemet's membrane.
- Deep corneal vascularization (Figures 5.9, 6.32)
- *Lens subluxation or luxation* (Figures 7.25, 7.26, 7.27, 7.28, 7.29, 7.30, 7.31, 7.32, 7.33, 7.34, 9.6, 9.8, 9.9, 9.10)
  - The stretching of the eye that occurs with buphthalmos results in rupture of the zonules.
- *Optic disc cupping* (Figures 8.46, 8.47, 9.11)
  - Increased IOP causes ischemic damage to the optic nerve and pushes it posteriorly.
- Tapetal hyperreflectivity (Figures 8.10, 8.11, 8.12, 8.13, 8.14, 8.15, 8.47)
  - Retinal ischemia results from increased IOP.
- Retinal vessel attenuation (Figures 8.10, 8.11, 8.12, 8.13, 8.14, 8.15, 8.46, 8.47)
  - Retinal ischemia is caused by elevated IOP.

In addition to acute and chronic signs, secondary glaucoma will also show signs of the concurrent ocular disease that led to glaucoma development.

- For example, clinical signs of uveitis (as per "Anterior uveitis" in Chapter 15), intraocular mass, cataract, lens subluxation or luxation, and retinal detachment.
- Iris bombé occurs when posterior synechiae form between the lens and the entire circumference of the pupillary zone of the iris, preventing aqueous humor from leaving the posterior chamber through the pupil (Figures 6.42, 6.54).
  - Occurs in the presence of anterior uveitis.
  - Buildup of aqueous humor in the posterior chamber pushes the iris anteriorly.
    - Except for the pupillary and ciliary zones, where the iris is anchored by synechiae (pupillary zone) and its root (ciliary zone).
  - Because aqueous humor cannot reach the anterior chamber and iridocorneal angle, the IOP rises.

Clinical significance
- Elevated IOPs are painful.
- Persistently elevated IOPs irreversibly damage the optic nerve and retina, causing blindness.
- *Primary glaucoma is a bilateral disease,* even if only one eye is affected at the time of initial diagnosis.

- Beginning treatment in the normotensive fellow eye can significantly delay onset of glaucoma in the fellow eye (Dees *et al.,* 2014; Miller *et al.,* 2000).
- Secondary glaucoma is associated with concurrent ophthalmic disease that requires therapy for control of glaucoma.
  - The concurrent ophthalmic disease may also be related to an underlying systemic disease.
  - Causes of secondary glaucoma include the following:
    - *Uveitis* (most common; can be due to underlying systemic disease)
    - Cataract
      - LIU
      - Intumescent cataract, which pushes the iris anteriorly, causing narrowing of the iridocorneal angle
    - Lens luxation
    - Intraocular neoplasia
    - Retinal detachment
  - This is the most common form of glaucoma in both cats and dogs.

Diagnosis
Diagnostics are aimed at making the diagnosis of glaucoma and then classifying it as primary or secondary glaucoma. If glaucoma is secondary, further diagnostics are also aimed at determining the underlying ocular and systemic causes.

Diagnosis of glaucoma
- Clinical signs should raise suspicion for glaucoma.
- Tonometry is used to confirm elevated IOP.
  - Tonometry should be performed in all ophthalmic examinations, especially if clinical signs (see aforementioned) compatible with glaucoma are present.
  - Glaucoma is diagnosed when clinical signs are present and IOP > 25 mm Hg.
  - Because uveitis is associated with low IOP, IOP within normal range in presence of intraocular inflammation can suggest glaucoma development.
  - Significant IOP difference between eyes can be suggestive of glaucoma in the eye with higher IOP.
- In cats, IOP difference >12 mm Hg between eyes should prompt further investigation (Miller *et al.,* 2001).

Classification of glaucoma
- If ophthalmic examination reveals evidence of a disease that can lead to glaucoma (i.e., uveitis, cataract, lens dislocation, intraocular tumor, retinal detachment), this suggests secondary glaucoma.
- The presentation of acute, unilateral, severe IOP elevation in a dog is most likely primary glaucoma, especially if the affected individual is of a predisposed breed.
- Gonioscopy (examination of the iridocorneal angle) should be performed for confirmation of glaucoma type.
  - Performed by a veterinary ophthalmologist.
  - This test determines whether goniodysgenesis is present.
  - If goniodysgenesis is present, it supports a diagnosis of primary glaucoma.

- Gonioscopy should be performed in all cases of glaucoma.
  - Identification of primary glaucoma facilitates treatment of the normal, fellow eye, which delays glaucoma development in that eye.

Identifying the cause of secondary glaucoma
- Ophthalmic examination should identify concurrent ophthalmic disease.
  - Specific underlying disease, if present, dictates further diagnostics.
  - For example, diagnostics to rule out systemic disease if uveitis is present (see "Anterior uveitis" in Chapter 15).

Treatment

Commonly used drugs include the following:
1 Cholinesterase inhibitors
   - Demecarium bromide 0.125% or 0.25% ophthalmic solution.
   - This drug induces miosis.
   - Most often used to delay glaucoma in the normotensive eye of a dog with primary glaucoma in the fellow eye.
   - Because of the potential for systemic side effects, be cautious with cats and small dogs and avoid in individuals already being treated with organophosphates.
2 Beta-blockers
   - Timolol 0.25%, 0.5% and betaxolol 0.25%, 0.5% ophthalmic solutions.
   - These drugs reduce aqueous humor production.
   - Uses
     - To delay glaucoma in the normotensive eye of a dog with primary glaucoma in the fellow eye.
     - In combination with carbonic anhydrase inhibitors (CAIs) to maintain normal IOP in glaucomatous eyes.
   - Because of the potential for systemic side effects, be cautious with cats and small dogs and avoid in individuals with pre-existing cardiac or respiratory disease.
3 CAIs
   - Dorzolamide 2% and brinzolamide 1% ophthalmic solutions and oral methazolamide.
   - These drugs reduce aqueous humor production.
   - Uses
     - To delay glaucoma in the normotensive eye of a dog with primary glaucoma in the fellow eye.
     - To maintain normal IOP in glaucomatous eyes, alone or in combination with beta-blockers.
   - Because of the potential for systemic side effects, ophthalmic administration is preferred over systemic; use caution with cats and small dogs; do not use oral form in cats.
     - Monitoring of electrolytes is recommended for cats being treated with CAIs due to potential for hypokalemia and associated clinical illness (Czepiel & Wasserman, 2021).
     - The efficacy of brinzolamide in cats is unclear (Gray *et al.*, 2003; Slenter *et al.*, 2020).

4 Prostaglandin analogs
   - Ophthalmic latanoprost 0.005%, travoprost 0.004%, bimatoprost 0.03%, and others.
   - These drugs reduce aqueous humor production and increase uveoscleral outflow.
   - Uses
     - Emergency management of acute glaucoma.
     - To maintain normal IOP in glaucomatous eyes.
   - Due to intense miosis, do not use in the presence of anterior lens luxation or significant uveitis.
   - The efficacy of commercially available prostaglandin analogs in cats is unclear (McDonald *et al.*, 2016).
5 Osmotic diuretics
   - Mannitol
   - This drug reduces fluid content of the eye.
   - Use
     - Emergency management of acute glaucoma.
   - Avoid in dehydrated patients and those with renal or cardiac disease.

Treatment protocols vary according to potential for vision and duration of IOP elevation. Three common situations with example treatment protocols are as follows:
1 Emergency management of acute glaucoma with marked IOP elevation.
   - The goals are to rapidly normalize IOP, restore comfort, and restore vision.
     - This is considered an emergency because there is a chance to regain functional vision if IOP is decreased rapidly.
   - This is the typical presentation for PACG in dogs, affecting one eye.
   - This situation is extremely uncommon in cats.
   - Secondary glaucoma can also present similarly.
   - **Step 1:** Begin therapy with topical prostaglandin analog or intravenous mannitol.
     - Prostaglandin analog: apply one drop to the glaucomatous eye. Repeat three to five times at 5-minute intervals.
       - Recheck IOP 45 minutes to 1 hour after administration.
         - The IOP should be decreased (although it may not yet be within normal range) by 1 hour.
     - IV mannitol: infuse 1–2 g/kg IV over 20 minutes.
       - Withhold water during treatment.
       - Recheck IOP at the end of infusion.
         - The IOP should be decreased by the end of the infusion.
   - **Step 2:** Begin treatment to maintain normal IOP in the glaucomatous eye.
     - Use CAI, prostaglandin analog, or both.
     - Ophthalmic CAI, alone or in combination with an ophthalmic beta-blocker for more pronounced IOP lowering.
       - Cats: ophthalmic dorzolamide 2% one drop to glaucomatous eye q12h–q8h.

- Dogs: ophthalmic dorzolamide 2% or brinzolamide 1% one drop to glaucomatous eye q8h.
  - If augmenting with beta-blockers, use one drop of timolol or betaxolol (0.25% or 0.5% ophthalmic solutions) applied to the glaucomatous eye once to twice daily or use a combination dorzolamide/timolol ophthalmic solution applied to the affected eye at a dose of one drop twice daily.
  - Use either ophthalmic or oral CAI, not both; there is no benefit to administering by both routes concurrently (Gelatt & MacKay, 2001a).
  - Oral CAI: methazolamide 2–5 mg/kg PO q12h–q8h (dogs only; do not use in cats).
  - Ophthalmic prostaglandin analog (latanoprost 0.005%, travoprost 0.004%, bimatoprost 0.03%).
    - Apply one drop to the glaucomatous eye q24h in the evening or q12h (Gelatt & MacKay, 2001b, 2001c, 2002).
    - Compared with once-daily application, twice-daily application is associated with less IOP fluctuation and a greater IOP decline (Gelatt & MacKay, 2001b, 2001c, 2002).
  - **Step 3:** If the patient is a dog of a breed predisposed to primary glaucoma, begin treatment to delay glaucoma in the fellow, normotensive eye.
    - Use demecarium bromide, a beta-blocker, or CAI, one drop into the normotensive eye q24h–q12h.
    - Use of an anti-inflammatory in conjunction with an antiglaucoma medication may be beneficial (Dees *et al.,* 2014; Miller *et al.,* 2000).
      - Prednisolone acetate 1% ophthalmic suspension or dexamethasone 0.1% solution, one drop to the normotensive eye q24h.
  - **Step 4:** Begin systemic analgesic therapy (e.g., veterinary NSAIDs, gabapentin, or opioids used at labeled doses).
  - **Step 5:** Arrange for recheck in 1–3 days.
  - **Step 6:** Arrange prompt referral to a veterinary ophthalmologist.
    - For ophthalmic examination, including gonioscopy to confirm or rule out primary glaucoma
    - For evaluation for suitability of surgical procedures to prolong vision
      - Cyclophotocoagulation
        - This is laser ablation of the ciliary body to reduce aqueous humor production.
      - Placement of anterior chamber shunt
        - This creates an alternative outflow pathway from the eye so that aqueous humor outflow is increased.
2 Mild to moderate IOP elevation in a visual eye
  - The goals are to normalize IOP, maintain vision, and maintain comfort.
    - Vision will not be retained if IOP is not controlled.
  - This situation is common with secondary glaucomas, affecting one or both eyes.

- This is a typical presentation for early POAG, affecting both eyes.
- **Step 1:** Begin therapy with CAI (with or without concurrent beta-blocker) (as mentioned earlier).
- **Step 2:** If signs of concurrent ocular disease are present (i.e., if there are signs of uveitis or other causes of secondary glaucoma), begin treatment for the concurrent disease.
  - As an example, if uveitis is present, begin treatment with prednisolone acetate 1% ophthalmic suspension, dexamethasone 0.1% solution, or an oral anti-inflammatory medication (see "Anterior uveitis" in Chapter 15).
- **Step 3:** Arrange recheck of IOP within 3–5 days.
  - If further IOP reduction is still needed at that time, add prostaglandin analog as mentioned earlier).
- **Step 4:** Arrange referral to a veterinary ophthalmologist.
  - For ophthalmic examination, including gonioscopy to classify as primary or secondary glaucoma
  - For evaluation for suitability of surgical procedures to prolong vision
    - Cyclophotocoagulation
      - This is laser ablation of the ciliary body to reduce aqueous humor production.
    - Placement of anterior chamber shunt
      - This creates an alternative outflow pathway from the eye so that aqueous humor outflow is increased.
3 Chronic IOP elevation in a blind eye
  - The goal is to restore comfort.
  - The eye is permanently blind and is also painful.
  - **Step 1:** Begin therapy with a topical or oral CAI (with or without concurrent beta-blocker), topical prostaglandin analog, or both classes of medication.
    - Doses as mentioned earlier.
  - **Step 2:** Begin systemic analgesic therapy (e.g., veterinary NSAIDs, gabapentin, or opioids used at labeled doses).
  - **Step 3:** If there is concurrent ocular disease, begin management for it.
    - For example, if uveitis is present, begin treatment with prednisolone acetate 1% ophthalmic suspension, dexamethasone 0.1% solution, or an oral anti-inflammatory medication (see "Anterior uveitis" in Chapter 15).
    - For example, if buphthalmos secondary to the chronic glaucoma has caused lagophthalmos and corneal exposure, begin therapy with an ophthalmic lubricant.
  - **Step 4:** Counsel owner on irreversible pain and blindness and recommend enucleation or other palliative procedures such as ciliary body ablation or evisceration with prosthesis.
  - **Step 5:** Arrange for referral to a veterinary ophthalmologist.
    - For ophthalmic examination, including gonioscopy to classify as primary or secondary glaucoma
    - For discussion of suitable palliative procedures

Prognosis

- Glaucoma cannot be cured.
- Primary glaucoma inevitably progresses to blindness.

◦ In addition to medications, veterinary ophthalmologists can surgically reduce aqueous humor production and/or increase its drainage (cyclophotocoagulation and anterior chamber shunt).

◦ These procedures delay, but do not stop, disease progression.

◦ The time course of progression is extremely variable.

- Without control of the underlying disease, secondary glaucomas also inevitably lead to blindness.

- Provided the underlying cause is controlled, control of IOP and vision maintenance for secondary glaucomas can be successful in the long term.

Additional information

- Consistently perform tonometry during each ophthalmic examination; this will minimize the potential for missing a diagnosis of glaucoma.

- Avoid pitfalls of tonometry.

  ◦ Measurement of IOP can be falsely elevated.

    ▪ Excessive restraint and collars can increase pressure around neck and therefore in the eyes (Pauli *et al.*, 2006).

    ▪ Excessive pressure applied to eyelids when opening eyes (Klein *et al.*, 2011).

    ▪ Body position can affect IOP readings; therefore, use consistent body positions for IOP measurement (Broadwater *et al.*, 2008; Rajaei *et al.*, 2018).

      ▫ Readings are most consistent in sternal recumbency (Broadwater *et al.*, 2008).

    ▪ There is variation between IOP readings obtained from different types of tonometers. Therefore, when tonometers of various types are available, the same type of tonometer should be used for each of a patient's IOP readings (von Spiessen *et al.*, 2015).

    ▪ Canine- and feline-specific Schiotz tables (for conversion of readings to IOP) are not accurate; human tables should be used (Miller & Pickett, 1992a, 1992b).

- Do not use Schiotz on delicate corneas (e.g., descemetoceles and recent intraocular surgery) due to risk of corneal rupture.

- Due to pressure around the neck causing increased IOP, harnesses should be used instead of neck collars in pets with glaucoma.

- Clinical presentation for cats often differs from dogs.

  ◦ Development of glaucoma is usually insidious and clinical signs are less visible.

    ▪ Therefore, cats often do not present until advanced stages of disease.

  ◦ Cats often retain vision even after development of buphthalmos.

- Signs of pain are often subtle in both cats and dogs.

  ◦ Pain often manifests as follows: patient is less playful, sleeps more, is less social, or less interested in food, or has minor alterations in posture (often interpreted as "just getting old").

  ◦ Therefore, many pet owners do not feel that glaucoma is causing pain.

◦ This makes enucleation difficult for many pet owners to accept.

◦ Many owners do not realize these signs are present until after a painful eye has been removed.

Further reading

Maggio, F. 2015. Glaucomas. *Topics in Companion Animal Medicine.* 30(3):86–96.

References

Broadwater, JJ, *et al.* 2008. Effect of body position on intraocular pressure in dogs without glaucoma. *American Journal of Veterinary Research.* 69(4):527–530.

Czepiel, TM & Wasserman, NT. 2021. Hypokalemia associated with topical administration of dorzolamide 2% ophthalmic solution in cats. *Veterinary Ophthalmology.* 24(1):12–19.

Dees, DD, *et al.* 2014. Efficacy of prophylactic antiglaucoma and anti-inflammatory medications in canine primary angle-closure glaucoma: a multicenter retrospective study (2004–2012). *Veterinary Ophthalmology.* 17(3):195–2000.

Gelatt, KN & MacKay, EO. 2001a. Changes in intraocular pressure associated with topical dorzolamide and oral methazolamide in glaucomatous dogs. *Veterinary Ophthalmology.* 4(1):61–67.

Gelatt, KN & MacKay, EO. 2001b. Effect of different dose schedules of latanoprost on intraocular pressure and pupil size in the glaucomatous beagle. *Veterinary Ophthalmology.* 4(4):283–288.

Gelatt, KN & MacKay, EO. 2001c. Effect of different dose schedules of travoprost on intraocular pressure and pupil size in the glaucomatous beagle. *Veterinary Ophthalmology.* 7(1):53–57.

Gelatt, KN & MacKay, EO. 2002. Effect of different dose schedules of bimatoprost on intraocular pressure and pupil size in the glaucomatous beagle. *Journal of Ocular Pharmacology and Therapeutics.* 18(6):525–534.

Gray, HE, *et al.* 2003. Effects of topical administration of 1% brinzolamide on normal cat eyes. *Veterinary Ophthalmology.* 6(4): 285–290.

Klein, HE, *et al.* 2011. Effect of eyelid manipulation and manual jugular compression on intraocular pressure measurement in dogs. *Journal of the American Veterinary Medical Association.* 238(10): 1292–1295.

McDonald, JE, *et al.* 2016. Effect of topical latanoprost 0.005% on intraocular pressure and pupil diameter in normal and glaucomatous cats. *Veterinary Ophthalmology.* 19(S1):13–23.

Miller, PE & Pickett, JP. 1992a. Comparison of the human and canine Schiotz tonometry conversion tables in clinically normal cats. *Journal of the American Veterinary Medical Association.* 201(7):1017–1020.

Miller, PE & Pickett, JP. 1992b. Comparison of the human and canine Schiotz tonometry conversion tables in clinically normal dogs. *Journal of the American Veterinary Medical Association.* 201(7): 1021–1025.

Miller, PE, *et al.* 2000. The efficacy of topical prophylactic antiglaucoma therapy in primary closed angle glaucoma in dogs: a multicenter clinical trial. *Journal of the American Animal Hospital Association.* 36(5):431–438.

Miller, PE, *et al.* 2001. Intraocular pressure measurements obtained as part of a comprehensive geriatric health examination from cats seven years of age or older. *Journal of the American Veterinary Medical Association.* 219(10):1406–1410.

Pauli, A, *et al.* 2006. Effects of the application of neck pressure by a collar or harness on intraocular pressure in dogs. *Journal of the American Animal Hospital Association.* 42(3):207–211.

Rajaei, SM, *et al.* 2018. Effect of body position, eyelid manipulation, and manual jugular compression on intraocular pressure in clinically normal cats. *Veterinary Ophthalmology.* 21(2):140–143.

Slenter, IJM, *et al.* 2010. The effects of topical dorzolamide 2% and brinzolamide 1%, either alone or combined with timolol 0.5%, on intraocular pressure, pupil diameter, and heart rate in healthy cats. *Veterinary Ophthalmology.* 23(1):16–24.

von Spiessen, L, *et al.*, 2015. Clinical comparison of the TonoVet® rebound tonometer and the Tono-Pen Vet® applanation tonometer in dogs and cats with ocular disease: glaucoma or corneal pathology. *Veterinary Ophthalmology.* 18(1): 20–27.

Index

Ablation, ciliary body, 217
Abscess, orbital, 4, 123, 126, 128–129, 132, 211
Accommodation, 183
Acyclovir, 159
Adenocarcinoma, 3, 30, 126, 142, 150, 151, 188
Adenoma
    iridociliary, 75, 188
    meibomian, 18–19, 142–144
Agenesis, eyelid, 16–17, 137–139, 183
Amlodipine, 210
Amoxicillin/clavulanic acid, 129, 131, 146, 175
Angiotensin-converting enzyme inhibitor
    benazepril, 210
    enalapril, 210
Anisocoria, 129, 185
Anterior chamber, 39, 59, 66–68, 73, 74, 76–79, 81, 94, 95, 119, 174, 180, 183–185, 189, 195–197, 214, 215, 217, 218
Anterior chamber shunt, 217, 218
Anterior synechia, 81, 184, 189
Anterior uvea, 65–83, 183–191
Anterior uveitis, 3, 39, 75–82, 94, 127, 162, 174, 176, 185, 186, 188–191, 194–197, 205–209, 211, 215–217
Antiviral medication
    acyclovir, 159
    cidofovir, 22, 159
    famciclovir, 33, 159
    ganciclovir, 159
    idoxuridine, 159
    trifluridine, 159
    valacyclovir, 159
Aphakic crescent, 93, 94, 96, 196, 198
Aqueous flare, 73, 77, 189
Aqueous humor, 76, 79, 162, 163, 183, 190, 193, 197, 200, 214–218
Asteroid hyalosis, 84, 114, 202, 203
Atapetal fundus, 99, 201
Atrophy
    iris, 69–71, 93, 185, 191
    optic nerve, 100, 102, 112, 128, 129, 202, 207, 211
    retinal, 194, 203–204
Atropine, 167, 171, 173, 175, 176, 178–180, 190, 191

Attenuation, avascular, 102, 215
Attenuation, vascular, 100, 101, 109, 202, 204, 205

Bacitracin, 131, 171, 178
Benazepril, 210
Beta-blocker
    betaxolol, 216, 217
    timolol, 216, 217
Betaxolol, 216, 217
Bimatoprost, 216, 217
Biopsy
    for diagnosis of eyelid neoplasia, 29, 142, 143, 150
    technique for conjunctiva, 29, 36, 153, 156, 160
    technique for third eyelid, 149, 150
Blepharitis, 21–23, 33, 143–145, 153, 154
Blepharospasm, 11, 125, 135–139, 141, 148, 153, 170, 178, 179, 189, 196, 214
Blindness, 124, 129, 131, 165, 167, 169, 174, 175, 177, 191, 195, 197, 203–205, 207, 208, 210, 211, 214, 215, 217, 218
Blood-aqueous barrier, 183, 188, 191
Blood-retinal barrier, xvii
Brachycephalic, 5, 6, 36, 43, 44, 124, 125, 130, 132, 136–138, 143, 148, 151, 152, 163, 165, 166, 168–170, 174, 177, 178, 180
Brachycephalic ocular syndrome, 5, 6, 43, 44, 124, 125, 136–138, 151, 166, 168–170, 177, 178, 180
Brinzolamide, 216, 217
Brunescence, 91, 194
Bulla, corneal, 43, 164
Buphthalmos, 3, 117, 119, 123, 215, 217, 218
Buprenorphine, 178–180, 191

Calcium channel blocker
    amlodipine, 210
Carbonic anhydrase inhibitor
    brinzolamide, 216, 217
    dorzolamide, 80, 119, 197, 216, 217
    methazolamide, 216, 217
Cartilage, third eyelid
    eversion, 26, 27, 147–149
    scrolled, 26, 27, 147, 148

Small Animal Ophthalmic Atlas and Guide, Second Edition. Christine C. Lim.
© 2023 John Wiley & Sons, Inc. Published 2023 by John Wiley & Sons, Inc.
Companion website: www.wiley.com/go/lim/atlas